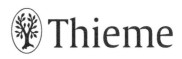

RadCases Plus Q&A Thoracic Imaging
Second Edition

Edited by

Carlos S. Restrepo, MD
Professor of Radiology
Vice Chair of Education
Section Chief, Cardio-Thoracic Radiology
University of Texas Health Science Center
San Antonio, Texas

Steven M. Zangan, MD
Associate Professor of Radiology
Associate Program Director, Interventional Radiology
   Residency
University of Chicago Medical Center
Chicago, Illinois

Series Editors

Jonathan M. Lorenz, MD, FSIR
Professor of Radiology
Section of Interventional Radiology
The University of Chicago
Chicago, Illinois

Hector Ferral, MD
Senior Medical Educator
NorthShore University HealthSystem
Evanston, Illinois

499 illustrations

Thieme
New York • Stuttgart • Delhi • Rio de Janeiro

Executive Editor: William Lamsback
Managing Editors: J. Owen Zurhellen IV & Kenneth Schubach
Editorial Assistant: Holly Bullis
Director, Editorial Services: Mary Jo Casey
Production Editor: Teresa Exley, Absolute Service, Inc.
International Production Director: Andreas Schabert
Editorial Director: Sue Hodgson
International Marketing Director: Fiona Henderson
International Sales Director: Louisa Turrell
Director of Institutional Sales: Adam Bernacki
Senior Vice President and Chief Operating Officer: Sarah Vanderbilt
President: Brian D. Scanlan
Printer: King Printing

Library of Congress Cataloging-in-Publication Data
Names: Restrepo, Carlos Santiago, editor. | Zangan, Steven M., editor.
Title: RadCases plus Q&A thoracic imaging / edited by
    Carlos S. Restrepo, Steven M. Zangan.
Other titles: Thoracic imaging (Restrepo) | RadCases plus Q and A
    thoracic imaging
Description: Second edition. | New York : Thieme, [2019] | Series:
    Radcases | Preceded by Thoracic imaging / edited by
    Carlos Santiago Restrepo, Steven M. Zangan. c2011. | Includes
    bibliographical references and index. |
    Identifiers: LCCN 2018038409 (print) | LCCN 2018038634
    (ebook) | ISBN 9781626238152 | ISBN 9781626238145 |
    ISBN 9781626238152 (e-book)
Subjects: | MESH: Radiography, Thoracic—methods | Tomography,
    Emission-Computed—methods | Diagnosis, Differential |
    Case Reports
Classification: LCC RC941 (ebook) | LCC RC941 (print) | NLM
    WF 975 | DDC 617.5/407572—dc23
LC record available at https://lccn.loc.gov/2018038409

Copyright © 2019 by Thieme Medical Publishers, Inc.
Thieme Publishers New York
333 Seventh Avenue, New York, NY 10001 USA
+1 800 782 3488, customerservice@thieme.com

Thieme Publishers Stuttgart
Rüdigerstrasse 14, 70469 Stuttgart, Germany
+49 [0]711 8931 421, customerservice@thieme.de

Thieme Publishers Delhi
A-12, Second Floor, Sector-2, Noida-201301
Uttar Pradesh, India
+91 120 45 566 00, customerservice@thieme.in

Thieme Publishers Rio de Janeiro, Thieme Publicações Ltda.
Edifício Rodolpho de Paoli, 25º andar
Av. Nilo Peçanha, 50 – Sala 2508
Rio de Janeiro 20020-906 Brasil
+55 21 3172-2297/+55 21 3172-1896
www.thiemerevinter.com.br

Cover design: Thieme Publishing Group
Typesetting by Absolute Service, Inc.
Printed in the United States by King Printing
5 4 3 2 1

ISBN 978-1-62623-814-5

Also available as an e-book:
eISBN 978-1-62623-815-2

Important note: Medicine is an ever-changing science undergoing continual development. Research and clinical experience are continually expanding our knowledge, in particular our knowledge of proper treatment and drug therapy. Insofar as this book mentions any dosage or application, readers may rest assured that the authors, editors, and publishers have made every effort to ensure that such references are in accordance with **the state of knowledge at the time of production of the book.**

Nevertheless, this does not involve, imply, or express any guarantee or responsibility on the part of the publishers in respect to any dosage instructions and forms of applications stated in the book. **Every user is requested to examine carefully** the manufacturers' leaflets accompanying each drug and to check, if necessary in consultation with a physician or specialist, whether the dosage schedules mentioned therein or the contraindications stated by the manufacturers differ from the statements made in the present book. Such examination is particularly important with drugs that are either rarely used or have been newly released on the market. Every dosage schedule or every form of application used is entirely at the user's own risk and responsibility. The authors and publishers request every user to report to the publishers any discrepancies or inaccuracies noticed. If errors in this work are found after publication, errata will be posted at www.thieme.com on the product description page.

Some of the product names, patents, and registered designs referred to in this book are in fact registered trademarks or proprietary names even though specific reference to this fact is not always made in the text. Therefore, the appearance of a name without designation as proprietary is not to be construed as a representation by the publisher that it is in the public domain.

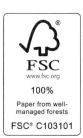

Dedicated to my wife, Marta, and to my children, Catalina, Juan, and Alejandro, with all my love.

– CSR

Dedicated to Tracie, Max, and Vincent.

– SMZ

Series Preface

As enthusiastic partners in radiology education, we continue our mission to ease the exhaustion and frustration shared by residents and the families of residents engaged in radiology training! In launching the second edition of the RadCases series, our intent is to expand rather than replace this already rich study experience that has been tried, tested, and popularized by residents around the world. In each subspecialty edition, we serve up 100 new, carefully chosen cases to raise the bar in our effort to assist residents in tackling the daunting task of assimilating massive amounts of information. RadCases second edition primes and expands on concepts found in the first edition with important variations on prior cases, updated diagnostic and management strategies, and new pathologic entities. Our continuing goal is to combine the popularity and portability of printed books with the adaptability, exceptional quality, and interactive features of an electronic case-based format. The new cases will be added to the existing electronic database to enrich the interactive environment of high-quality images that allows residents to arrange study sessions, quickly extract and master information, and prepare for theme-based radiology conferences.

We owe a debt of gratitude to our own residents and to the many radiology trainees who have helped us create, adapt, and improve the format and content of RadCases by weighing in with suggestions for new cases, functions, and formatting. Back by popular demand is the concise, point-by-point presentation of the Essential Facts of each case in an easy-to-read, bulleted format, and a short, critical differential starting with the actual diagnosis. This approach is easy on exhausted eyes and encourages repeated priming of important information during quick reviews, a process we believe is critical to radiology education. New since the prior edition is the addition of a question-and-answer section for each case to reinforce key concepts.

The intent of the printed books is to encourage repeated priming in the use of critical information by providing a portable group of exceptional core cases to master. Unlike the authors of other case-based radiology review books, we removed the guesswork by providing clear annotations and descriptions for all images. In our opinion, there is nothing worse than being unable to locate a subtle finding on a poorly reproduced image even after one knows the final diagnosis.

The electronic cases expand on the printed book and provide a comprehensive review of the entire specialty. Thousands of cases are strategically designed to increase the resident's knowledge by providing exposure to a spectrum of case examples—from basic to advanced—and by exploring "Aunt Minnies," unusual diagnoses, and variability within a single diagnosis. The search engine allows the resident to create individualized daily study lists that are not limited by factors such as radiology subsection. For example, tailor today's study list to cases involving tuberculosis and include cases in every subspecialty and every system of the body. Or study only thoracic cases, including those with links to cardiology, nuclear medicine, and pediatrics. Or study only musculoskeletal cases. The choice is yours.

As enthusiastic partners in this project, we started small and, with the encouragement, talent, and guidance of Timothy Hiscock and William Lamsback at Thieme Publishers, we have further raised the bar in our effort to assist residents in tackling the daunting task of assimilating massive amounts of information. We are passionate about continuing this journey and will continue to expand the series, adapt cases based on direct feedback from residents, and increase the features intended for board review and self-assessment. First and foremost, we thank our medical students, residents, and fellows for allowing us the privilege to participate in their educational journey.

Jonathan M. Lorenz, MD, FSIR
Hector Ferral, MD

Preface

Imaging of the thorax, from conventional radiographs to more complex modalities, comprises the key workload in contemporary radiology departments. Proper observation, analysis, and interpretation of such imaging requires thorough understanding of the pathophysiology and imaging manifestations of a broad range of diseases. In this second edition, the essential imaging details of core thoracic imaging cases are reinforced and a variety of new conditions, common and uncommon, are introduced. We trust that this concise review of imaging findings, differential diagnoses, essential facts, and pearls and pitfalls will prepare you well for exams, patients, and a lifelong career in radiology.

Case Authorship

Cases 1 to 50 were authored by Steven M. Zangan, and cases 51 to 100 were authored by Carlos S. Restrepo.

Acknowledgments

We thank Drs. Heber MacMahon, Steven Montner, and Jonathan Chung for kindly sharing their voluminous teaching files and offering some of the pearls that have made their way into RadCases.

Case 1

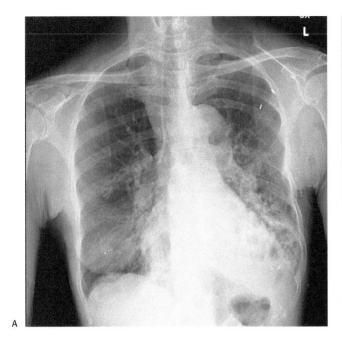

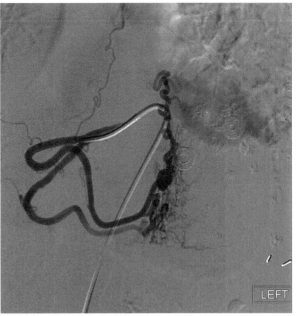

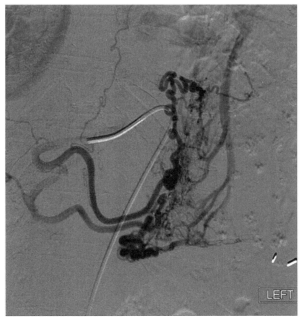

■ Clinical Presentation

A 55-year-old woman presents with recurrent pneumonia.

■ Imaging Findings

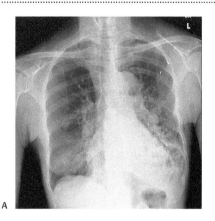 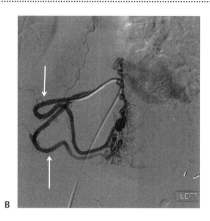 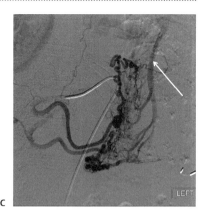

A   B   C

(A) Chest radiograph demonstrates dense consolidation in the left lower lobe. **(B)** Conventional catheter angiogram shows hypertrophied nonbronchial systemic arteries supplying the left lower lobe mass (*arrows*). **(C)** Delayed venous phase image shows pulmonary venous drainage (*arrow*).

■ Differential Diagnosis

- ***Intralobar pulmonary sequestration:*** Bronchopulmonary sequestration is a mass of lung tissue with airway and alveolar elements; it lacks communication with the tracheobronchial tree, and receives arterial blood supply from the systemic circulation. Intralobar sequestrations lack their own visceral pleura and demonstrate pulmonary venous drainage.
- *Pulmonary arteriovenous malformation (AVM):* Pulmonary AVMs are abnormal communications between pulmonary arteries and veins.
- *Extralobar pulmonary sequestration:* Extralobar sequestrations have their own visceral pleura and demonstrate systemic venous drainage.
- *Congenital pulmonary airway malformation (CPAM):* Previously known as congenital cystic adenomatoid malformation, CPAMs are hamartomatous developmental malformations of the lower respiratory tract comprising cystic and adenomatoid elements. CPAMs have connections with the tracheobronchial tree. The arterial and venous supply almost always arises from the pulmonary circulation.

■ Essential Facts

- Intralobar sequestrations are more common and are usually diagnosed later in childhood or early adulthood.
- Some cases of intralobar sequestration may be acquired.
- Extralobar sequestrations are typically diagnosed in the prenatal or neonatal period. A large number of these are associated with other abnormalities such as diaphragmatic hernia and congenital heart disease.

- Imaging options:
  - Chest radiographs typically show a dense pulmonary mass in the lower chest, often on the left.
  - Contrast-enhanced CT image can show the parenchymal abnormalities to advantage. Air-fluid levels may develop due to anomalous airway connections, collateral air drift via the pores of Kohn, and recurrent infections. The systemic arterial supply to the mass can often be identified.
  - MRI and ultrasonography can be useful in the prenatal workup of suspected extralobar sequestration.
- Treatment options:
  - Symptomatic patients can be cured with surgical excision. This typically requires lobectomy or segmental resection.
  - In asymptomatic patients, resection is considered for those at high risk for developing complications. In others, conservative management with observation may be sufficient.

✓ Pearls and ✗ Pitfalls

✓ The arterial supply is usually from the lower thoracic or upper abdominal aorta.
✓ Most intralobar sequestrations are located in the posterobasal segment of the left lower lobe.
✓ Arterial embolization has been described in selected cases.
✗ Pulmonary arterial supply is always absent in intralobar sequestration but may be present in extralobar sequestration.
✗ The systemic venous drainage from extralobar sequestrations may be via the azygos vein, hemiazygos system, or inferior vena cava.

Case 2

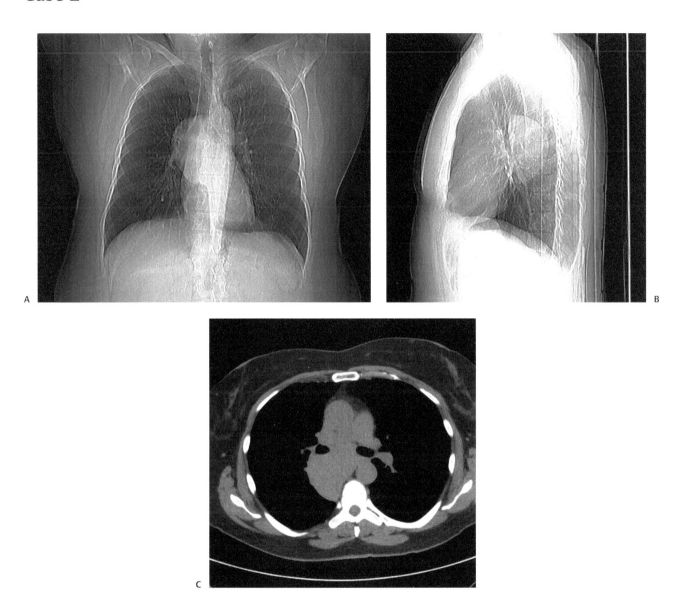

■ Clinical Presentation

A 35-year-old man with a positive purified protein derivative test.

■ Imaging Findings

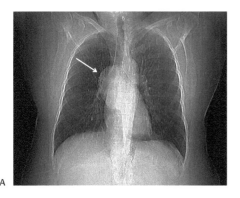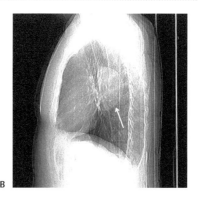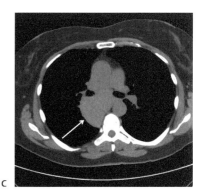

(A) Frontal projection from CT scout image demonstrates a smoothly marginated mediastinal mass protruding toward the right hilum (*arrow*). **(B)** Lateral projection from CT scout image shows the smooth posterior margin to advantage (*arrow*). **(C)** Unenhanced chest CT image shows a homogeneous smoothly marginated subcarinal mass of near water density (*arrow*).

■ Differential Diagnosis

- **Bronchogenic cyst:** A cystic subcarinal mass is typical of a bronchogenic cyst.
- *Lymphadenopathy:* Nodes are typically of higher density, although low-density nodes can be seen with extensive necrosis, lymphoma, and some infections such as tuberculosis. The presence of contrast enhancement would help differentiate because a cyst should not enhance.
- *Pericardial cyst:* The most common location of a pericardial cyst is in the right cardiophrenic angle.
- *Small-cell lung cancer:* Small-cell lung cancer can have a central location, although smooth margins, homogeneous near water density, lack of local invasion or symptoms, and the patient's age all argue against malignancy.

■ Essential Facts

- Bronchogenic cysts are the most common cystic masses of the mediastinum.
- These congenital anomalies result from abnormal ventral budding or branching of the tracheobronchial tree during embryologic development.
- They are lined by respiratory epithelium and their walls usually contain cartilage and smooth muscle.
- Most are near the carina.
- Approximately 15% of bronchogenic cysts occur within the lung parenchyma.

- Bronchogenic cysts are usually incidental findings and require no treatment. Surgical excision is considered for symptomatic patients.
- Imaging options:
  - Chest radiographs typically show a well-defined solitary mass with homogeneous opacity.
  - On CT imaging, a bronchogenic cyst appears as a single, smooth, usually round mass with an imperceptible wall and uniform attenuation. No enhancement should be present.
  - T2-weighted MR image almost always shows high signal intensity. On T1-weighted series, the signal intensity is variable because the cyst may contain protein, hemorrhage, or mucoid material.

✓ Pearls and ✗ Pitfalls

- ✓ Calcification may develop in the wall of the cyst.
- ✓ Cysts may increase in size due to hemorrhage or infection.
- ✓ Esophageal (enteric) duplication cysts can appear almost identically, although they are usually adjacent to or within the esophageal wall.
- ✗ Air within the cyst is uncommon and suggestive of secondary infection and communication with the tracheobronchial tree.
- ✗ Although typically low attenuation, cyst content may have a Hounsfield unit value > 100 due to high protein level or calcium oxalate.

Case 3

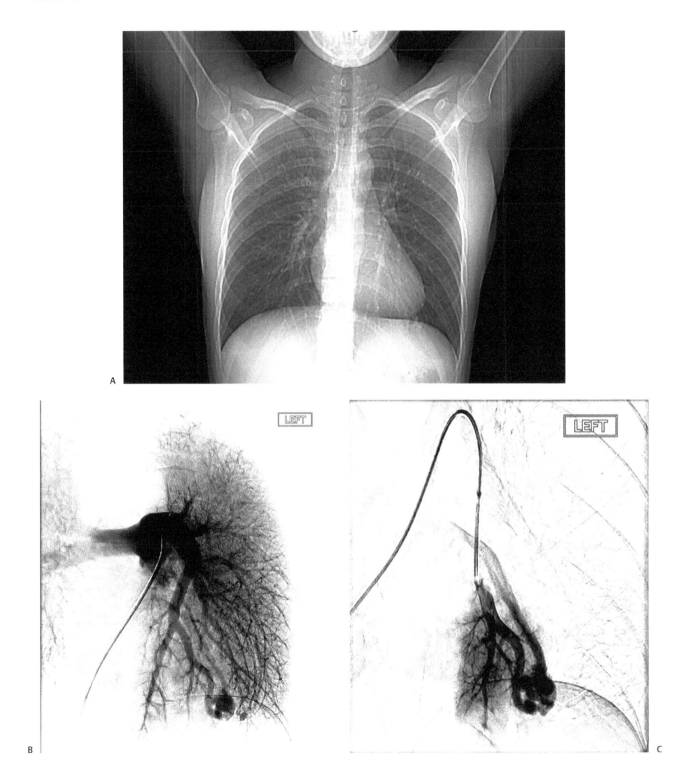

■ Clinical Presentation

A 37-year-old woman with ischemic stroke.

■ Imaging Findings

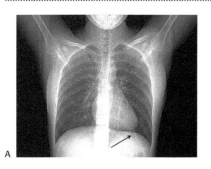 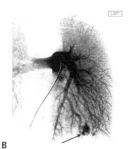 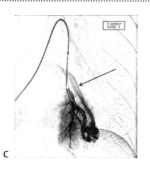 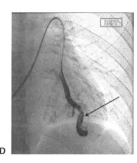

(A) Frontal projection from CT scout image shows a left lower lobe nodule (*arrow*). **(B)** Left pulmonary angiogram shows a left lower lobe pulmonary arteriovenous malformation (AVM; *arrow*). **(C)** Selective left lower lobe angiogram shows the AVM to advantage. Note the enlarged draining vein (*arrow*). **(D)** Following diagnosis, the patient underwent embolotherapy. This image, not shown previously, demonstrates no further filling of the AVM after deployment of multiple coils (*arrow*).

■ Differential Diagnosis

- ***Arteriovenous malformation (AVM):*** A vascular sac with a feeding pulmonary artery and draining pulmonary vein is compatible with a pulmonary AVM.
- *Carcinoid:* A carcinoid tumor may enhance avidly but is not expected to have a feeding artery and draining vein.
- *Septic emboli:* Often have a feeding vessel, although a dilated draining vein is not expected. When larger, cavitation may be seen. Intense enhancement is not expected.
- *Pulmonary varix:* A pulmonary varix is an abnormal dilatation of a pulmonary vein with no abnormal arteriovenous communication or shunt. They may be congenital or secondary to long-standing pulmonary hypertension, partial anomalous pulmonary venous return, or mitral regurgitation.

■ Essential Facts

- Pulmonary AVMs can be classified as simple (solitary feeding artery and draining vein) or complex (more than one feeding artery).
- Results in a right-to-left shunt and hypoxia.
- Orthodeoxia refers to hypoxemia in an upright position; this is due to the fact that most AVMs are in the lower lobes and there is more shunting when upright.
- Can present with hemoptysis, hemorrhage, or paradoxic embolism.
- Over 90% of multiple AVMs are associated with hereditary hemorrhagic telangiectasia (HHT; Osler–Weber–Rendu syndrome), an autosomal-dominant disorder.
- The four main criteria for the diagnosis of HHT are 1) spontaneous and recurrent epistaxis, 2) multiple mucocutaneous telangiectasias, 3) visceral involvement with AVMs, and 4) first-degree relative with HHT. When at least three of these criteria are met, HHT is definitively diagnosed.

- There is an association between HHT and pulmonary hypertension. This is mediated by mutations of activin receptor–like kinase type 1 (ALK1), which is found in abundance in vascular endothelial cells.
- On radiograph, an AVM manifests as a lobulated but sharply defined pulmonary nodule, mostly in the lower lobes.
- CT is the preferred screening study for AVMs because it is more sensitive than radiography or angiography. The feeding artery and draining vein are shown to advantage.
- Embolotherapy is recommended for AVMs with feeding arteries > 3 mm in diameter.
- Following embolotherapy, AVMs typically decrease in size.
- Acquired AVMs can occur in patients with hepatopulmonary syndrome.
- Pulmonary telangiectasia is an uncommon malformation characterized by innumerable small fistulas.

■ Other Imaging Findings

- Up to 15% of patients with HHT have intracerebral and/or hepatic AVMs.
- Contrast echocardiography is useful to identify small right-to-left shunts.
- Tc-99m macroaggregated albumin can help estimate the size of the right-to-left shunt.

✓ Pearls and ✗ Pitfalls

✓ Multiple AVMs are seen in 35% of cases.
✓ Consider HHT when pulmonary AVMs are identified.
✗ Although rare, life-threatening complications including stroke and pulmonary AVM hemorrhage can manifest during pregnancy.
✗ After hemorrhage, the AVM may be obscured.
✗ Special intravenous tubing and filters are advisable in patients with HHT, given the potential for paradoxical air embolism.

Case 4

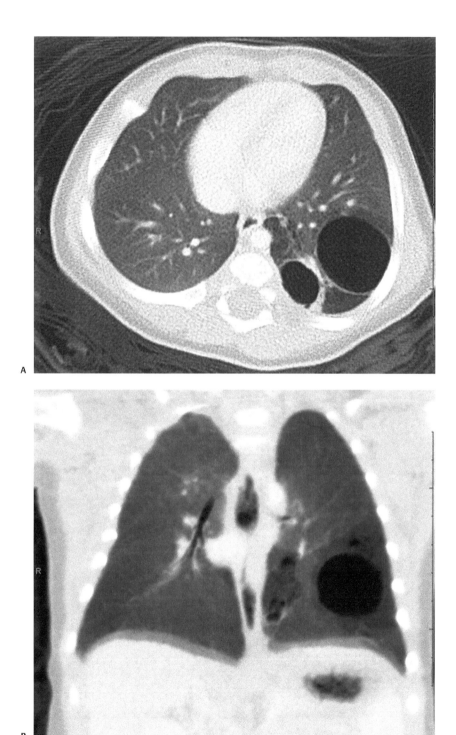

A

B

■ Clinical Presentation

A 3-week-old boy with respiratory distress and decreased breath sounds in the left hemithorax.

■ Imaging Findings

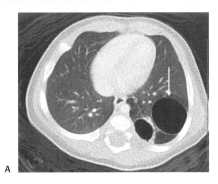 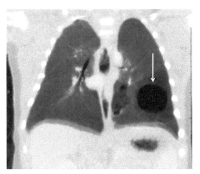

(A) Contrast-enhanced chest CT image (lung window) demonstrates large thin-walled cysts in the left lower lobe (*arrow*). (B) Coronal minimum intensity projection shows the cystic lesion to advantage (*arrow*).

■ Differential Diagnosis

- ***Congenital pulmonary airway malformation (CPAM):***
  Previously known as congenital cystic adenomatoid
  malformation, CPAMs are hamartomatous
  developmental malformations of the lower respiratory
  tract comprising cystic and adenomatoid elements.
  CPAMs have connections with the tracheobronchial tree.
- *Lymphangioma/cystic hygroma:* This usually involves the
  neck and thoracic inlet. Mediastinal involvement can be
  seen as a cystic lesion.
- *Intralobar pulmonary sequestration:* Bronchopulmonary
  sequestration is a mass of lung tissue with airway and
  alveolar elements; it lacks communication with the
  tracheobronchial tree and receives arterial blood supply
  from the systemic circulation. Intralobar sequestrations
  lack their own visceral pleura and demonstrate
  pulmonary venous drainage.

■ Essential Facts

- CPAMs result from adenomatous overgrowth of the
  terminal bronchioles and consequent reduced alveolar
  growth during abnormal embryogenesis of the
  bronchoalveolar tissue early in the first trimester.
- If not detected antenatally, most are discovered by
  2 years of age.
- CPAMs are classified into five types according to cyst size
  and histology.
- Only three types of CPAMs are distinguished at imaging:
  - Type I—large cyst (> 2 cm), comprising 50 to 70%
    of CPAMs.
  - Type II—small cyst/macrocystic, comprising < 40%
    of cases.
  - Type III—microcystic or solid type (cysts < 5 mm with
    no discernible cystic spaces) has the worst prognosis
    and comprises < 10% of CPAMs.
- May communicate with the proximal airways.
- Blood supply is via the pulmonary artery with
  pulmonary venous drainage.
- Most commonly localized to a single lobe.

- When large, the lesion may compress the esophagus
  or lung and cause polyhydramnios or pulmonary
  hypoplasia, respectively.
- More than half of affected children present with
  respiratory distress.
- Postnatal radiograph of large-cyst CPAM shows variable
  density in the region of the mass depending on the
  fluid contents of the cysts. It may gradually fill with air,
  resulting in well-defined air-filled cysts with thin walls
  or air-fluid levels.
- Small-cyst CPAM is seen as an echogenic mass on
  prenatal ultrasound image. The T2-weighted MR image
  has variable appearance depending on the cystic and
  solid components. CT may allow better characterization
  of a heterogeneous mass with small cysts.
- Microcystic CPAM is predominantly solid-appearing
  and echogenic on ultrasound, and a homogeneously
  hyperintense solid mass on T2-weighted MR image.
- Treatment is surgical resection. Open fetal surgical
  resection has been described in extreme cases.
- Minimally invasive fetal surgery and creation of a
  thoracoamniotic shunt may decrease the size of the
  CPAM by draining fluid out of the large cysts.
- Ex utero intrapartum treatment procedure consists
  of surgical resection of the mass while the fetus is
  maintained on placental circulation, and this has been
  described in hydropic fetuses.
- Resection of asymptomatic CPAMs is controversial.

✓ Pearls and ✗ Pitfalls

- ✓ On fetal ultrasound or MR image, demonstration of
  the normally positioned stomach and visualization of
  the diaphragm help exclude congenital diaphragmatic
  hernia as an etiology of an abnormal mass in the thorax.
- ✓ A small percentage of CPAMs detected prenatally get
  smaller or completely resolve.
- ✗ Hybrid lesions can have a systemic blood supply, similar
  to sequestrations.
- ✗ Malignant transformation into rhabdomyosarcoma,
  bronchoalveolar carcinoma, and pleuropulmonary
  blastoma can occur.

Case 5

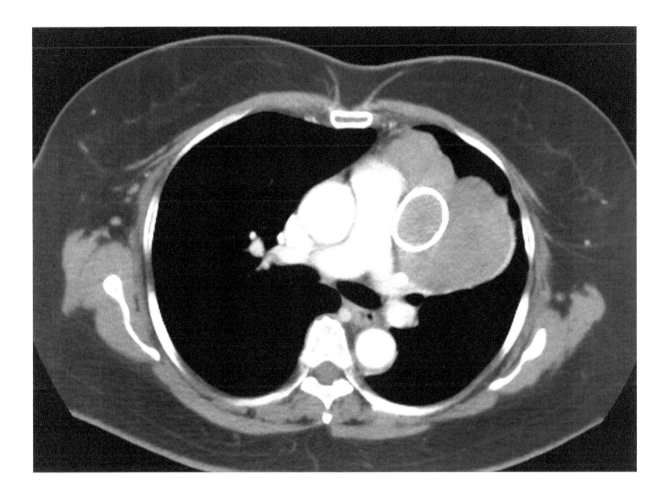

∎ Clinical Presentation

A 25-year-old woman with a mediastinal mass.

■ Imaging Findings

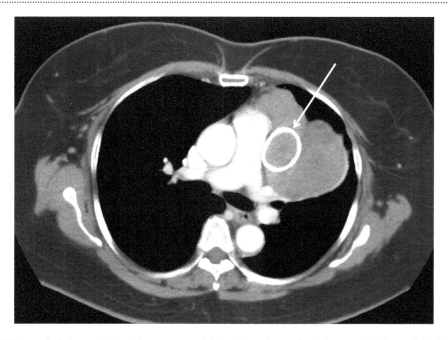

(A) Contrast-enhanced CT image (soft tissue windows) demonstrates a lobulated anterior mediastinal mass with a focus of circular calcification (*arrow*).

■ Differential Diagnosis

- **Teratoma:** Most commonly multilocular with cystic components. The presence of calcium and the patient's age support this diagnosis.
- *Thymoma:* Smoothly marginated anterior mediastinal mass. Often in older patients and associated with paraneoplastic syndromes in 40%.
- *Lymphoma:* Involvement of other lymph node groups is common. Enhancement may be heterogeneous. Systemic clinical symptoms may be present.
- *Nonseminomatous germ cell neoplasm:* Can be heterogeneous and calcification has been described, although it is rare. However, in patients of this age, nonseminomatous germ cell neoplasms occur almost exclusively in men.

■ Essential Facts

- The most common location for extragonadal germ cell neoplasms is the anterior mediastinum. Less than 10% of teratomas occur in the posterior mediastinum.
- Primitive germ cells are thought to be misplaced along midline structures during their migration from the yolk endoderm to the gonad during early embryogenesis.
- Mature teratoma is the most common mediastinal germ cell tumor.
- Occurs in young adults with equal gender predilection.

- Immature teratomas consist of > 10% immature neuroectodermal and mesenchymal tissue and have a low potential for malignancy.
- Teratoma with additional malignant components is rare and represents an aggressive malignancy. This was formerly termed *malignant teratoma.*
- Teratomas are mostly asymptomatic, although they may present due to mass effect or rupture.
- On CT imaging, internal foci of fat are seen in 75%.
- Calcification is uncommonly seen on chest radiographs; however, it can be detected on CT imaging in 50% of cases. The presence of bone or teeth is rare.
- The mass may be adherent to mediastinal structures.
- Soft tissue and rim enhancement can be seen.
- Complete excision of mature teratoma is curative, with 5-year survival approaching 100%.
- MR image may show fat within the lesion to better advantage.

✓ Pearls and ✗ Pitfalls

- ✓ Rupture into the pleural or pericardial space may occur. Rupture into the lung or tracheobronchial tree can result in lipoid pneumonia or expectoration of oily substances or hair.
- ✓ The presence of a fat-fluid level is virtually diagnostic of teratoma but is seen in only 11% of cases.
- ✗ The presence of soft tissue elements is expected; however, a solid teratoma is uncommon.

Case 6

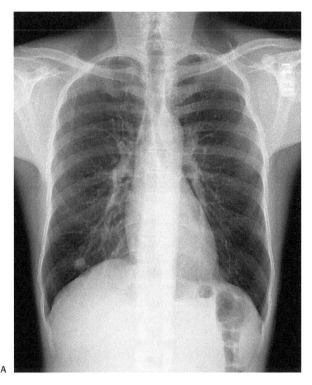

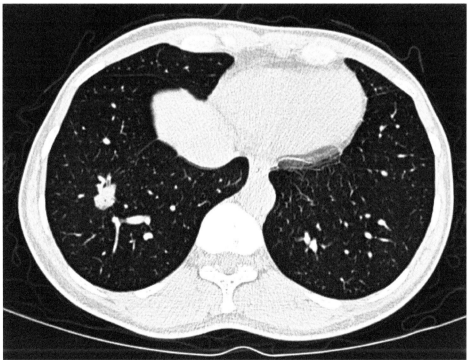

■ Clinical Presentation

A 60-year-old man with cough.

■ Imaging Findings

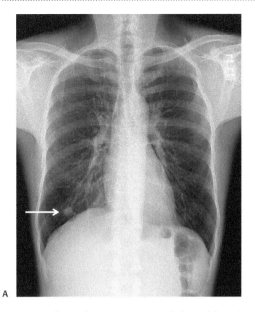 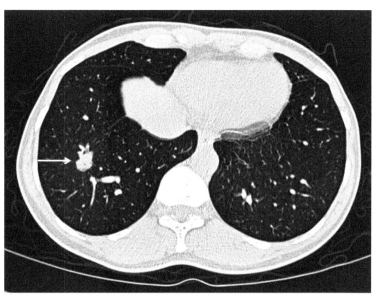

(A) Chest radiograph demonstrates a right lower lobe pulmonary nodule (*arrow*). **(B)** CT image shows a spiculated right lower pulmonary nodule (*arrow*).

■ Differential Diagnosis

- ***Lung cancer presenting as a solitary pulmonary nodule (SPN):*** A spiculated, noncalcified pulmonary nodule in an adult patient should be considered lung cancer until proven otherwise.
- *Tuberculoma:* An active tuberculoma can present as a round, indeterminate pulmonary nodule, similar in appearance to lung cancer.
- *Round pneumonia:* Several infections, bacterial or nonbacterial in etiology, may present as spherical parenchymal consolidation in the form of an indeterminate SPN.

■ Essential Facts

- An SPN is defined as a focal, spherical lesion in the lung parenchyma, surrounded by aerated lung, measuring < 3 cm in diameter.
- A nodule that is not calcified in a benign pattern and that has not shown to be stable for longer than 2 years is referred to as an indeterminate nodule.
- An SPN may be detected on chest radiograph or CT image either in the evaluation of a symptomatic patient or as an incidental finding.
- A wide variety of benign and malignant conditions can present as an SPN.
- Although many SPNs are benign, as many as 40% can be malignant in older cohorts. One fourth to one third of lung cancers initially present as an SPN.
- The most common cause of malignant SPN is adenocarcinoma (50%), followed by squamous cell carcinoma (25%).

- The most common causes of benign indeterminate SPNs are nonspecific granulomas (25%), infectious granulomas (15%), and hamartomas (15%).
- A lobulated contour reflects uneven growth and has been associated with malignancy.
- Nodules with an irregular or spiculated margin or a sunburst appearance (corona radiata sign) are more likely to be malignant.
- An air bronchogram within an SPN has also been associated with malignancy.
- Positron emission tomography/CT and dynamic contrast-enhanced CT evaluation of nodule vascularity help differentiate benign from malignant SPNs. Enhancement of more than 25 Hounsfield units favors malignancy.

✓ Pearls and ✗ Pitfalls

- ✓ Malignant SPNs are potentially curable; more than 60% of patients with clinical stage IA cancers will survive 5 years after treatment.
- ✓ The smaller the nodule, the greater chance that it is benign; 80% of benign nodules are < 2 cm in diameter. The likelihood of malignancy in nodules < 5 mm is < 1%.
- ✗ More than half of nodules detected on conventional chest radiographs are false-positive findings and not confirmed on CT imaging.
- ✗ Calcification is rare in lung cancers presenting as SPNs (6%). Whereas diffuse, popcorn, central, and laminated calcifications are benign patterns of calcification, stippled and eccentric calcifications are indeterminate.

Case 7

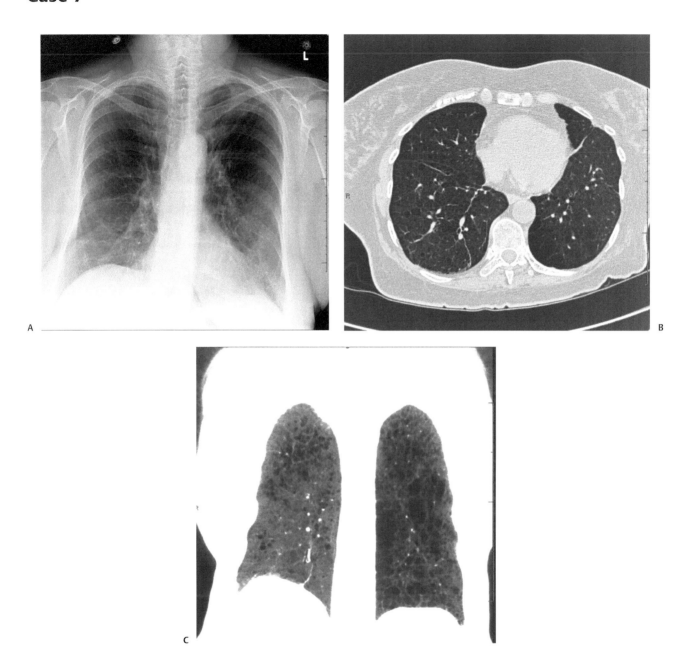

■ Clinical Presentation

A 58-year-old woman with chronic dyspnea and shortness of breath.

■ Imaging Findings

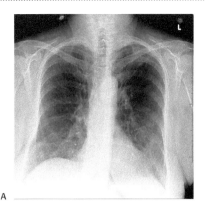
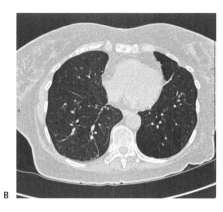
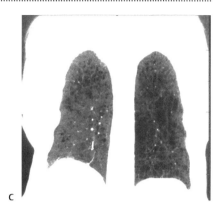

(A) Posteroanterior chest radiograph demonstrates large lung volumes consistent with chronic obstructive pulmonary disease. **(B)** Chest CT image (lung windows) shows panlobular emphysema with extensive lower lobe involvement. **(C)** Coronal minimum intensity projection shows the lower lobe involvement to advantage.

■ Differential Diagnosis

- **α_1-Antitrypsin (AAT) deficiency:** Panlobular emphysema, characterized by more extensive involvement of the lower lobes and segments in young adults, is suggestive of AAT deficiency.
- *Centrilobular emphysema:* The typical distribution of centrilobular emphysema is upper lobe predominant with characteristic morphology of smaller lucencies and an imperceptible wall.
- *Cystic lung diseases:* Cytic lung diseases such as lymphangioleiomyomatosis and pulmonary Langerhans cell histiocytosis may manifest as thin-walled lucencies.

■ Essential Facts

- AAT deficiency is a hereditary condition in which absent or reduced serum levels of the AAT enzyme lead to the early development of pulmonary emphysema and effects on other organs and systems. The prevalence is about 1 in 3500 live births.
- AAT deficiency is inherited by autosomal-codominant transmission, meaning that affected individuals have inherited an abnormal *AAT* gene from each parent.
- AAT is a protease inhibitor that prevents enzymes such as elastase from degrading normal host tissue. In patients with severe deficiency, the neutrophil elastase acts unopposed, resulting in damage to the lower respiratory tract.
- AAT deficiency occurs in people who inherit two protease inhibitor deficiency alleles of the *AAT* gene, located on chromosome 14.
- Panlobular/panacinar emphysema is the principal resulting clinical anomaly and the major cause of morbidity and mortality in affected patients.

- In panlobular emphysema, the pulmonary lobules are uniformly destroyed from the level of the respiratory bronchioles to the level of the distal alveoli.
- The second most common and most significant complication is liver disease (cholestasis and cirrhosis).
- Cirrhosis and carcinoma of the liver develop in up to 40% of patients with AAT deficiency who are older than 50 years of age.
- Smoking is the most significant additional risk factor for the rapid deterioration of pulmonary function.
- Supportive therapy for patients with AAT-related emphysema follows the usual guidelines for chronic obstructive pulmonary disease.
- Intravenous augmentation with pooled human AAT, lung volume reduction surgery, and lung transplantation are potential treatments in selected cases.

✓ Pearls and ✗ Pitfalls

- ✓ The obstructive airway disease in AAT manifests on pulmonary function tests as a reduced ratio of the forced expiratory volume in 1 second to the forced vital capacity and is due mainly to the loss of elastic recoil as a consequence of parenchymal destruction.
- ✓ AAT deficiency should be suspected in subjects who have an early onset of emphysema, emphysema in the absence of recognized risk factors, lower lobe–predominant emphysema, emphysema with unexplained liver disease, or clinical history of panniculitis.
- ✓ The basal predominance is likely due to the gravitational distribution of blood flow.
- ✗ Associated centrilobular emphysema may be present in the upper lobes.
- ✗ Diffuse cystic bronchiectasis has been reported in 10 to 40% of patients with AAT deficiency.

Case 8

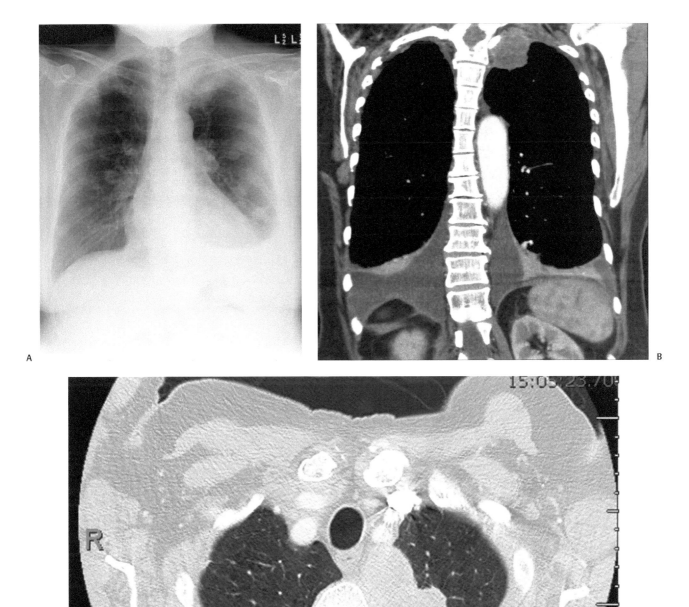

A

B

C

■ Clinical Presentation

A 63-year-old female smoker with shoulder pain.

■ **Imaging Findings**

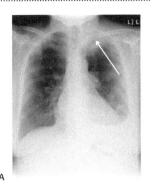 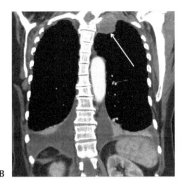 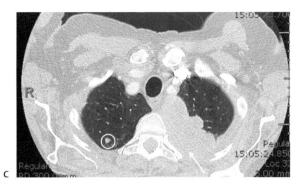

A   B   C

(A) Frontal chest radiograph demonstrates a mass in the left apex *(arrow)*. Pulmonary nodules are seen bilaterally. **(B)** Contrast-enhanced coronal reformat image (soft tissue window) confirms a left superior sulcus tumor. **(C)** Axial CT image (lung window) shows chest wall extension *(arrow)*. A metastatic nodule is seen on the right *(circle)*.

■ **Differential Diagnosis**

- **Superior sulcus tumor:** The presence of an apical mass with chest wall extension in a patient of this age makes superior sulcus tumor the best choice. Additional pulmonary nodules are highly suggestive of malignancy.
- *Tuberculosis (TB):* Reactivation TB can present as an apical lung mass, although typically other findings such as bronchiectasis, cavitation, and scarring are also present. Calcification may be present. Can be associated with rib destruction, although not as commonly as with malignancy.
- *Nerve sheath tumor:* The most common cause of a posterior mediastinal mass. Can extend over the lung apex. Would expect widening of the neural foramen.
- *Mesothelioma:* Often presents with unilateral pleural thickening with volume loss and extension into the fissure, especially in a patient with a significant asbestos exposure history. May be associated with a pleural effusion.

■ **Essential Facts**

- Non–small cell lung carcinoma arising from the lung apex and invading the chest wall or soft tissues of the thoracic inlet.
- Can be associated with Pancoast syndrome, which was originally described as shoulder and arm pain, atrophy of the hand muscles, and Horner syndrome (ptosis, miosis, and anhidrosis due to sympathetic nerve involvement) in association with an apical lung mass. Because not all cases of apical lung tumors result in Pancoast syndrome, the term *superior sulcus tumor* is preferred.
- Represents 3% of primary lung cancers, with adenocarcinomas and squamous cell carcinomas accounting for most cases.

- Because the tumors are peripheral, the usual symptoms of lung cancer may be absent. Patients may present with shoulder pain or other musculoskeletal or neurologic complaints.
- An asymmetrical apical cap, with a convex margin > 5 mm, especially when increased compared to previous radiographs, is suggestive of a superior sulcus tumor.
- Osseous destruction is seen in one third of cases.
- A lordotic radiograph may better depict the lung apex.
- On CT imaging, rib destruction and encasement of nerves or blood vessels are signs of chest wall invasion.

✓ **Pearls and ✗ Pitfalls**

✓ MRI is more accurate for evaluating brachial plexus and subclavian artery involvement. Spinal extension is also usually better depicted. Cardiac and respiratory gating can be used to minimize motion and pulsation artifacts.

✓ Superior sulcus tumors are at least stage IIB because of extrathoracic soft tissue invasion.

✓ Brachial plexus invasion above T1, vertebral body invasion > 50%, invasion of the esophagus or trachea, distant metastases, or N2/N3 nodal metastases are considered absolute contraindications to surgical resection.

✓ Because T1 sagittal sequences often provide the most information, these should be performed first in case the study cannot be completed.

✗ In patients who have undergone resection, a cerebrospinal fluid leak due to a subarachnoid-pleural fistula may develop.

✗ Often missed on initial chest radiographs.

Case 9

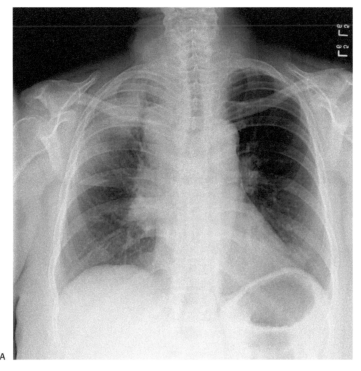

A

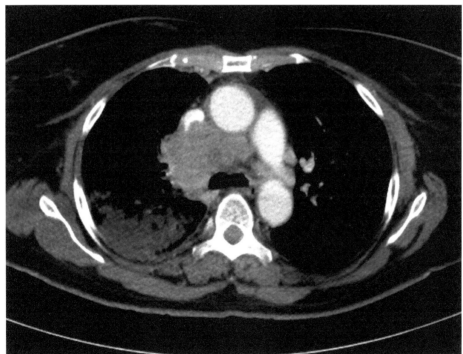

B

■ Clinical Presentation

A 58-year-old woman with cough and dysphagia.

■ Imaging Findings

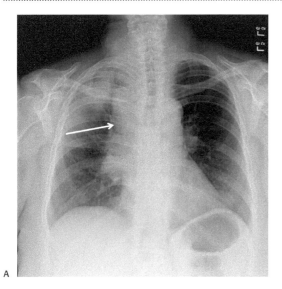
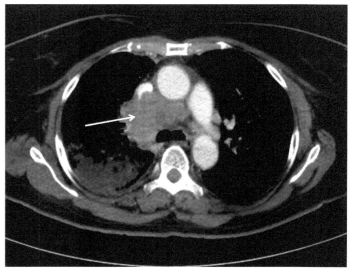

(A) Chest radiograph demonstrates a mediastinal mass (*arrow*) and nonspecific right upper lobe opacity. **(B)** Contrast-enhanced CT image shows a large irregularly marginated mediastinal mass invading the superior vena cava (*arrow*). There is patchy right upper lobe opacity.

■ Differential Diagnosis

- **Small-cell lung cancer (SCLC):** The most common imaging presentation is a large mediastinal mass, generally without imaging evidence of a lung parenchymal lesion.
- *Lymphoma:* A large mediastinal mass may also be the initial presentation of a lymphoma. The presence of airway obstruction helps in the differentiation between lymphoma and SCLC. Bronchial narrowing or an intraluminal mass is more common in lung cancer than in lymphoma.
- *Metastasis:* A wide variety of intra- and extrathoracic malignancies with mediastinal dissemination may present as a large mediastinal mass.

■ Essential Facts

- SCLC, also known as oat cell lung cancer, accounts for 20% of all primary lung cancers.
- Most SCLCs arise from the epithelium of the proximal airways (neuroendocrine cells), demonstrate rapid growth, and metastasize early.
- SCLCs are considered a type of neuroendocrine carcinoma.
- The incidence of SCLC is higher in males. It occurs almost exclusively in cigarette smokers and presents at a younger age than non–small-cell lung cancers.
- SCLC is aggressive with a poor prognosis and < 5% survival rate 5 years after diagnosis.

- The majority of patients have advanced disease at the time of diagnosis.
- Common imaging findings include a large, bulky mediastinal mass; a hilar mass; bronchial arrowing or obstruction; and postobstructive pneumonitis.
- A minority (< 5%) presents as limited disease (solitary pulmonary nodule).
- Common manifestations of SCLC include obstructive symptoms (cough, hemoptysis), dyspnea, dysphagia, hoarseness (recurrent laryngeal nerve involvement), and superior vena cava (SVC) syndrome.
- Positron emission tomography/CT is superior to CT for staging SCLC because it better identifies occult, advanced, or distant disease.

✓ Pearls and ✗ Pitfalls

- ✓ Collateral circulation with prominent neck and chest wall veins may be seen in patients with SCLC who present with SVC syndrome (12%).
- ✓ Disease is typically classified as limited or extensive. Limited disease is confined to one hemithorax, the mediastinum, and one ipsilateral supraclavicular node. Only 20% have limited disease at presentation.
- ✗ SCLC, like other neuroendocrine tumors, may produce metabolically active substances (e.g., adrenocorticotropic hormone, parathyroid hormone, antidiuretic hormone, calcitonin) that manifest clinically before the lung cancer is diagnosed.

Case 10

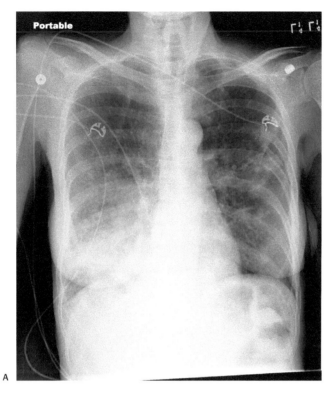

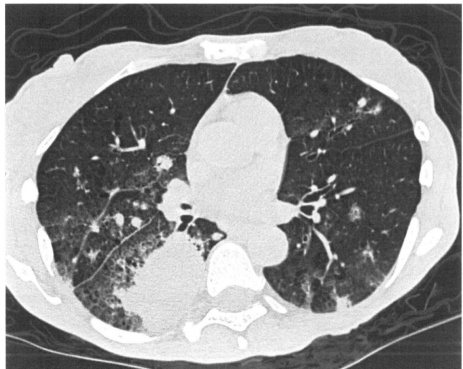

■ Clinical Presentation

A 50-year-old woman with progressive cough for 3 months.

■ Imaging Findings

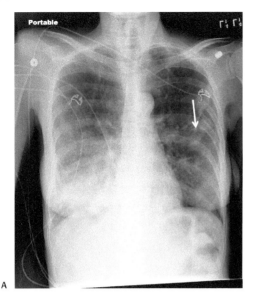
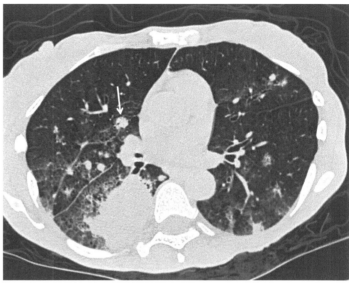

(A) Chest radiograph demonstrates right lower lung consolidation and multiple pulmonary nodules (*arrow*). **(B)** Noncontrast chest CT (lung windows) shows dense consolidation and right lower lobe with septal thickening. Multiple solid and subsolid pulmonary nodules are noted (*arrow*).

■ Differential Diagnosis

- *Lepidic predominant adenocarcinoma:* Lepidic predominant adenocarcinoma should be considered with a chronic, nonresolving consolidation in an adult.
- *Pneumonia:* The spectrum of infectious pneumonia can be quite variable, ranging from minimal parenchymal opacity to ill-defined ground glass density to complete lobar or multifocal air space consolidation. Atypical pneumonia (*Legionella, Mycoplasma, Chlamydia*), as well as viral and pneumocystic pneumonia, may present as ground glass opacities.
- *Interstitial pneumonia:* Some of the different types of interstitial pneumonia (desquamative interstitial pneumonia, nonspecific interstitial pneumonia) may present as extensive areas of ground glass opacity. Other differential diagnoses include pulmonary edema, drug toxicity, and alveolar hemorrhage.

■ Essential Facts

- Invasive mucinous adenocarcinoma is a variant of invasive adenocarcinoma, which was formerly known as mucinous bronchoalveolar carcinoma.
- Lepidic predominant adenocarcinoma describes invasive adenocarcinoma with a predominant lepidic pattern and > 5 mm of invasion. This was formerly referred to as nonmucinous bronchoalveolar carcinoma.
- Tumor cells are arranged in a single layer without producing pulmonary architectural destruction (lepidic growth pattern).
- When there is lepidic growth in the majority of the tumor but < 5 mm of invasion, the subtype is termed *minimally invasive adenocarcinoma.*

- Two types of preinvasive glandular proliferations are atypical adenomatous hyperplasia and adenocarcinoma in situ.
- In general, tumors that demonstrate only lepidic growth tend to be indolent, and the prognosis is better than with tumors that have solid invasive components.
- The incidence of this subtype of lung cancer has increased in the last several decades.
- The tumor cells may secrete intra-alveolar mucus or surfactant-like proteinaceous fluid, which can be significant in volume.
- The most common presentation is a peripheral, solitary, well-circumscribed pulmonary nodule (60%) followed by ill-defined areas of ground glass opacity or consolidation, mimicking pneumonia.
- When large amounts of mucin are present, the opacity can have low attenuation on CT imaging.
- An atypical appearance is that of multiple pulmonary nodules.

✓ Pearls and ✗ Pitfalls

- ✓ Bronchial wall thickening proximal to the lesion and pleural thickening associated with the lesion favor pneumonia. In contrast, deformity of the air-filled bronchus within the area of consolidation (stretching, squeezing, widening of the branching angle) or bulging of the interlobar fissure favor malignancy.
- ✓ Cavitating pulmonary metastases can occur rarely. This has been termed the "Cheerios sign."
- ✗ Positron emission tomography scanning in lepidic predominant adenocarcinoma has a lower sensitivity and a higher false-negative rate than in other types of lung carcinoma.

Case 11

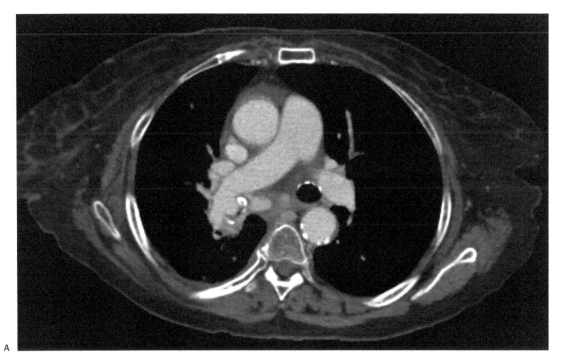

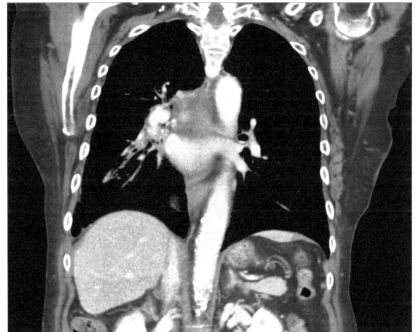

■ Clinical Presentation

A 50-year-old man with history of tuberculosis and massive hemoptysis.

■ Imaging Findings

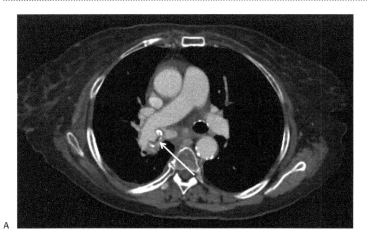
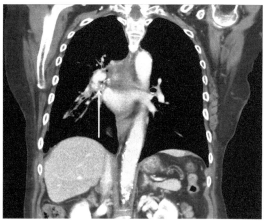

(A) Contrast-enhanced CT image shows a right pulmonary artery pseudoaneurysm extending into the bronchus (*arrow*). **(B)** Coronal CT reformat image shows the inflammatory hilar mass consistent with tuberculosis to advantage (*arrow*).

■ Differential Diagnosis

- ***Rasmussen aneurysm:*** Infectious aneurysms in a pulmonary artery secondary to pulmonary tuberculosis (TB) are referred to as Rasmussen aneurysms. Although not clearly seen in this case, they characteristically develop as a result of weakening of a pulmonary artery wall adjacent to a TB cavity.
- *Infectious pulmonary aneurysm (mycotic aneurysm):* Mycotic aneurysms of a pulmonary artery result from septic pulmonary embolism, typically in patients with infective endocarditis, or from direct arterial wall involvement in patients with necrotizing pneumonia. Syphilis was one culprit organism. In this case, direct arterial wall involvement from a central lung cancer can also be considered.
- *Traumatic pseudoaneurysm:* In patients who have sustained a penetrating lung injury, a traumatic pseudoaneurysm may develop, but it is more often in a peripheral pulmonary artery. Similarly, a pseudoaneurysm may develop secondary to endovascular injury from an intravascular catheter.

■ Essential Facts

- Hemoptysis in patients with TB may originate from either the bronchial arteries or the pulmonary arteries.
- Rasmussen aneurysms are pseudoaneurysms, considered to develop as a result of direct continuity with a focus of chronic fibrocaseous pulmonary parenchymal TB infection that directly invades or erodes a pulmonary artery.

- The mechanism is different from that seen in septic thromboembolism, in which the infective organism gains access to the arterial wall from a septic endovascular embolism that usually originates in an infected tricuspid valve in intravenous drug users.
- Localized dilatation of the medium size pulmonary arteries contiguous with the fibrous capsule of the wall of a chronic TB cavity has been described in 4% of patients with chronic cavitary TB.
- Rasmussen aneurysms of the pulmonary arteries result from destruction of the media of segmental pulmonary arteries by infection-induced granulation tissue.
- Catheter angiography helps to delineate the origin of the bleeding when clinically significant hemoptysis develops as a complication of pulmonary TB. In addition, endovascular embolization may be used to control the bleeding.

✓ Pearls and ✗ Pitfalls

✓ Massive hemoptysis (> 300 mL/24 h) is a well-known complication of chronic cavitary TB and can be life-threatening in as many as 20% of cases.

✓ Congenital cardiac anomalies leading to pulmonary hypertension, pulmonary valve stenosis, and pulmonary vasculitides such as Behçet disease and Hughes–Stovin syndrome can also case pulmonary aneurysms.

✗ Contrast-enhanced CT may be limited in defining whether a pulmonary parenchymal aneurysm or pseudoaneurysm originates from the pulmonary arterial circulation or from the bronchial systemic vasculature.

Case 12

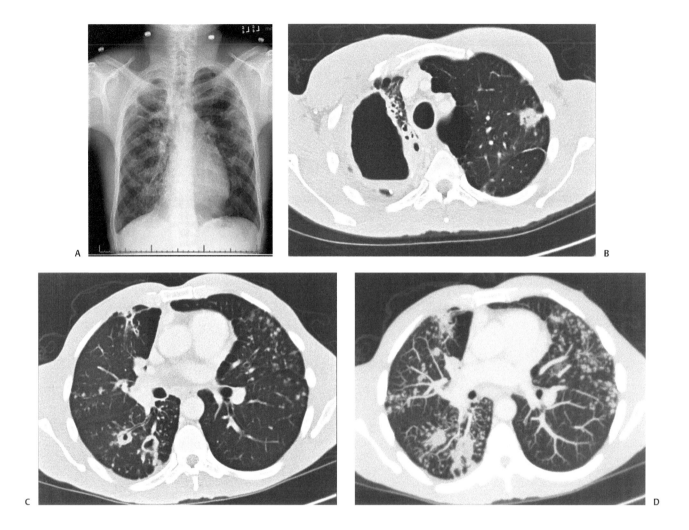

■ Clinical Presentation

A 44-year-old man with productive cough and night sweats.

■ **Imaging Findings**

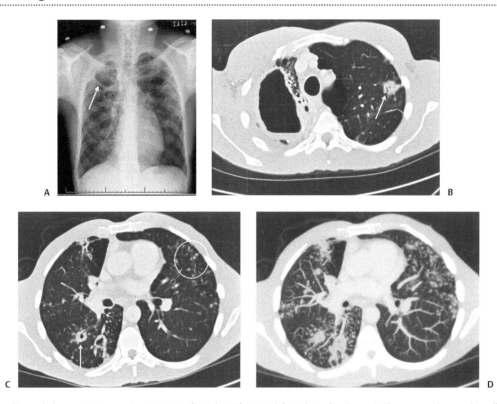

(A) Frontal chest radiograph demonstrates a cavitary mass on the right with upper lobe volume loss (*arrow*). There are widespread small pulmonary nodules and bronchial wall thickening. **(B)** Contrast-enhanced CT (lung window) shows the cavitary right upper lobe lesions to advantage. There is also an ill-defined nodule on the right (*arrow*). **(C)** Axial CT image (lung window) through the mid thorax shows multiple centrilobular nodules (*circle*) as well as thick-walled cavitary nodules (*arrow*). Mild bronchial wall thickening and bronchiectasis is also seen. **(D)** Maximum intensity projection image shows the centrilobular nodules and "tree-in-bud" opacity to advantage.

■ **Differential Diagnosis**

- **Postprimary tuberculosis:** Upper lobe volume loss with cavitary lesions, centilobular nodules, tree-in-bud opacity, and lack of adenopathy in this clinical setting make tuberculosis (TB) the diagnosis of exclusion.
- *Bronchogenic carcinoma:* Primary lung cancer can mimic TB in cases with cavitation, adenopathy, and chronic lung opacity. In this case, the patient's age and bilateral nature of findings make primary lung cancer unlikely.
- *Sarcoidosis:* End-stage sarcoidosis can result in upper lobe volume loss and small nodules. However, multiple thick-walled cavitary nodules would not be expected.

■ **Essential Facts**

- TB is usually confined to the respiratory system.
- Primary TB is seen in patients not previously exposed to the organism. It typically manifests as middle or lower lobe consolidation.
- Miliary disease is usually seen in the elderly, infants, and immunocompromised people. It can occur in primary and postprimary TB.
- Postprimary TB refers to both reinfection and reactivation TB.

- Postprimary TB manifests as consolidation, usually in the apical and posterior segments of the upper lobes. Cavitation is seen in 50%.
- Lymphadenopathy is rare in postprimary TB.
- In primary TB, lymphadenopathy is commonly seen in children but only in roughly half of adults.
- With primary infection, a pleural effusion, often with septations, can be seen.
- Endobronchial spread results in tree-in-bud opacity.
- Airway involvement can lead to bronchial stenosis.

✓ **Pearls and** ✗ **Pitfalls**

✓ Cavitation is the hallmark of postprimary disease.
✓ Rasmussen aneurysm refers to a pulmonary artery aneurysm due to adjacent cavitary TB.
✓ A Ghon focus refers to residual parenchymal scarring at a site of prior consolidation.
✗ Tuberculomas usually show uptake at fluorodeoxyglucose-positron emission tomography.
✗ Aspergillomas can develop in cavities.
✗ Broncholithiasis, pericardial involvement, fibrosing mediastinitis, fibrothorax, and chest wall involvement are additional sequelae of TB.

Case 13

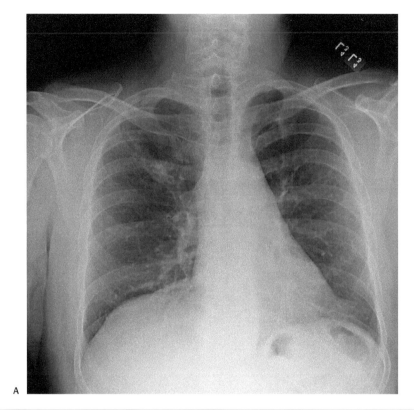

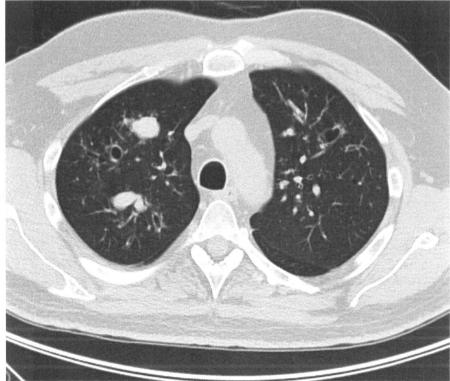

■ Clinical Presentation

A 29-year-old man with asthma and productive cough.

■ Imaging Findings

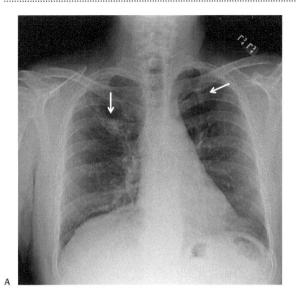 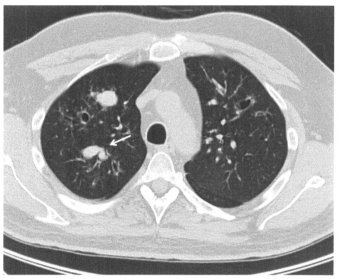

(A) Chest radiograph demonstrates upper lobe predominant bronchiectasis and branching tubular opacities (*arrows*). **(B)** Contrast-enhanced chest CT image (lung windows) demonstrates to advantage the branching, dilated bronchi with inspissated mucus (*arrow*).

■ Differential Diagnosis

- **Allergic bronchopulmonary aspergillosis (ABPA):** Fingerlike densities in a bronchial distribution are the characteristic finding of ABPA. The structures represent mucus plugs, more significantly involving the upper lobes, as well as bronchiectasis, and are occasionally associated with atelectasis.
- *Cystic fibrosis:* Bronchiectasis with mucoid impaction is relatively common in patients with cystic fibrosis. Usually, other findings such as bronchiolar impaction (tree-in-bud opacities), emphysema, abscess, and bullous formations are also present.
- *Bronchial atresia:* Mucoid impaction associated with bronchial atresia is common but characteristically involves a single lobe or segment.

■ Essential Facts

- ABPA results from a hypersensitivity reaction to *Aspergillus* spp., in particular *A. fumigatus.*
- The fungus does not invade tissue (bronchial or pulmonary).
- Marked local and systemic eosinophilia is characteristic of this condition.
- ABPA is a complication of persistent asthma (1–2%) and cystic fibrosis (5–15%), in part related to the excessive production of viscous mucus and abnormal mucociliary clearance.
- Inhaled *Aspergillus* spp. spores colonize and multiply in preexisting mucus inducing an allergic reaction with increased inflammation and further production of mucus.

- Histopathology reveals central bronchiectasis, eosinophilic pneumonitis, bronchocentric granulomatosis, bronchiolitis, and hyphae-laden microabscesses.
- Clinical manifestations include chronic cough, bronchorrhea, brown plugs containing *Aspergillus* spp. hyphae in the sputum, and wheezing.
- Imaging findings include central bronchiectasis (> 80%), predominantly in the upper lobes, toothpaste, gloved-finger or V/Y–shaped mucoid impaction, and pulmonary consolidation, which may represent eosinophilic alveolar infiltrates (eosinophilic pneumonia).
- Atelectasis due to retained secretions, which tend to shift over time from one part of the lung to another and may be segmental or lobar or affect an entire lung, is an additional common finding.

✓ Pearls and ✗ Pitfalls

✓ In some patients with ABPA (25%), the inspissated mucus plugs in the dilated bronchi may have a CT density higher than that expected for soft tissues. Similarly, high-density material is known to occur in the sinuses of patients with chronic allergic fungal sinusitis. It is believed to be secondary to high calcium and/or metallic content in the mucus.

✗ The sensitivity of plain films for the detection of bronchiectasis, which is one of the most significant features of ABPA, is limited (50%). Thin-slice CT should always be used to detect this abnormal finding.

Case 14

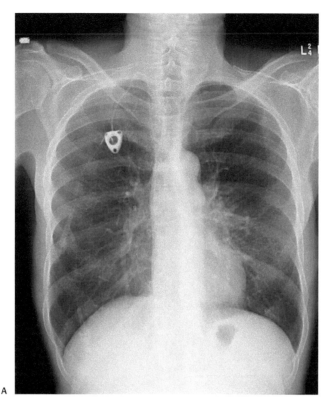

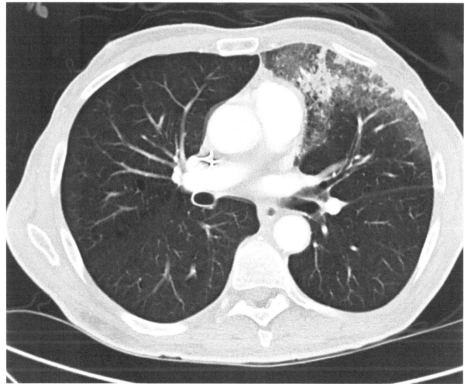

■ Clinical Presentation

A 32-year-old man with fever and cough.

■ Imaging Findings

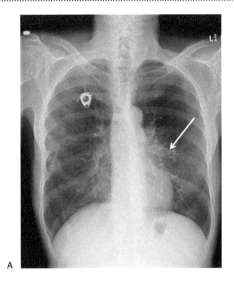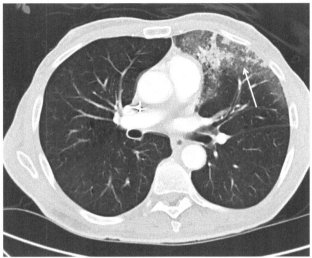

(A) Chest radiograph demonstrates lingular consolidation with loss of the silhouette of the left heart border (*arrow*). **(B)** Contrast-enhanced chest CT image (soft tissue windows) demonstrates patchy ground-glass and solid coalescing nodular opacities (*arrow*).

■ Differential Diagnosis

- **Klebsiella pneumonia:** This gram-negative bacillus, as well as other gram-negative organisms (*Escherichia coli* and *Pseudomonas aeruginosa*), are important causes of nosocomial pneumonia and are more likely than other organisms to cause necrotizing disease and cavity formation.
- *Tuberculosis (TB):* Reactivation TB also tends to involve the posterior segment of the upper lobes and to present with necrosis and cavitation. Lobar consolidation of the surrounding parenchyma is less common.
- *Necrotizing lung cancer:* In adults, lung cancer should always be considered in the differential diagnosis of a cavitary lesion in the upper lobes, especially if it is thick walled.

■ Essential Facts

- Gram-negative bacilli, including *Klebsiella pneumoniae*, *P. aeruginosa*, *Enterobacter*, and *E. coli*, are important causes of nosocomial and community-acquired pneumonia.
- With some variation among medical centers, the most common pathogens isolated in patients with nosocomial pneumonia are gram-negative organisms and *Staphylococcus aureus*.
- Important risk factors include intubation, mechanical ventilation, enteral nutrition, reduced level of consciousness, and increased gastric pH (achlorhydria or the administration and anti-acid medications).
- Between 50 and 70% of cases of ventilator-associated nosocomial pneumonia in intensive care units are caused by gram-negative bacilli.

- *K. pneumoniae* is the most common infective agent seen in the elderly, people with alcoholism, and debilitated men.
- The source or pulmonary infection is commonly aspirated infected oral secretions.
- The infectious process typically involves the posterior segment of the right upper lobe or the posterior lower lobes.
- Parapneumonic pleural effusion and empyema are common complications in these patients (> 60%).
- Lobar consolidation is more typical of *Klebsiella* pneumonia, whereas bronchopneumonia, manifesting as multifocal opacities (80%), is more common with *E. coli* and *P. aeruginosa* infection.
- *Klebsiella* pneumonia tends to present with lobar expansion and bulging of the interlobar fissures (30%) more than with pneumococcal consolidation (10%). This finding is known as the bulging fissure sign.

✓ Pearls and ✗ Pitfalls

✓ Pneumatoceles differ from lung abscesses associated with gram-negative or anaerobic bacteria. Pneumatoceles are thin-walled, gas-filled spaces seen in areas of air space disease and consolidation in patients with pneumonia. They develop from the acute infection and resolve in weeks or months.

✗ Partially resolved *Klebsiella* pneumonia, in which the bulk of the consolidation resolves leaving an upper lobe cavity and scarring, may have imaging findings similar to those seen in reactivation TB.

Case 15

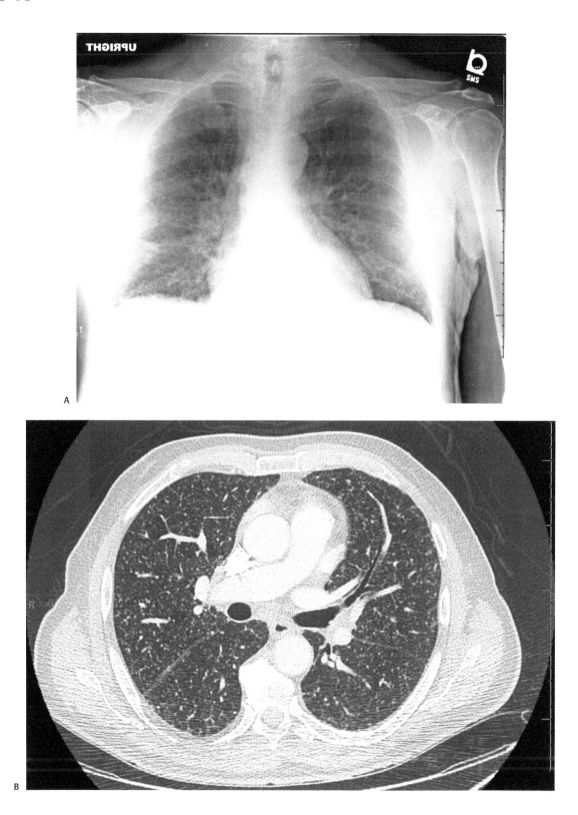

A

B

■ Clinical Presentation

A 42-year-old man with skin rash, shortness of breath, and fever.

■ Imaging Findings

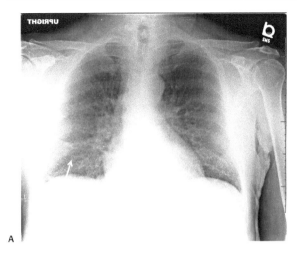
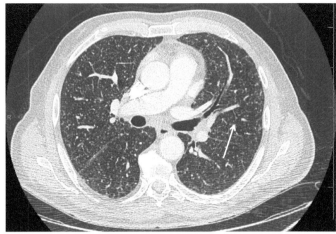

(A) Portable chest radiograph demonstrates multiple bilateral small nodular opacities (*arrow*). **(B)** Contrast-enhanced chest CT image (lung windows) demonstrates innumerable punctate nodular opacities in a miliary pattern (*arrow*).

■ Differential Diagnosis

- ***Varicella pneumonia:*** The association of the typical skin rash with multiple pulmonary nodules scattered throughout the lung parenchyma should raise the question of varicella-zoster virus (VZV) pneumonia.
- *Other viral pneumonias (cytomegalovirus [CMV], influenza, measles):* Several viral pneumonias in adult patients may present with a combination of irregular patchy opacities and nodular ground-glass densities in the lung parenchyma.
- *Hemorrhagic pulmonary metastases:* Hemorrhagic pulmonary metastases from choriocarcinoma or angiosarcoma may present as multiple ground-glass pulmonary nodules.

■ Essential Facts

- Viral pneumonias in adult patients may present in two different clinical settings: in an otherwise healthy host (so-called atypical pneumonia) or in an immunocompromised host.
- Most cases of varicella pneumonia in adults occur in patients with lymphoma or who are immunocompromised.
- The proportion of viral infections in cases of community-acquired pneumonia varies from 10 to 50%, depending on the age of the population, geography, and diagnostic criteria.
- Common viral infectious agents in immunocompetent hosts includes influenza A and B viruses, adenoviruses, Epstein–Barr virus, and hantaviruses.
- The most common viral infectious agents in immunocompromised patients include CMV, herpes simplex viruses, VZV, measles virus, and adenoviruses.

- Imaging manifestations in viral pneumonias usually reflect the combination of interstitial and air space disease, with multifocal, poorly defined areas of patchy consolidation, ground-glass opacities, centrilobular nodules, reticular opacities resulting from interlobular septal thickening, and lobular consolidation.
- With varicella, common findings include multiple small nodular opacities (some with a surrounding halo), patchy ground-glass opacities, and coalescence of nodules. A miliary pattern may also be seen.
- Lesions can calcify and persist as punctate, randomly scattered dense nodules.
- Lobar consolidation is less common in viral pneumonia than in bacterial infection.
- Interstitial opacities can be seen in both bacterial and viral pneumonias.
- The differentiation between bacterial and viral pneumonias on clinical grounds or laboratory findings is limited; the proportions of patients with an elevated white cell count or elevated erythrocyte sedimentation rate are similar in bacterial and viral pneumonias.
- In some viral pneumonias, particularly in children, significant bronchial wall thickening with overinflation and atelectasis are the dominant imaging findings.

✓ Pearls and ✗ Pitfalls

✓ Pneumonia is a common and serious complication of VZV infection (chickenpox) in adults, with significant morbidity and mortality.

✗ Pleural effusion is not exclusively a complication of bacterial pneumonias. A significant amount of parapneumonic pleural fluid can be associated with different viral pneumonias.

Case 16

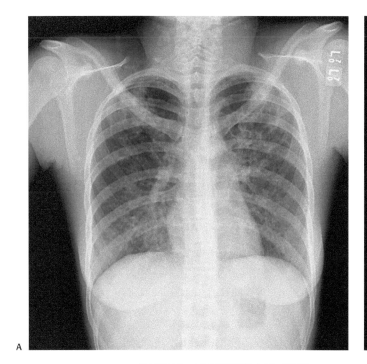

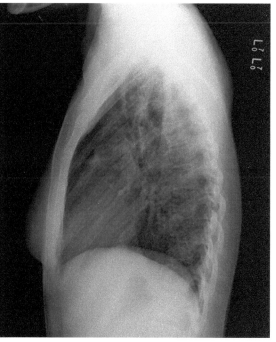

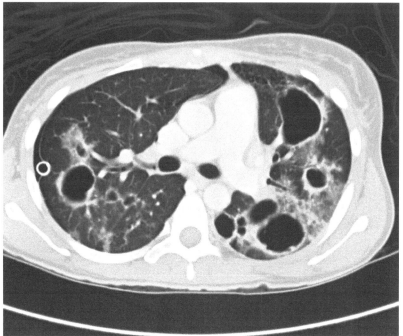

■ Clinical Presentation

A 44-year-old man with AIDS and progressive shortness of breath.

■ Imaging Findings

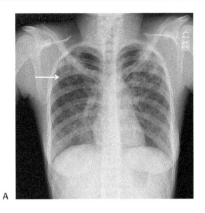
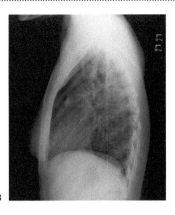
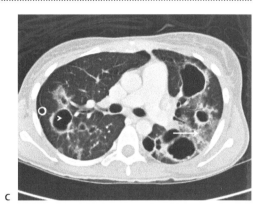

(A) Frontal chest radiograph demonstrates bilateral diffuse opacity with upper lobe predominant cavitary lesions. A small right pneumothorax is present (*arrow*). **(B)** Lateral chest radiograph shows increased opacity with no significant pleural effusions. **(C)** Axial chest CT image (lung window) confirms ground-glass opacity (*arrow*) and thick irregular cysts (*arrowhead*). A chest tube has been placed on the right for treatment of a spontaneous pneumothorax.

■ Differential Diagnosis

- **Pneumocystis pneumonia:** Multifocal ground-glass opacities more confluent in the upper lobes associated with cystic changes in a patient with AIDS are highly suggestive of *Pneumocystis* pneumonia.
- *Cytomegalovirus (CMV) pneumonia:* Ground-glass opacities with a multifocal distribution may also be seen in immunocompromised patients with CMV infection. Pulmonary nodules are often associated.
- *Pulmonary edema:* Diffuse ground-glass opacity and interlobular septal thickening are very common imaging findings in pulmonary edema. When progressive, pleural effusions may develop; pleural effusions are typically not found in *Pneumocystis* pneumonia.

■ Essential Facts

- *Pneumocystis* pneumonia is an infection caused by *Pneumocystis jirovecii*, an opportunistic fungal pathogen.
- *Pneumocystis* is the most prevalent opportunistic infectious agent in patients with HIV. It is responsible for 25% of cases of pneumonia in patients with HIV and is one of the most common causes of death among patients with AIDS.
- Affected patients typically have profound T-cell immunosuppression, with a CD4 count of < 200 cells/mm³.
- Affected patients typically present with fever, nonproductive cough, dyspnea, hypoxemia, and elevated lactic dehydrogenase levels.
- Bilateral diffuse or multifocal ground-glass opacities are a characteristic finding.

- When the ground-glass opacities are associated with interlobular septal thickening, "crazy paving" is the dominant imaging pattern.
- Severe cases may present with dense air space consolidation.
- CT image reveals ground-glass opacities in the perihilar regions and upper lobes.
- Pleural effusions and lymphadenopathy are uncommon.
- *Pneumocystis* infection less commonly presents in patients with forms of immunosuppression other than AIDS, such as transplant recipients (10%), patients with solid tumors, and patients with collagen vascular disease receiving steroid therapy (2%).
- *Pneumocystis* pneumonia demonstrates increased activity on gallium scans.

✓ Pearls and ✗ Pitfalls

- ✓ In humans, *Pneumocystis* infection is caused by *P. jirovecii*. This is different from *Pneumocystis carinii*, which causes infections in other mammals.
- ✓ Pulmonary cysts, one of the complications of *Pneumocystis* infection (10–30%), may result in spontaneous pneumothorax.
- ✓ *Pneumocystis* pneumonia is exceedingly rare in immunocompetent patients.
- ✗ *Pneumocystis* is a well-known cause of pneumonia in patients with normal findings on chest radiographs (10–30%). However, it is extremely rare for patients with *Pneumocystis* pneumonia to have normal findings on CT imaging.
- ✗ HIV-positive patients with CD4 counts > 200 cells/mm³ account for 10% of cases.

Case 17

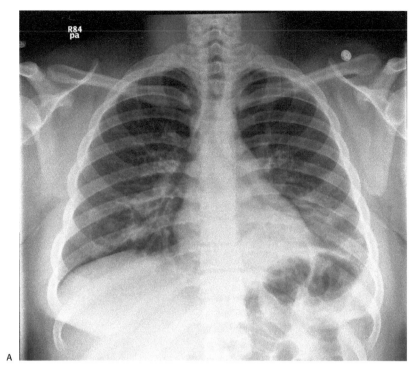

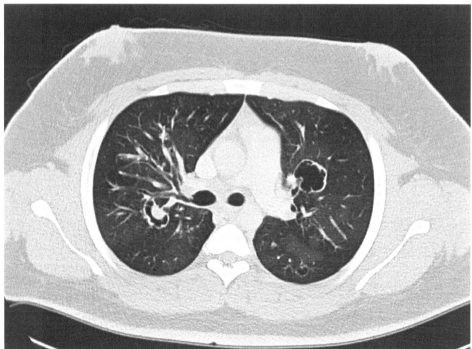

■ Clinical Presentation

A 19-year-old woman with chronic cough and wheezing.

■ Imaging Findings

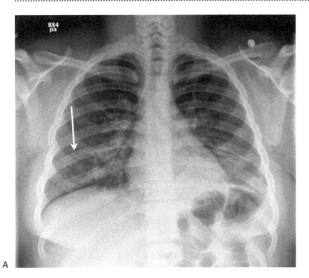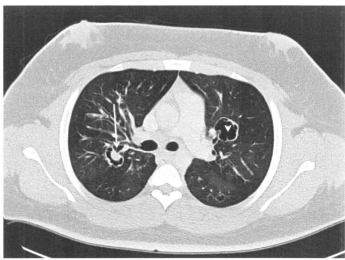

A   B

(A) Chest radiograph demonstrates multiple cavitary lesions. The mass in the right lower lobe has a thin wall (*arrow*). **(B)** Conventional enhanced CT image on lung window shows a thin-walled cavity in the left upper lobe (*arrowhead*) and a cavitating nodule in the right upper lobe (*arrow*).

■ Differential Diagnosis

- **Pulmonary papillomatosis:** The patient's age and the presence of multiple nodules and cavities favor papillomatosis.
- *Pulmonary Langerhans cell histiocytosis (PLCH):* PLCH can also present with nodules and cysts, but typically the lung volumes are large and the upper lobes are more affected. There is a strong association with cigarette smoking.
- *Lymphangioleiomyomatosis (LAM):* LAM is characterized by diffusely distributed thin-walled cysts. It occurs exclusively in women.

■ Essential Facts

- Also termed *tracheobronchial papillomatosis* and *pulmonary papillomatosis.*
- Results from human papillomavirus infection (types 6, 11, 16, and 18) of the upper respiratory tract, most commonly as the child passes through an infected birth canal.
- Adult sexual transmission can occur.
- Most cases remain limited to the trachea and can result in focal or diffuse nodular airway narrowing.
- Lung disease develops in 1% of cases, typically 10 years after laryngeal disease.

- Lung involvement may be secondary to implantation of inhaled fragments from the larynx or multifocal viral infection.
- Lung disease is characterized by multiple well-defined perihilar and posteriorly located nodules, which eventually cavitate.
- Demonstrate extremely slow growth, measured in decades.
- Laser therapy, antiviral medications, and surgical excision have been used to treat papillomatosis.
- Progression of disease can lead to respiratory failure.
- Large intrabronchial lesions may cause obstructive atelectasis, pneumonia, or bronchiectasis.
- Solitary papillomas are rare and typically occur in adult male smokers.

✓ Pearls and ✗ Pitfalls

- ✓ Malignant degeneration to squamous cell carcinoma occurs in 10% of cases.
- ✓ The presence of an air-fluid level suggests superinfection.
- ✓ Any new or enlarging nodule should be evaluated further to exclude malignancy.
- ✗ Cavities may represent cavitary nodules, necrotic squamous cell carcinoma, or abscess secondary to obstructive pneumonitis.

Case 18

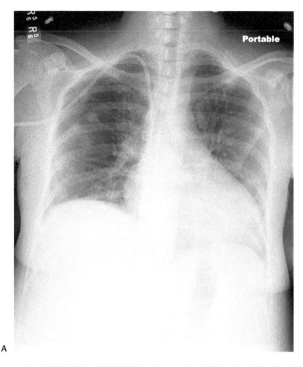

A

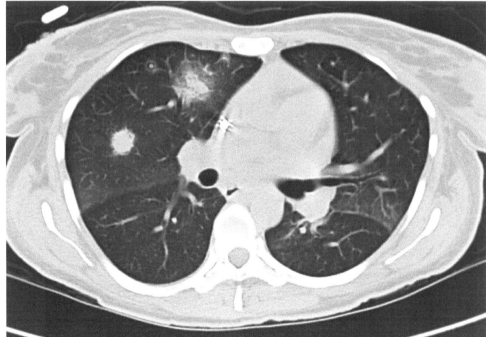

B

■ Clinical Presentation

A 40-year-old woman with neutropenic fever.

■ Imaging Findings

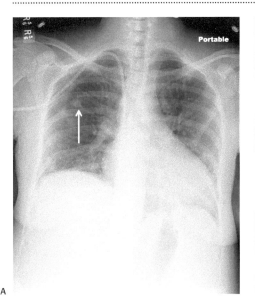 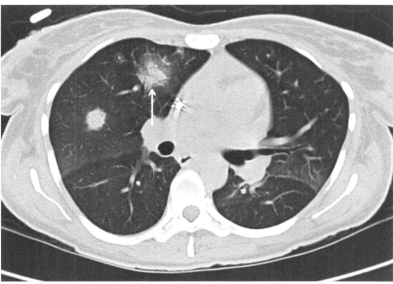

A

B

(A) Chest radiograph demonstrates multiple pulmonary nodules on the right (*arrow*). **(B)** Contrast-enhanced chest CT image (lung windows) demonstrates pulmonary nodules with irregular margins. Note the surrounding ground-glass halo of lesser density (*arrow*).

■ Differential Diagnosis

- **Angioinvasive aspergillosis with the halo sign:** In an immunocompromised patient, a dense nodule surrounded by a ground-glass halo is highly suggestive of angioinvasive aspergillosis.
- *Hemorrhagic tumor:* Neoplasms with bleeding may present with a dense nodule and a ground-glass rim of hemorrhage.
- *Vasculitis:* Pulmonary changes due to vasculitis may also manifest with a central dense nodular opacity and a peripheral halo. Cavitation may also be present.

■ Essential Facts

- The halo sign consists of a halo of ground-glass attenuation, which represents alveolar hemorrhage, surrounding a central denser nodule, which corresponds to a focus of infarction.
- This imaging sign was originally described in patients with invasive aspergillosis.
- In immunosuppressed patients, the halo sign is suggestive of aspergillosis, mucormycosis (*Rhizopus*), candidiasis, coccidioidomycosis, or infection with other fungi.
- The prevalence of the halo sign varies with disease evolution. It is more prevalent (> 90%) early in the course of the disease and less prevalent (< 20%) after 2 weeks.
- Approximately half of the nodules may evolve to cavitation, which has been associated with the recovery of white blood cell count.

- When the central necrotic lung separates away from the surrounding parenchyma, an air crescent can be seen.
- Risk factors for angioinvasive aspergillosis include immunosuppression with severe neutropenia after treatment for hematologic malignancies (high-dose chemotherapy, stem cell or bone marrow transplant) as well as immunosuppression after solid organ transplant and with chronic corticosteroid therapy for autoimmune disease.

✓ Pearls and ✗ Pitfalls

- ✓ Besides nodules, angioinvasive aspergillosis may also manifest as wedge-shaped areas of peripheral parenchymal consolidation.
- ✓ High-resolution CT pulmonary angiography may help in differentiating among various conditions presenting with the halo sign by detecting vascular occlusion in angioinvasive aspergillosis.
- ✗ Angioinvasive pulmonary aspergillosis has a high mortality rate (> 30%) in immunocompromised patients.
- ✗ Besides opportunistic infection, the halo sign has been demonstrated in other conditions associated with pulmonary hemorrhage, including metastases (angiosarcoma, choriocarcinoma), Kaposi sarcoma, vasculitis, organizing pneumonia, and lung injury.

Case 19

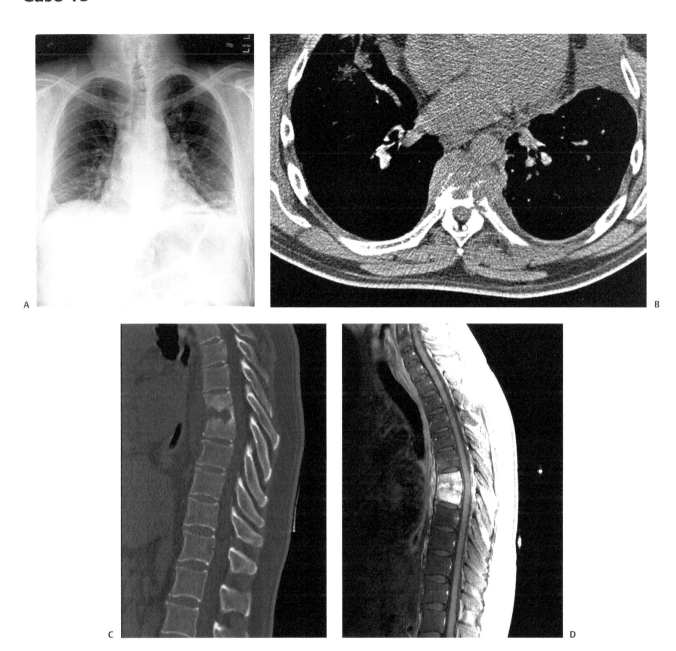

■ Clinical Presentation

A 45-year-old man with back pain and fever.

■ **Imaging Findings**

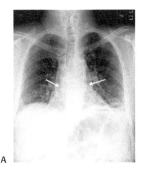 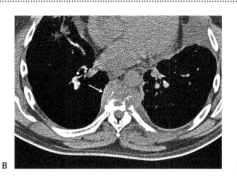 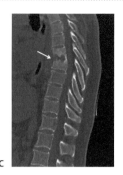 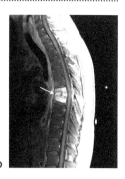

(A) Portable chest radiograph demonstrates widening of the paravertebral stripes at the mid thoracic level (*arrows*). (B) Noncontrast spine CT image shows an osteolytic lesion and fluid density with a paraspinal low-density mass (*arrow*). (C) Noncontrast spine CT sagittal reformat image shows that osteolysis to advantage (*arrow*). (D) Postcontrast sagittal MR image shows avid enhancement of the disk and adjacent vertebral bodies (*arrow*).

■ **Differential Diagnosis**

- ***Bacterial spondylodiskitis (vertebral osteomyelitis):***
  Vertebral body destruction and paraspinal fluid (abscess) are characteristic findings of bacterial infection of the vertebral bodies and disk.
- *Osteolytic tumor:* Primary (e.g., plasmacytoma, lymphoma) or secondary (e.g., metastasis from lung cancer, breast cancer) tumors may also present as vertebral body erosion, pathologic fracture, and paraspinal hemorrhage.
- *Vertebral body fracture:* Trauma with vertebral body fracture may present with paraspinal and posterior mediastinal hematoma.

■ **Essential Facts**

- Bacterial spondylodiskitis is the infection of an intervertebral disk space and the adjacent vertebral bodies.
- The infectious process is believed to begin at the vertebral body end plate as the consequence of hematogenous dissemination from a distant source (urinary tract infection, skin, prostatitis, endocarditis).
- Important risk factors include intravenous drug abuse, diabetes, malnutrition, renal failure, steroid therapy, HIV infection, and other causes of immunosuppression.
- *Staphylococcus aureus* accounts for > 50% of cases of pyogenic spondylodiskitis.
- Other infectious microorganisms include *Streptococcus viridans*, *Escherichia coli*, *Staphylococcus epidermidis*, and other gram-negative bacteria such as *Proteus* and *Pseudomonas*.
- In some parts of the world, *Mycobacterium tuberculosis* is still a common cause of spinal infection (Pott disease), second only to *S. aureus*.
- Clinical manifestations include back pain (90%), fever, night sweats, anemia, and, in advanced stages, neurologic manifestations of spinal cord compression.
- Inflammatory markers such as CRP and ESR are typically elevated.
- The thoracic or thoracolumbar spine is affected in nearly 45% of cases.

- Compression fractures and epidural abscess may result in significant neurologic complications.
- One in every three to four cases is complicated by an epidural abscess.
- Conventional radiography may reveal collapse of a vertebral body or an intervertebral disk space.
- CT image may show more obvious vertebral body destruction, disk space obliteration, and paraspinal abscess.
- Typical findings of spondylodiskitis on MR images are low signal intensity of the disks and adjacent vertebral bodies on T1-weighted images and hyperintensity on T2-weighted and fat-suppressed sequences.
- Contrast-enhanced MR images show inhomogeneous enhancement of the disks and adjacent vertebral bodies, and of the epidural and paravertebral soft tissue.
- Enhancing areas represent granulation tissue, whereas nonenhancing areas represent necrosis and the central portion of an abscess.
- Pathologic intraspinal and paravertebral soft tissue and epidural abscess, when present, can also be better appreciated with contrast-enhanced MR image.
- Fluorodeoxyglucose–positron emission tomography (PET) scan has a high sensitivity for spondylodiskitis, although it is nonspecific. With a negative PET scan, infectious spondylodiskitis can usually be excluded.

✓ **Pearls and** ✗ **Pitfalls**

✓ MRI is the imaging modality of choice for the diagnosis of infective spondylodiskitis, particularly in the early stages of the disease when other imaging modalities yield negative results.

✓ In children, infection may start in the intervertebral disk itself due to direct blood supply.

✓ Diffusion-weighted MR image shows hyperintensity in the acute stage, which eventually becomes hypointense.

✗ In the early stage of infective spondylodiskitis, the findings on conventional radiography and CT may be normal.

✗ In untreated cases, osseous sclerosis may appear after 10 to 12 weeks.

Case 20

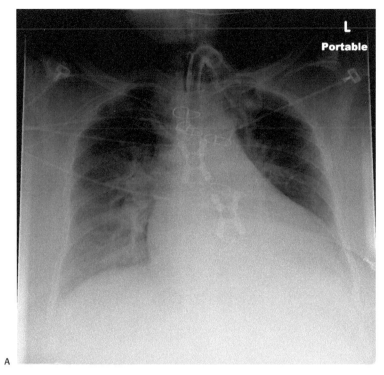

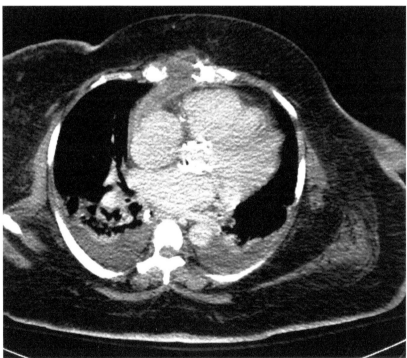

■ Clinical Presentation

A 60-year-old man with fever 3 weeks after cardiac surgery.

■ Imaging Findings

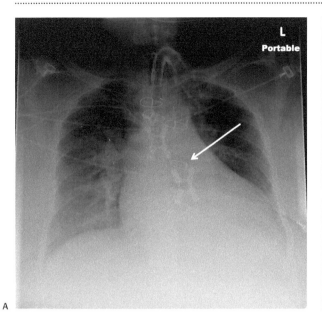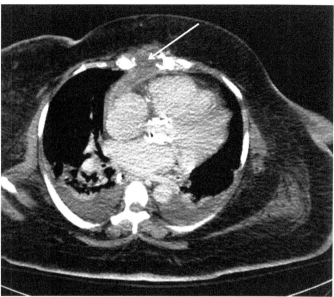

A   B

(A) Portable chest radiograph demonstrates displacement of multiple sternal wires and sideplate and screw-fixation devices (*arrow*). **(B)** Contrast-enhanced chest CT image (soft tissue windows) through the sternum demonstrates a sternal abscess (*arrow*) extending to the pericardium.

■ Differential Diagnosis

- ***Sternal dehiscence with abscess and mediastinitis:*** The presence of displaced sternal wires in association with a large fluid collection and soft tissue stranding in the anterior mediastinum make sternal dehiscence with abscess and mediastinitis the best answer.
- *Seroma:* In the first 14 days following surgery, a fluid collection may be normal. The time frame and associated findings in this case make a simple fluid collection unlikely.
- *Tuberculosis (TB):* Chest wall involvement of TB is uncommon, although when present, chest wall abscess and sinus tract formation is seen in 25% of cases. It would be highly unlikely to manifest as a postoperative complication.

■ Essential Facts

- Poststernotomy complications occur in < 5% of cases.
- The mortality of sternal wound infection with mediastinitis is > 50%.
- Sternal dehiscence, mediastinitis, and osteomyelitis are the most notable poststernotomy complications.

- Complications usually manifest 1 to 2 weeks after surgery.
- The presence of localized mediastinal fluid and pneumomediastinum is sensitive but nonspecific for mediastinitis in the first 14 days after surgery. The specificity increases significantly after 14 days.
- Sternal dehiscence is defined as complete separation of the sternum and is frequently associated with infection, most often *Staphylococcus aureus*.
- In sternal dehiscence, the wires are typically displaced. Rotation and disruption of wires can also occur.
- Debridement and flap closure are usually necessary.
- Following chest tube removal, there may be spontaneous evacuation of the sterile drain from the surgical site.

✓ Pearls and ✗ Pitfalls

- ✓ The term "wandering wires" has been used to describe the characteristic radiographic appearance of sternal wires in dehiscence.
- ✗ Sternal wire fracture by itself is usually not clinically significant.

Case 21

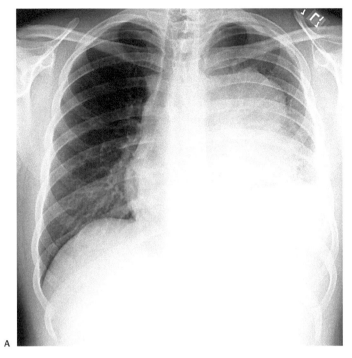

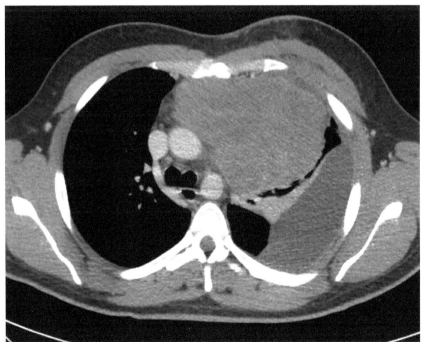

■ Clinical Presentation

A 30-year-old woman with fatigue.

■ **Imaging Findings**

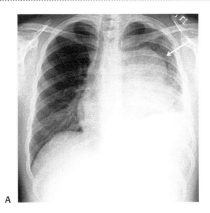 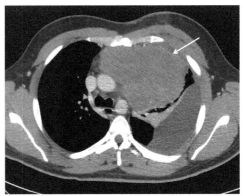

(A) Frontal chest radiograph demonstrates a large mass in the medial left hemithorax (*arrow*). There is loss of the left heart border, but the left hilar structures project through the mass (hilum overlay sign). **(B)** CT image with contrast confirms the anterior location of the mass (*arrow*) causing displacement of mediastinal structures. Note the left pleural effusion.

■ **Differential Diagnosis**

- **Lymphoma:** The presence of a solitary noncalcified anterior mediastinal mass separate from the thymus in a patient of this age is suggestive of lymphoma. Although this patient had large B-cell non-Hodgkin lymphoma, Hodgkin disease (HD) would be the most likely diagnosis because most mediastinal lymphoma is HD.
- *Thymoma:* Slow-growing anterior mediastinal mass. Typically occurs in older patients and shows calcification or cystic changes in one third of cases. The presence of a normal thymus separate from this mass argues against a thymic lesion.
- *Teratoma:* Mature teratomas frequently demonstrate cystic components, fat, and/or calcium. However, seminoma, the most common primary malignant germ cell tumor of the mediastinum, typically presents as a homogeneous, well-marginated soft tissue mass in which cystic components and calcification are uncommon.
- *Castleman disease:* Also called angiofollicular or giant lymph node hyperplasia. More typically a middle mediastinal and hilar mass with multiple enlarged lymph nodes which may show intense enhancement. Calcification is seen in 10%.

■ **Essential Facts**

- May present with cough or chest pain.
- "B symptoms" comprise weight loss, fever, and night sweats.
- Mediastinal lymphoma is more likely to be HD than non-Hodgkin lymphoma.
- HD has a bimodal age distribution and demonstrates intrathoracic involvement in 85% of cases.
- Nodular sclerosing is the most common subtype of HD, and there is a strong predilection for the anterior mediastinum.
- Intrathoracic involvement is seen in 50% of cases of non-Hodgkin lymphoma.

- Non-Hodgkin lymphoma commonly presents with bulky asymmetric mediastinal and hilar lymphadenopathy.
- Diffuse large B-cell lymphoma is seen in young adult females. Other large-cell lymphomas present in older patients, with a slight male predominance.
- Calcification is rarely seen prior to treatment.
- Posttransplant lymphoproliferative disorder (PTLD) occurs in 5% of solid organ transplants. The peak incidence is 3 to 4 months after treatment. Most cases are B-cell non-Hodgkin lymphoma.
- Mild enhancement is seen on CT and MR images.
- Pleural, pericardial, and lung parenchymal involvement is rare.
- Signal intensity on T1-weighted MR image is similar to that of muscle.
- Low signal intensity on T2-weighted MR image is seen in successfully treated lesions.
- High signal intensity on T2-weighted MR image may represent active disease, inflammation, cystic change, or immature fibrosis.
- Gallium-67 scintigraphy was historically used to differentiate residual disease from posttreatment fibrosis but has been largely replaced by positron emission tomography.

✓ **Pearls and** ✗ **Pitfalls**

✓ When the normal hilar structures project through a mass (hilum overlay sign), the mass is assumed to be located anterior or posterior to the hilum.

✓ On a posteroanterior radiograph, when the cephalic border of a mediastinal mass is obscured at or below the clavicles, it is located in the anterior mediastinum (cervicothoracic sign). If the mass is clearly delineated on all borders above the clavicles, the mass is posterior to the trachea.

✓ Lymphoma is more likely to displace mediastinal structures rather than invade them.

✗ Following radiation therapy, up to 20% of cases will show calcification.

Case 22

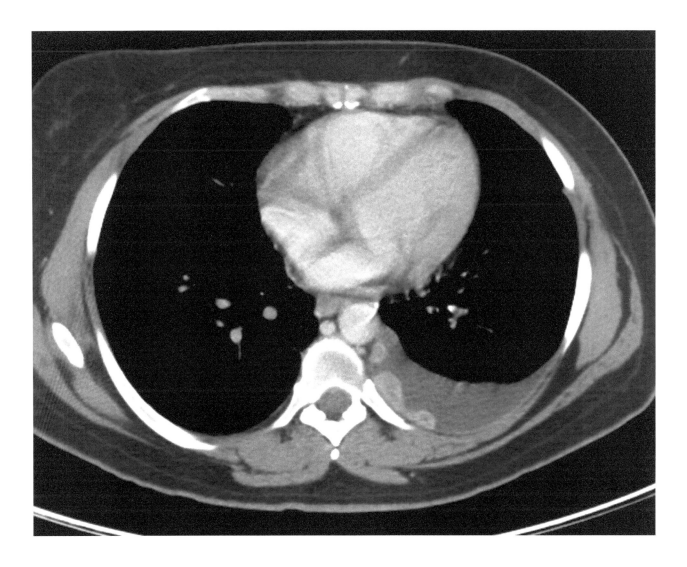

■ **Clinical Presentation**

A 30-year-old woman with fatigue.

■ Imaging Findings

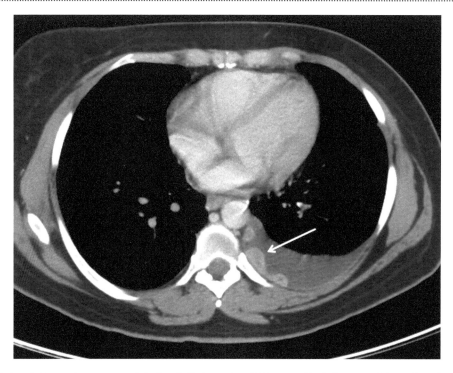

(A) Contrast-enhanced chest CT image demonstrates a left pleural effusion with multiple areas of high-density nodularity along the pleural surface (*arrow*).

■ Differential Diagnosis

- ***Pleural metastases:*** The presence of a pleural effusion and pleural-based nodules in a patient with a history of thyroid cancer make pleural metastases the most likely diagnosis.
- *Invasive thymoma:* Pleural metastases are very common with invasive lesions. There may be extension into the abdomen or retroperitoneum. An anterior mediastinal mass would support this diagnosis.
- *Mesothelioma:* The most common findings are unilateral pleural effusion and pleural thickening. Extension into the interlobar fissures, which is not seen in this case, is common. Calcified pleural plaques are seen in 10 to 20% of cases. Often associated with hemithoracic volume loss.
- *Splenosis:* Autotransplantation of splenic tissue following trauma or surgery typically results in multiple small pleural masses in the inferior posterior left hemithorax. Splenosis is not associated with lymphadenopathy or pleural effusion. Nuclear medicine tests such as sulfur colloid liver-spleen scan or tagged red blood cell scan are confirmatory.

■ Essential Facts

- Primary tumors account for < 5% of pleural neoplasms.
- Metastases develop via lymphangitic, vascular, or direct invasion.
- The visceral pleura is most commonly involved.

- Adenocarcinoma is the most common tumor to metastasize to the pleura, with lung (35%) and breast (25%) cancer accounting for the majority of cases.
- A pleural effusion, mostly hemorrhagic, is seen in 60% of patients.
- Solid tumor deposits or "pleural studding" can be seen.
- The masses are usually well defined, with angles obtuse to the chest wall.
- Metastases may also appear as a solitary implant on the costal, diaphragmatic, or mediastinal pleura or within the interlobar fissures.
- Pleural lymphoma can manifest as a solitary nodule or diffuse tumor infiltration with associated pleural effusion.

✓ Pearls and ✗ Pitfalls

✓ Circumferential pleural thickening, disseminated pleural nodularity, a parietal pleural thickness exceeding 1 cm, and mediastinal pleural involvement favor a neoplastic process.

✗ Mesothelioma has both radiologic and histologic similarity to metastatic adenocarcinoma, making distinction difficult when there is no known primary tumor.

✗ Epithelioid hemangioendothelioma, synovial sarcoma of the pleura, and primary leiomyosarcoma are rare tumors resulting in pleural nodularity and effusion, which can mimic pleural metastases.

Case 23

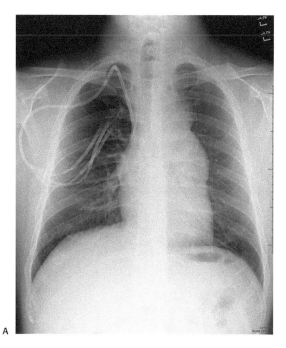

A

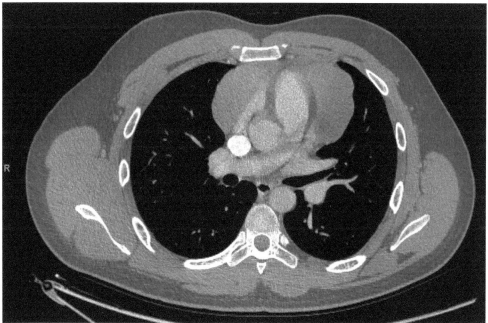

B

■ Clinical Presentation

A 23-year-old man with fatigue, anemia, and easy bruising.

■ Imaging Findings

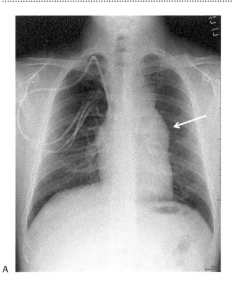 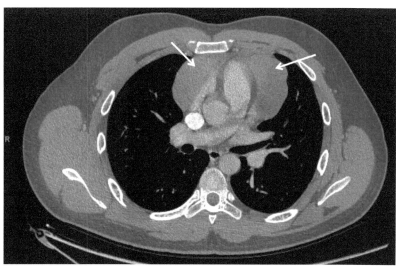

(A) Chest radiograph shows a mediastinal mass (*arrow*). **(B)** Contrast-enhanced chest CT image shows an infiltrative mediastinal mass of low density (*arrows*).

■ Differential Diagnosis

- ***Leukemia (acute lymphocytic leukemia [ALL]):*** Abnormally enlarged mediastinal lymph nodes or diffuse mediastinal masses are commonly seen in acute and chronic leukemias.
- *Lymphoma:* Both Hodgkin and non-Hodgkin lymphomas may present with extensive mediastinal involvement as well as pleural and pericardial effusions.
- *Small-cell lung cancer:* An extensive mediastinal mass may be seen at the initial presentation or during the course of disease in small-cell lung cancer.

■ Essential Facts

- Four major types of leukemia are recognized, depending on type of cell (myelogenous or lymphocytic) and type of clinical presentation and evolution (acute or chronic): ALL, chronic lymphocytic leukemia (CLL), acute myelogenous leukemia (AML), and chronic myelogenous leukemia.
- Most cases of leukemia present in adults (average age at diagnosis is 67 years); leukemia is 10 times more common in adults than in children.
- CLL is the most common type of leukemia in adults, whereas ALL is the most common type in children.
- Generalized lymphadenopathy is a common finding in some types of leukemia (e.g., adult T-cell leukemia, ALL, CLL) and is seen in > 50% of cases in some series.
- Pleural effusion or plaquelike pleural thickening is reported in as many as one third of patients with leukemia in autopsy series but is less commonly seen in these patients clinically (10%).
- The frequency of respiratory involvement in patients with acute leukemia is high. Respiratory involvement results either from pulmonary infiltration by leukemia or from pulmonary hemorrhage.

- The most common imaging findings in the lung parenchyma are ground-glass attenuation, centrilobular nodules, and interlobular septal thickening. Lymphocyte infiltration occurs along the interstitium and the alveolar spaces.
- Patients with leukemia who have undergone bone marrow transplant may also present with pulmonary complications such as bacterial pneumonia or opportunistic infections (e.g., *Pneumocystis* pneumonia, cytomegalovirus infection, *Aspergillus* infection).
- More than 60% of deaths of patients with leukemia are due to infectious disease, which tends to occur after chemotherapy or in the neutropenic stage after bone marrow transplant.
- Granulocytic sarcomas or chloromas are tumors formed by immature granulocytes, derived from myeloid precursors, that can be seen in AML or ALL. The most common locations in the thorax are in the subperiosteal region of the ribs or sternum, or in relation to the thoracic vertebral bodies. Occasionally, these tumors may also be seen in the soft tissues or skin.

✓ Pearls and ✗ Pitfalls

- ✓ In the majority of patients with leukemic pulmonary infiltrates, pulmonary disease is strongly associated with an elevated number of blast cells (peripheral blast count > 40%).
- ✗ Thoracic imaging findings in patients with leukemia are nonspecific. In particular, the imaging findings in the lung parenchyma may represent leukemic infiltration, drug toxicity, pulmonary edema, or infection.

Case 24

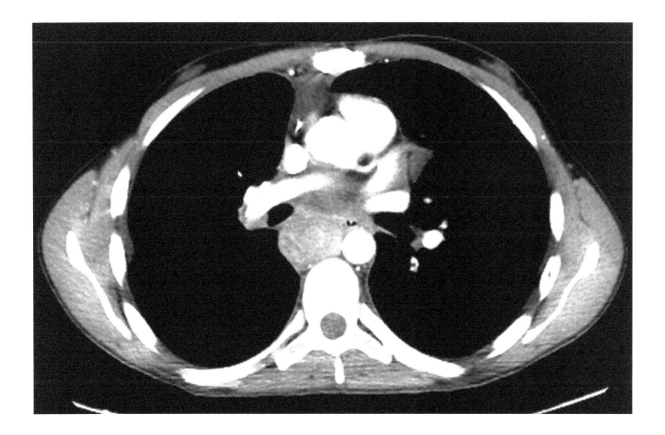

■ Clinical Presentation

A 24-year-old man with cough.

■ Imaging Findings

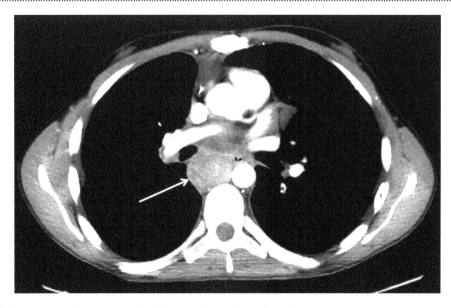

(A) Contrast-enhanced chest CT image demonstrates a high-density subcarinal mass (*arrow*).

■ Differential Diagnosis

- ***Castleman disease:*** The size, density, and enhancement of the mass make Castleman disease a leading consideration.
- *Bronchogenic cyst:* Although the location is a common site for bronchogenic cysts, the density and enhancement make this diagnosis unlikely.
- *Lymphoma:* Involvement of other lymph node groups is common. It can be difficult to distinguish from Castleman disease. Lymphoma typically does not demonstrate intense contrast enhancement.

■ Essential Facts

- Also known as angiofollicular mediastinal lymph node hyperplasia or benign giant lymph node hyperplasia.
- 70% of cases occur in the thorax.
- Unicentric or multicentric proliferation of hyperplastic lymph nodes.
- Unicentric disease is typically a benign entity occurring in young adults. There is a female predominance.
- Multicentric disease typically occurs in older adults and is more strongly associated with human herpesvirus 8, HIV infection, and lymphoma. It is more commonly symptomatic and has a worse prognosis.
- Two main histologic variants: hyaline vascular and plasma cell. Hyaline vascular variant is the most common, accounting for > 90% of cases.
- All types are associated with marked interfollicular vascular proliferation, which can result in bronchial encasement or mural erosion by enlarged, hypervascular lymph nodes.

- Unicentric disease is associated with a smooth, intensely enhancing large mass most commonly in the middle mediastinum or hilum.
- Calcification is seen in up to 10%.
- Multicentric disease is typified by multiple smaller masses in multiple mediastinal compartments.
- Compared to unicentric disease, enhancement in multicentric disease is not as robust.
- Unicentric disease is treated with excision, whereas multicentric disease is treated with chemotherapy and antiretroviral therapy.
- Hyperintense on T1- and T2-weighted MR images.
- Angiography image demonstrates a hypervascular mass with intense blush and enlarged feeding vessels.
- In addition to the bronchial arteries, the intercostal and internal mammary arteries may supply the mass.
- Multicentric disease is more likely to occur outside of the thorax.

✓ Pearls and ✗ Pitfalls

- ✓ The most common manifestation of Castleman disease is an intensely enhancing large mediastinal mass.
- ✓ Kaposi sarcoma and Castleman disease can occur concurrently in patients with AIDS.
- ✓ On MR image, flow voids may be present around the mass, representative of enlarged feeding vessels.
- ✗ Necrosis or fibrosis may result in diminished contrast enhancement.
- ✗ Pulmonary involvement is rare; however, multicentric disease may be associated with lymphocytic interstitial pneumonia.
- ✗ Fine needle aspirate is typically nondiagnostic. Core biopsy can be complicated by substantial hemorrhage.

Case 25

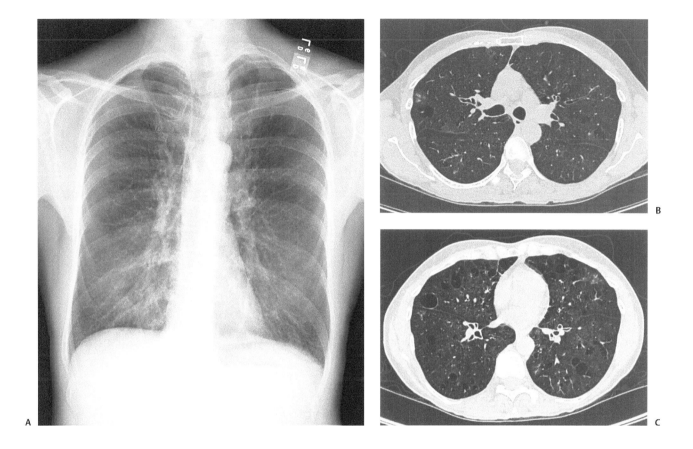

A

B

C

■ Clinical Presentation

A 45-year-old man with Sjögren disease and chronic dyspnea.

■ Imaging Findings

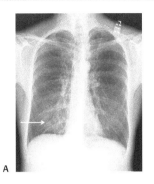
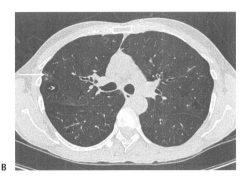
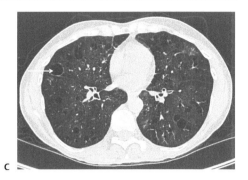

(A) Chest radiograph demonstrates a fine interstitial opacity at the bases (*arrow*). **(B)** Chest CT image (lung windows) at the level of the carina shows randomly distributed thin-walled cysts (*arrowhead*). There are scattered small centrilobular nodules and ground-glass opacity (*arrow*). **(C)** Chest CT image (lung windows) at the bases shows more thin-walled cysts (*arrow*).

■ Differential Diagnosis

- ***Lymphocytic interstitial pneumonia (LIP):*** The presence of scattered ground-glass opacity and random thin-walled cysts in a patient with Sjögren syndrome is highly suggestive of LIP.
- *Nonspecific interstitial pneumonia (NSIP):* Although ground-glass opacities and a micronodular pattern may be seen, thin-walled cysts are not typically present in NSIP.
- *Hypersensitivity pneumonitis (HP):* Although ground-glass attenuation and small centrilobular nodules are seen in HSP, the presence of thin-walled cysts argues against this diagnosis. Although not always present, an appropriate exposure to a specific antigen may be evident.

■ Essential Facts

- Rare benign lymphoproliferative disorder.
- Most commonly associated with Sjögren syndrome, AIDS, lupus, and Castleman disease.
- More common in women.
- Slowly progressive cough and dyspnea.

- Variable response to corticosteroids.
- Very rarely evolves into B-cell lymphoma.
- Lower lobe predominant centrilobular nodular opacities.
- Bilateral ground-glass opacities.
- Randomly distributed thin-walled cysts.
- Mild lymphadenopathy is seen in the majority of cases.
- Thickened bronchovascular bundles and interlobular septal thickening seen on high-resolution CT imaging.
- Fibrosis and honeycombing are rare.
- Except for the cysts, the radiologic abnormalities may resolve with successful treatment.

✓ Pearls and ✗ Pitfalls

- ✓ Nodules are more common in patients with HIV.
- ✓ Cysts are thought to develop due to obstruction of bronchioles by lymphocytic infiltrate.
- ✗ Differentiation of LIP from *Pneumocystis* pneumonia can be difficult in patients with AIDS. Although both result in ground-glass opacities and cysts, the presence of interlobular septal thickening and lymphadenopathy favors LIP.
- ✗ LIP is an AIDS-defining illness in children but not in adults.

Case 26

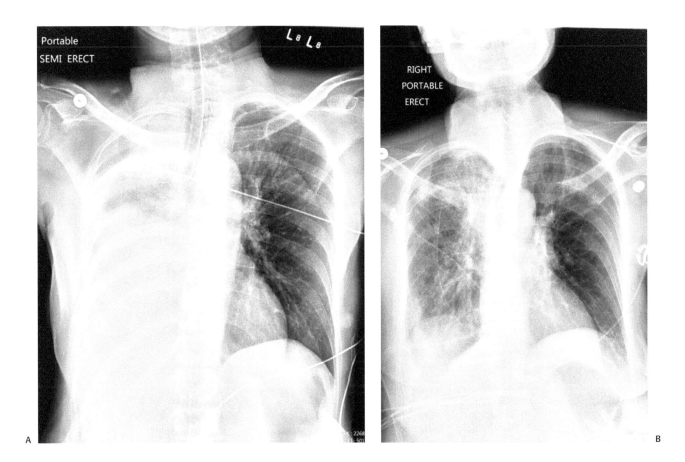

■ Clinical Presentation

A 28-year-old man with persistent hypoxia following chest tube placement for pneumothorax.

■ Imaging Findings

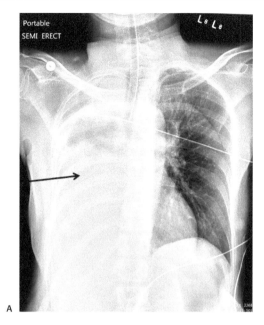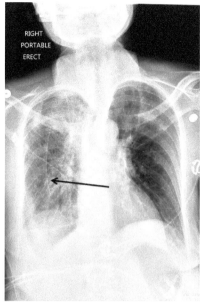

(A) Portable chest radiograph demonstrates a large right pleural effusion (*arrow*) with compressive atelectasis. An endotracheal tube is present. (B) Portable chest radiograph following placement of a right pleural drain (*arrow*) shows considerable decrease in right pleural effusion. Note the asymmetric interstitial opacity consistent with reexpansion pulmonary edema.

■ Differential Diagnosis

- ***Reexpansion pulmonary edema (RPE):*** The development of diffuse pulmonary parenchymal opacities after reexpansion of a lung collapsed from pneumothorax or drainage of a large pleural effusion is consistent with RPE.
- *Pulmonary contusion:* In trauma patients with unilateral posttraumatic pneumothorax, ipsilateral or bilateral parenchymal opacity may result from pulmonary contusion.
- *Pneumocystis pneumonia:* Diffuse unilateral parenchymal opacity may represent pneumonia. Infections with agents such as *Pneumocystis jirovecii* may present with spontaneous pneumothorax resulting from the rupture of pulmonary cysts.

■ Essential Facts

- RPE was first described after the rapid drainage of large pleural effusions.
- Later, RPE after reexpansion of a lung collapsed from pneumothorax was also described.
- Multiple mechanisms for the development of RPE have been postulated. A rapid increase in blood flow to the lung during reexpansion causes an abrupt increase in capillary pressure leading to liquid and protein overflow to the lung interstitium and air space. Surfactant production is also reduced.

- Currently, two major mechanisms are considered responsible: an alteration of capillary permeability and an increase in hydrostatic pressure.
- More than 80% of cases of RPE occur in patients with prolonged pulmonary collapse (> 72 hours). Other risk factors include large pneumothorax, large-volume pleural drainage (> 3 liters), and young patients.
- Inflammatory mediators (polymorphonuclear cells, interlukin-8, and monocyte chemotactic protein) are additional factors in the development of RPE.
- In ~7% of cases, the pulmonary edema is bilateral.
- Imaging findings in RPE vary from interstitial edema with septal lines to alveolar edema with air space consolidation.
- Edema may persist for up to 1 week.
- The mortality rate associated with RPE can exceed 20%.

✓ Pearls and ✗ Pitfalls

- ✓ The speed of pulmonary reexpansion is more significant than the use of negative pressure in the development of RPE.
- ✗ Other causes of unilateral pulmonary edema include atypical cardiogenic pulmonary edema, contralateral pulmonary embolism, pulmonary vein stenosis, and mitral valve regurgitation.

Case 27

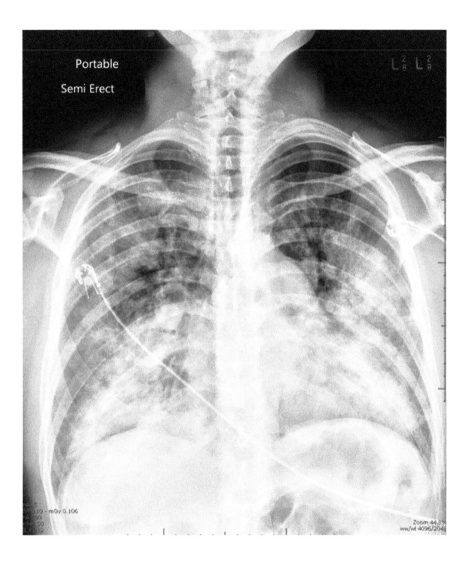

■ Clinical Presentation

A 40-year-old woman with a history of intravenous substance use disorder presents with hypoxia and altered mental status.

■ **Imaging Findings**

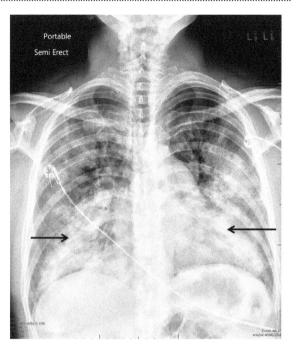

(A) Chest radiograph demonstrates diffuse perihilar alveolar and interstitial opacity (*arrows*).

■ **Differential Diagnosis**

- ***Heroin-induced pulmonary edema:*** Bilateral parenchymal opacities in a patient with a history of heroin overdose are a common presentation of heroin-induced pulmonary edema.
- *Pneumonia:* People with substance use disorders are at increased risk of community-acquired pneumonia and opportunistic infections, which may present with a multifocal and bilateral distribution.
- *Aspiration:* The altered mental status of a patient with heroin overdose is associated with an increased risk of aspiration.

■ **Essential Facts**

- Heroin use and heroin-related visits to the emergency department have increased dramatically.
- Heroin overdose is a serious condition with significant mortality, often related to cardiopulmonary pathology.
- Pulmonary edema develops in a minority of patients with heroin overdose (2%), but pulmonary edema is commonly seen in those who die.
- Altered mental status, pinpoint pupils, and severely decreased respiratory drive are a common clinical triad in heroin overdose.
- The initial management of these patients includes the administration of naloxone and oxygen supplementation.

- Pulmonary edema secondary to heroin overdose should be suspected if there is persistent hypoxia after the respiratory rate has normalized and if fluffy alveolar opacities are seen on chest radiographs.
- The majority of respiratory symptoms resolve within 24 hours.
- As many as one third of patients require intubation and mechanical ventilation.
- Imaging findings consist of bilateral parenchymal opacities.
- Increased capillary permeability, not heart failure, is considered to be the cause of heroin-induced pulmonary edema.
- Patchy atelectasis and nodular opacities may also be seen in patients with heroin-induced pulmonary edema.

✓ **Pearls and ✗ Pitfalls**

✓ Approximately half of patients presenting to the emergency department with heroin overdose test positive for cocaine and/or alcohol. Cocaine is known to produce both cardiogenic and noncardiogenic pulmonary edema.

✓ Other causes of noncardiogenic pulmonary edema include near-drowning, negative pressure/reexpansion, acute respiratory distress syndrome, transfusion-related effects, high altitude, reperfusion, and neurogenic effects.

✗ As many as one fourth of patients who have heroin-induced pulmonary edema present with unilateral disease on imaging examinations.

ng: 55

Case 28

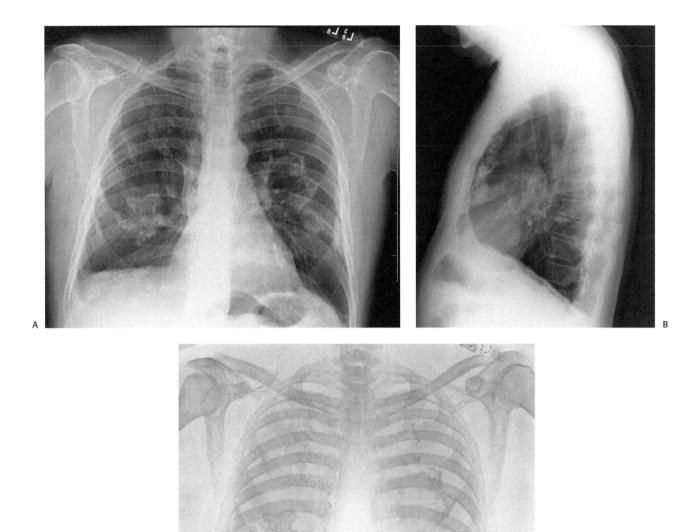

Clinical Presentation

An 80-year-old man with cough and dyspnea.

■ Imaging Findings

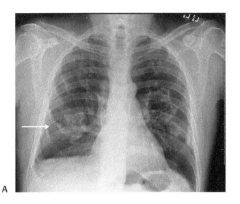
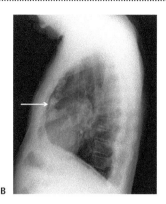
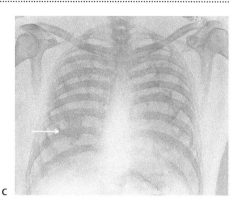

(A) Posteroanterior (PA) chest radiograph demonstrates bilateral, irregularly shaped areas of calcification (*arrow*). The diaphragmatic surfaces are also involved. **(B)** Lateral radiograph shows the calcification along the anterior pleura (*arrow*) and diaphragmatic surface. **(C)** Energy-subtracted views from the PA radiograph show the calcification to advantage (*arrow*).

■ Differential Diagnosis

- ***Calcified pleural plaque secondary to asbestos exposure:*** Bilateral thin calcified pleural plaques in this distribution are compatible with calcified pleural plaques, which are highly suggestive of asbestos exposure.
- *Pleural calcification secondary to previous hemothorax:* This is often associated with imaging evidence of previous trauma or surgery and is usually unilateral.
- *Mesothelioma:* Typically manifests as unilateral pleural thickening > 1 cm and is associated with a pleural effusion. Circumferential involvement and ipsilateral hemithoracic volume loss may be present.

■ Essential Facts

- Asbestos is a naturally occurring, fire-resistant silicate that has been used in insulation, brake pads, floor tiles, and electric wiring. The biohazard arises from inhalation of the fibers during mining and processing. Amphibole fibers are more hazardous due to their durability and geometry.
- Asbestos exposure can result in pleural effusion, pleural plaques, diffuse pleural thickening, asbestosis, malignant mesothelioma, and bronchogenic carcinoma.
- Benign pleural effusion is the earliest pleural-based finding. It is usually self-limited.

- Pleural plaques are discrete areas of fibrosis involving the parietal pleura and are the most common manifestation of asbestos exposure. They typically occur 20 to 30 years after exposure. Patients are usually asymptomatic even with widespread plaques. The plaques are not associated with malignant mesothelioma.
- Pleural plaques are typically bilateral and multifocal. They preferentially involve the posterolateral parietal pleural, the dome of the diaphragm, and the mediastinal pleura. The apices and costophrenic angles are usually spared.
- Approximately 15% of plaques are calcified. The amount of calcification can increase with time.

✓ Pearls and ✗ Pitfalls

- ✓ When viewed in profile, a linear band of attenuation is seen. However, when seen en face, the plaque assumes an irregular "holly leaf" configuration.
- ✓ A "hairy plaque" describes a visceral pleural plaque with radiating short interstitial lines in the adjacent lung parenchyma.
- ✓ The incomplete border sign results from a well-defined inner margin tangential to the X-ray beam and a tapering outer margin which is indistinct as it is en face to the beam.
- ✗ Asbestosis refers to lung fibrosis caused by asbestos and may not be associated with pleural fibrosis.

Case 29

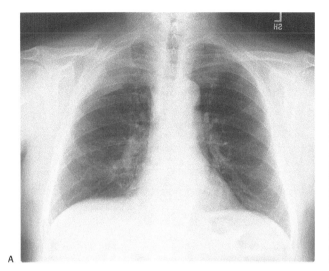

A

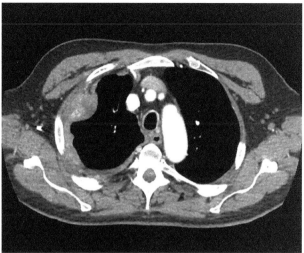

B

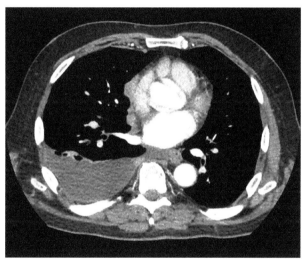

C

■ Clinical Presentation

A 65-year-old male mechanic with progressive dyspnea.

■ **Imaging Findings**

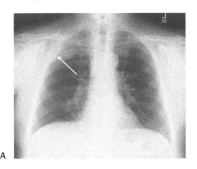 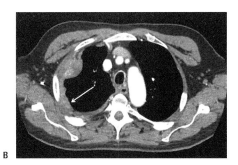 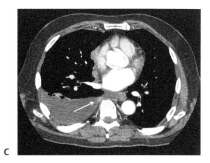

A   B   C

(A) Chest radiograph demonstrates right hemithoracic volume loss and pleural thickening (*arrow*). **(B)** Contrast-enhanced CT image (soft tissue windows) demonstrates circumferential right-sided pleural thickening (*arrow*). The left hemithorax is normal. **(C)** Contrast-enhanced CT image (soft tissue windows) shows a right pleural effusion. Note the nodularity along the heart border and the pleural studding (*arrow*).

■ **Differential Diagnosis**

- **Mesothelioma:** Unilateral pleural thickening with volume loss is suggestive of mesothelioma, especially in a patient with a significant asbestos exposure history.
- *Metastatic adenocarcinoma:* Adenocarcinoma metastatic to the pleura cannot be reliably differentiated from mesothelioma based on imaging alone. Pleural effusion is slightly less common with metastases.
- *Empyema:* Although pleural effusion and thickening are seen in both empyema and pleural effusion, circumferential distribution, nodularity, thickening of > 1 cm, and involvement of the mediastinal pleura are findings that favor malignancy.

■ **Essential Facts**

- Most common primary neoplasm of pleura. Occurs in up to 10% of individuals exposed to asbestos, a risk factor of 30 compared to the general population.
- Although all types of asbestos have been linked to mesothelioma, crocidolite (an amphibole fiber) is the most carcinogenic due to its aspect ratio (length/diameter) and durability in tissue. The incidence of mesothelioma is highest in those with the longest and most severe exposure. There is no association with cigarette smoking.
- High-risk occupations include insulation work, asbestos manufacturing, heating trades, shipyard work, and automotive brake lining manufacture and repair.
- The latency period is 30 to 40 years.
- Histologically divided into epithelioid, sarcomatous, and biphasic variants. The parietal pleura is involved to a much greater degree.
- Unilateral pleural and fissural thickening associated with pleural effusion are the hallmark imaging findings.
- Circumferential encasement involving all pleural surfaces is a late manifestation.
- Chest wall invasion manifests radiographically as periosteal reaction or rib erosion/destruction but is

identified in only 20% of cases. CT adds sensitivity, and obliteration of extrapleural fat plane and invasion of intercostal muscles may also be demonstrated.
- Lung parenchymal and hilar/mediastinal nodal metastases are evidence of advanced disease.
- Transdiaphragmatic extension is suggested by encasement of the hemidiaphragm and loss of clear fat planes with the abdominal organs.
- MR can help detect invasion of the diaphragm or chest wall. Lesions are usually minimally hyperintense to muscle on T1 and moderately hyperintense on T2.
- Fluorodeoxyglucose–positron emission tomography may aid the preoperative evaluation because of its high sensitivity in detecting extrathoracic metastases. It can also provide information about metabolically active areas and therefore determine the most appropriate area for biopsy.
- Extrapleural pneumonectomy is performed in selected cases but has significant morbidity and mortality. Radiation therapy and chemotherapy have had disappointing results. The median survival for mesothelioma is 10 months.

✓ **Pearls and** ✗ **Pitfalls**

✓ A "frozen hemithorax" describes the lack of contralateral mediastinal shift in association with massive pleural effusion due to encasement of the lung and fissures by neoplasm.
✓ Despite asbestos exposure, calcified pleural plaques are seen in only 20% of cases.
✗ The term "benign mesothelioma" has been used to describe a localized fibrous tumor of the pleura. This nomenclature is discouraged because these lesions are a separate entity and are histologically benign. There is no association with asbestos exposure.
✗ Pleural fluid cytology and fine needle aspiration are not sufficient for diagnosis. Video-assisted thoracoscopic surgery can result in chest wall seeding in 50% of patients. This can be prevented with local postoperative radiation therapy.

Case 30

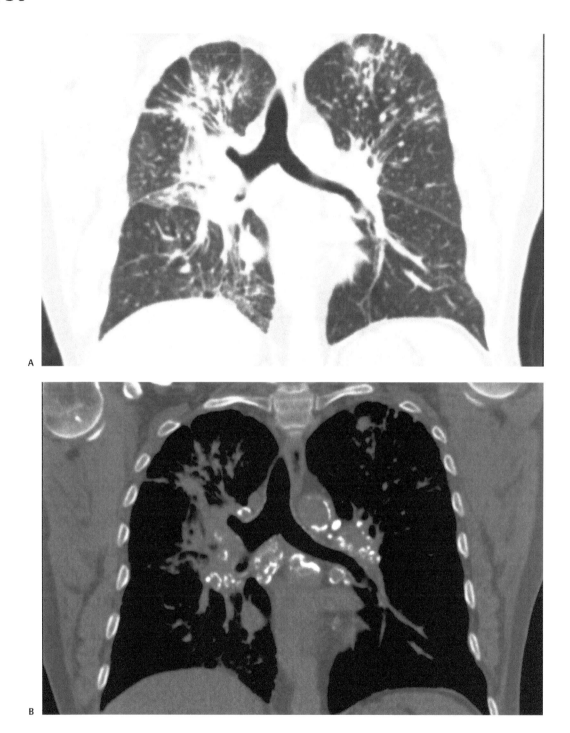

A

B

■ Clinical Presentation

A 52-year-old man with progressive dyspnea on exertion.

■ Imaging Findings

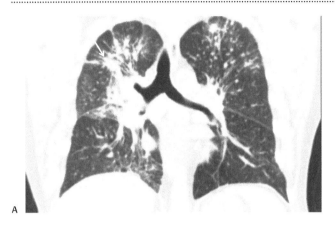 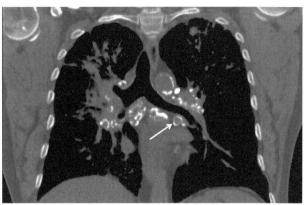

(A) CT coronal reformat image (lung windows) demonstrates peripherally calcified mediastinal and hilar lymph nodes. Note the upper lobe–predominant nodules with areas of coalescence and fibrosis *(arrow)*. **(B)** CT coronal reformat image (soft tissue windows) shows the nodal "eggshell" calcification to advantage *(arrow)*.

■ Differential Diagnosis

- **Silicosis:** Complicated silicosis (progressive massive fibrosis) is characterized by masslike opacities resulting from the coalescence of fibronodular fibrosis. It is usually upper lobe predominant. "Eggshell" calcification can affect the lymph nodes.
- *Tuberculosis (TB):* Upper lobe–predominant apical opacities with cavitation, pleural thickening, and volume loss may be seen in reactivation TB.
- *Sarcoidosis:* Upper lobe–predominant reticulonodular opacities with lymphadenopathy can be seen in sarcoidosis.

■ Essential Facts

- Silicosis is the most prevalent pneumoconiosis.
- It is an occupational disease resulting from chronic aspiration of free crystalline silica dust, a major component of Earth's crust.
- Silicone dioxide, in the form of small particles that deposit in the respiratory bronchioles, is the chemical compound responsible for inducing the inflammatory lung reaction.
- Occupations such as mining, tunneling, quarrying, sandblasting, polishing, stonecutting, and the like are most commonly associated with this condition.
- There is a predilection for the upper lobes and superior segments of the lower lobes.
- Simple silicosis is characterized by the presence of multiple small (1–10 mm), well-defined pulmonary nodules, uniform in shape and mainly peripheral in distribution.
- The small nodules have a posterior and centrilobular distribution.

- Complicated silicosis, also known as progressive massive fibrosis, is characterized by confluent nodular opacities > 1 cm in diameter and an increased amount of fibrosis, occasionally with dystrophic calcification and cavitation.
- Foci of irregular, cicatricial emphysema are often seen adjacent to confluent fibrosis.

✓ Pearls and ✗ Pitfalls

- ✓ Calcification of the small nodules is seen in < 20% of cases.
- ✓ Eggshell calcification of hilar and mediastinal lymph nodes is commonly seen.
- ✓ Caplan syndrome, also known as rheumatoid pneumoconiosis, is a rare variant of silicosis, coal worker pneumoconiosis, and other pneumoconiosis that is seen in patients with rheumatoid disease and lung involvement. It is characterized by large necrobiotic nodules superimposed on a background of multiple pulmonary nodules.
- ✗ Acute silicosis, or silicoproteinosis, is a rare form of the disease associated with massive exposure to silica dust, usually in enclosed spaces. It develops after a relatively short exposure (usually months), progresses rapidly, and has a poor prognosis.
- ✗ Coal worker pneumoconiosis results from the aspiration of a mixture of inorganic dusts, including coal, mica, kaolin, and silica, and is not the same condition as silicosis. The two entities have a different clinical course; in coal worker pneumoconiosis, there is significantly less fibrosis. However, the imaging presentations may be similar and include innumerable small pulmonary nodules.

Case 31

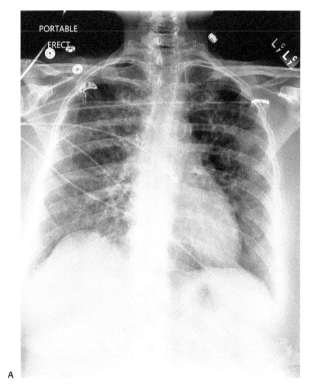

A

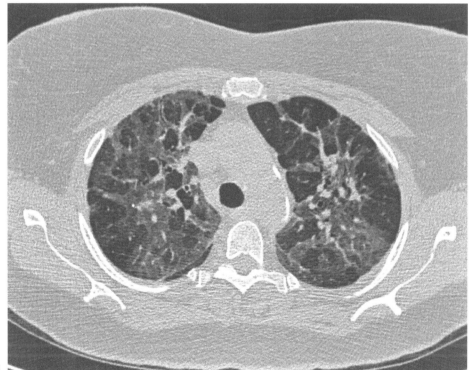

B

■ **Clinical Presentation**

A 50-year-old woman with chronic cough and dyspnea.

■ Imaging Findings

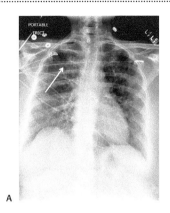
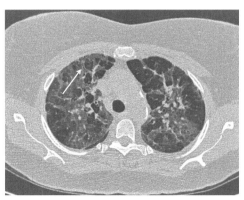

(A) Chest radiograph demonstrates faint upper lobe opacity (*arrows*). **(B)** Chest CT image (lung windows) demonstrates patchy upper lobe ground-glass opacities, with intervening normal areas, as well as an area of traction bronchiectasis (*arrow*).

■ Differential Diagnosis

- **Hypersensitivity pneumonitis (HP):** Centrilobular ground-glass nodules and patchy areas of ground-glass opacity are commonly seen in HP.
- *Atypical infection:* Viral infection and infection with *Mycoplasma* or *Chlamydia* may present as ground-glass centrilobular nodules and patchy ground-glass opacities.
- *Diffuse alveolar hemorrhage:* Goodpasture syndrome and different forms of vasculitis may present with diffuse alveolar hemorrhage that manifests as ground-glass nodules and opacities.

■ Essential Facts

- HP, or extrinsic allergic alveolitis, is a complex and heterogeneous group of disorders that result from the inhalation of various airborne organic particles.
- In a susceptible host, the particles induce an immune-mediated reaction in the airways and pulmonary parenchyma.
- Although symptoms may develop after weeks of contact with the allergen, most cases of HP occur following months or years of continuous or intermittent inhalation of the agent.
- Causative particles may be bacteria, fungi, avian proteins, wood dusts, and certain chemical compounds.
- Histopathologic features of HP include neutrophilic infiltration, cellular bronchiolitis, lymphocytic infiltrates, small, noncaseating granulomas, and areas of organizing pneumonia.
- In a large number of cases, the offending agent is never identified.
- The clinical presentation includes fever, chills, dyspnea, cough, weight loss, and fatigue.
- Three major forms of HP are recognized: acute, subacute, and chronic.
- Recurrent subacute episodes of HP may lead to pulmonary fibrosis.

- Typical imaging findings in the acute phase are centrilobular ground-glass nodules and ground-glass patchy opacities.
- Lung cysts due to bronchiolar obstruction are sometimes seen.
- Mild lymphadenopathy is seen in the minority of patients.
- The middle and lower lung zones may be more significantly affected.
- Chronic exposure to the antigen can result in interstitial pulmonary fibrosis with reticulation, traction bronchiectasis, and some degree of honeycombing that resembles nonspecific interstitial pneumonia (NSIP).
- The finding of fibrosis on CT is associated with increased mortality and a poor prognosis.
- Air trapping on expiratory high-resolution CT (HRCT) may also be seen and reflects the presence of respiratory bronchiolitis, a common histopathologic feature in HP.
- Fluid from bronchoalveolar lavage usually demonstrates an increased number of white cells, at least 20 to 30% of which are lymphocytes.

✓ Pearls and ✗ Pitfalls

- ✓ The best-known forms of hypersensitivity pneumonitis include farmer lung, bird fancier lung, and hot tub lung.
- ✓ The combination of patchy ground-glass opacities, normal regions, and air trapping on CT image is referred to as the headcheese sign.
- ✗ During acute and subacute episodes of HP, findings on conventional chest radiographs are commonly normal. A significant number of symptomatic patients with normal chest radiographs will have abnormal findings on HRCT.
- ✗ Upper lung predominance of fibrosis sometimes occurs in hypersensitivity pneumonitis, but it is uncommon in idiopathic pulmonary fibrosis and NSIP.

Case 32

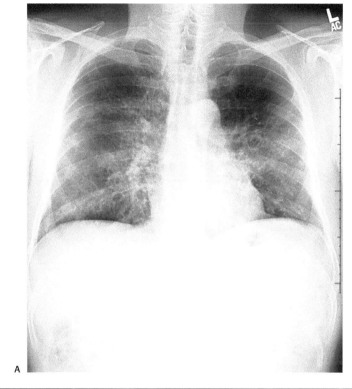

A

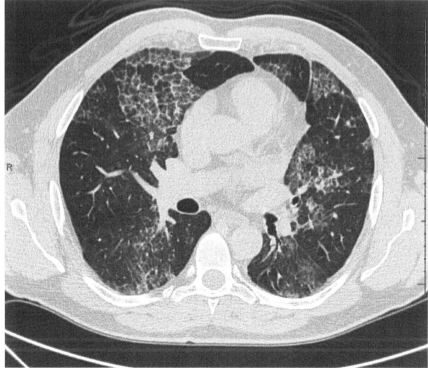

B

■ Clinical Presentation

A 36-year-old male smoker with gradual onset of mild dyspnea.

■ Imaging Findings

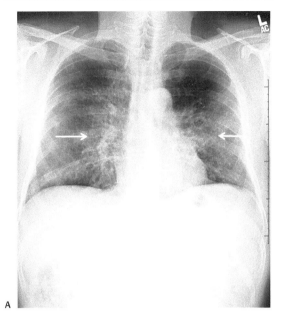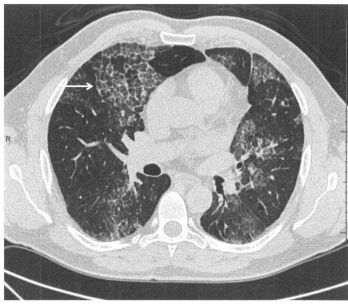

(A) Chest radiograph demonstrates central bilateral ground-glass and linear interstitial opacity (*arrows*). **(B)** Contrast-enhanced CT image (lung windows) shows geographic ground-glass opacity with interlobular septal thickening (*arrow*) sharply demarcated from normal lung.

■ Differential Diagnosis

- **Pulmonary alveolar proteinosis:** The central geographic pattern, lack of adenopathy, and mild symptoms favor alveolar proteinosis.
- *Pulmonary edema:* Typically also associated with cardiomegaly and pleural effusions. The presentation is usually more acute.
- *Pneumocystis jirovecii pneumonia:* Typically presents with fever and hypoxia. Patients are immunosuppressed. Cysts may be present.

■ Essential Facts

- The "crazy paving sign" represents thickened interlobular septa superimposed on a background of ground-glass opacity. The pattern resembles paving stones of various shapes.
- "Crazy paving" was first reported with alveolar proteinosis but can be seen with other diseases with air-space and interstitial components.
- Opacities are typically bilateral and central with relative sparing of the apices and costophrenic angles.

- Ground-glass opacity represents alveoli filled with periodic acid–Schiff–positive phospholipid material.
- *Nocardia asteroides* is the most common complicating superinfection.
- Diagnosed and treated with bronchoalveolar lavage.
- Alveolar proteinosis can show uptake on gallium scan.
- Secondary (due to hematologic malignancy, inhalational lung disease, and immunodeficiency) and congenital (due to specific gene mutations) account for < 10% of cases of alveolar proteinosis.

✓ Pearls and ✗ Pitfalls

- ✓ "Crazy paving" is classic but is not specific for pulmonary alveolar proteinosis.
- ✗ Retained lavage fluid may falsely worsen the imaging findings in the acute posttreatment period.
- ✗ Mucinous carcinoma can have a similar appearance but may be more focal and associated with lymphadenopathy.
- ✗ Exogenous lipoid pneumonia can manifest with the "crazy paving" pattern. If concomitant consolidation is present, however, it is typically low in attenuation.

Case 33

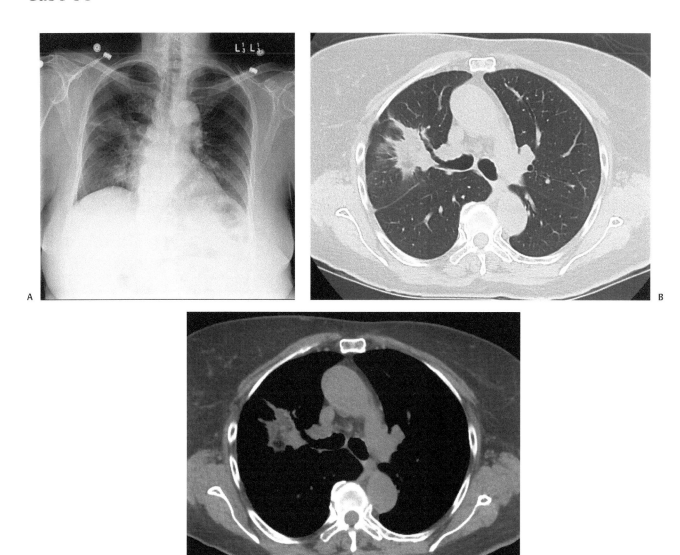

■ Clinical Presentation

A 70-year-old woman with chronic cough.

■ Imaging Findings

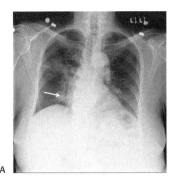
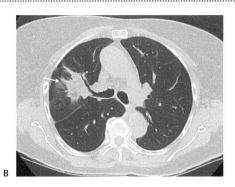
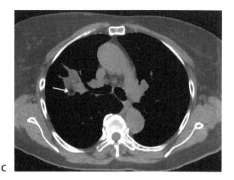

(A) Chest radiograph demonstrates consolidation in the right lower lung (*arrow*). **(B)** CT chest image (lung windows) shows a dense right middle lobe consolidation (*arrow*). **(C)** CT chest image (soft tissue windows) shows the low density to advantage. Note the fat density along the posterior aspect of the opacity (*arrow*).

■ Differential Diagnosis

- ***Exogenous lipoid pneumonia:*** Masslike consolidation with low areas of attenuation support the diagnosis of lipoid pneumonia.
- *Pneumonia:* Community-acquired pneumonia can result in consolidation but low/fat density within the opacity is not expected. The clinical course is typically acute.
- *Lung cancer:* Certain lung cancer histologies, such as mucinous adenocarcinoma, may present with a chronic consolidation.

■ Essential Facts

- Lipoid pneumonia can be classified as exogenous or endogenous, depending on the source and origin of the intra-alveolar lipid.
- Exogenous lipoid pneumonia results from the acute or chronic aspiration of inhalation of oily substances like mineral, vegetable, or animal oil into the air spaces.
- Mineral oil is relatively inert and ingested by macrophages. With chronic aspiration, a foreign body inflammatory reaction results with fibrosis and formation of a mass (paraffinoma).
- The most common cause of exogenous lipoid pneumonia in the elderly is the aspiration of mineral oil used as a laxative. Inhalation of mineral oil nose drops used for chronic rhinitis also can result in lipoid pneumonia.

- A consolidation with low density on CT (-30 to -120 Hounsfield units) is highly suggestive of intrapulmonary fat and lipoid pneumonia. The prevalence of this finding is variable, reported in 15 to 70% of patients with exogenous lipoid pneumonia.
- The distribution is typically bilateral, lower lobe, and posterior.
- Management is incumbent upon preventing additional exposure.
- The masslike consolidation is typically stable over many months or years but can show regression.
- Exogenous lipoid pneumonia is a cause of the crazy-paving pattern on CT images.

✓ Pearls and ✗ Pitfalls

- ✓ The diagnosis of exogenous lipoid pneumonia is based on the history of exposure, the presence of an opacity on images, and the demonstration of lipid-laden macrophages on bronchoalveolar lavage or biopsy.
- ✗ Endogenous lipoid pneumonia results from the degeneration of alveolar cell walls distal to an airway obstruction, usually from lung cancer.

Case 34

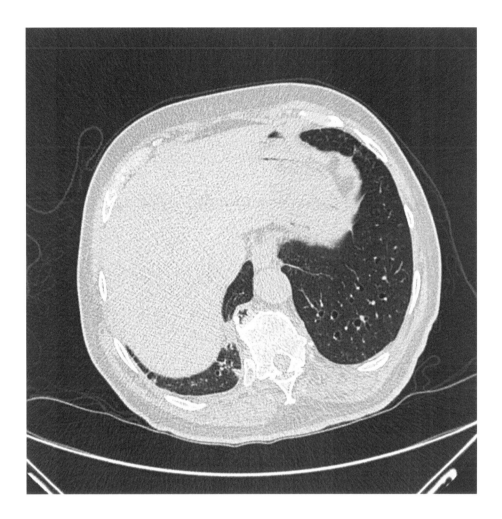

■ Clinical Presentation
....

A 52-year-old woman with head and neck cancer and chronic cough.

■ Imaging Findings

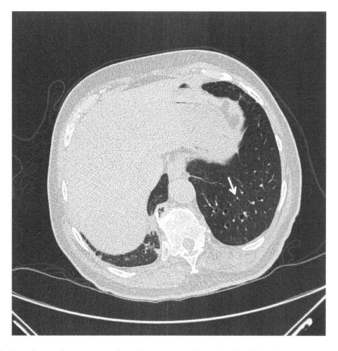

(A) Noncontrast chest CT image at the lung bases demonstrates bronchiectasis and bronchial wall thickening. Note the dilation of the airway in relation to the pulmonary artery. This appearance has been dubbed the "signet ring sign" (*arrow*).

■ Differential Diagnosis

- ***Bronchiectasis due to chronic aspiration:*** Patients with chronic aspiration can develop bronchiectasis.
- *Cystic fibrosis:* Bronchiectasis is usually upper lobe predominant. Cystic fibrosis is typically more severe and progressive and patients present earlier in life.
- *Williams–Campbell syndrome:* A congenital disorder of defective cartilage in fourth to sixth bronchial generations, either diffusely or in one focal area of lung. The lung distal to the bronchiectasis may be emphysematous.

■ Essential Facts

- Typically manifests clinically as a chronic productive cough.
- Cystic fibrosis, ciliary dyskinesia, Mounier–Kuhn syndrome, Williams–Campbell syndrome, allergic bronchopulmonary aspergillosis (ABPA), postinfectious chronic aspiration, toxic inhalation, and yellow nail syndrome are all causes of bronchiectasis.
- Bronchiectasis is classified into three categories: cylindrical, varicose, and cystic.
- Radiographic findings include linear atelectasis and dilated and thickened airways.
- Tram lines are often best seen on lateral projection.
- Ring shadows are evident when the bronchi are seen in cross-section.

- Irregular peripheral opacities may represent mucopurulent plugs.
- The "signet ring sign" refers to visualization of a dilated bronchus adjacent to the pulmonary artery in cross-section.
- Mucopurulent debris results in a "tree-in-bud" pattern when small airways are affected.
- Clustered cysts are a feature of more destructive bronchiectasis.

✓ Pearls and ✗ Pitfalls

✓ Central distribution suggests ABPA, upper lobe distribution suggests cystic fibrosis, and lower lobe predominance is typical of idiopathic and postinfectious/aspiration bronchiectasis.

✓ Kartagener syndrome is a subgroup of primary ciliary dyskinesia in which situs inversus, sinusitis, and bronchiectasis occur together.

✓ Lack of bronchial tapering or visualization of bronchi within 1 cm of the pleura may be an early finding of bronchiectasis on high-resolution CT images.

✗ Patients with hemoptysis may require bronchial artery embolization.

✗ Pulmonary Langerhans cell histiocytosis, lymphangiomyomatosis, lymphocytic interstitial pneumonia, and other cystic lung diseases may mimic cystic bronchiectasis.

Case 35

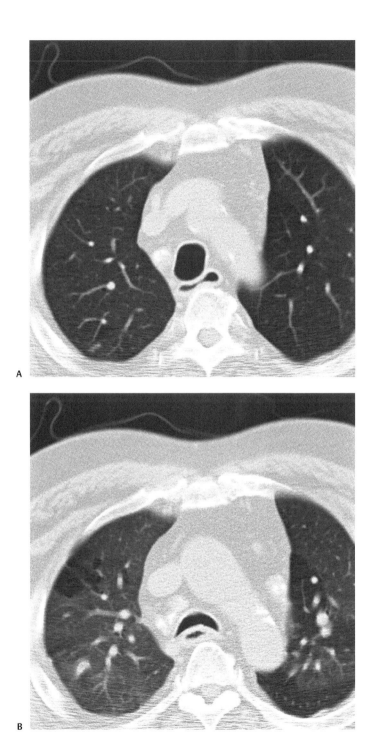

A

B

▪ Clinical Presentation

A 51-year-old morbidly obese woman with shortness of breath and stridor.

■ Imaging Findings

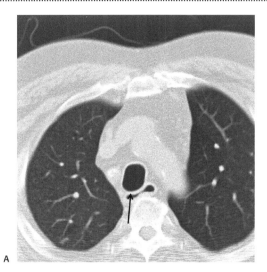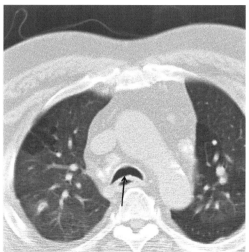

(A) Dynamic chest CT image (lung windows) during inspiration shows enlarged tracheal area and with a convex posterior membrane (*arrow*). **(B)** Dynamic chest CT image (lung windows) during exhalation shows an excessive airway collapsibility creating a crescent-shaped or "frown sign" appearance (*arrow*).

■ Differential Diagnosis

- **Tracheobronchomalacia (TBM):** Excessive airway collapsibility secondary to weakness of the airway wall is known as TBM.
- *Tracheobronchial stenosis:* A fundamental difference between tracheobronchial stenosis and several different pathologic conditions (amyloidosis, sarcoidosis, relapsing polychondritis) is the fixed nature of the airway narrowing.
- *Tracheal diverticulum:* A tracheal diverticulum may be seen as an abnormal collection of air in the right paratracheal region. The remainder of the trachea is typically normal and would not be associated with collapsibility.

■ Essential Facts

- Tracheomalacia (TM) is abnormal weakness of the tracheal wall causing increased collapsibility. TBM is the same process but with involvement of the upper airways, not only the trachea. The two terms are commonly used interchangeably.
- TM was originally described in children who presented with airway collapse in expiration and clinical manifestations of dyspnea, stridor, and cyanosis.
- In children, TM/TBM may be congenital/primary (often associated with prematurity) or acquired/secondary (often associated with protracted intonation or vascular rings).
- In adults, acquired forms of TBM may result from any condition that damages and weakens the tracheal or bronchial wall: intubation, external trauma, surgery

(tracheostomy, lung transplantation), vascular rings and mediastinal tumors (goiter), and inflammation (relapsing polychondritis).
- It has been suggested that cigarette smoking and general chronic inflammation contribute to the development of TBM. Of adult patients with TBM, > 20% have chronic bronchitis.
- TBM has been reported in as many as 20% of patients in a bronchoscopy series.
- Images in expiration show significant anterior bowing of the posterior membranous part of the tracheal wall, bringing the anterior and posterior parts of the tracheal wall closer and creating a crescent appearance (frown sign). Both dynamic CT and MRI have been shown to provide good visualization of tracheal collapsibility.
- On inspiratory CT, a dilated trachea (> 3 cm) due to increased compliance, especially with posterior bowing of the membranous portion, may suggest the diagnosis.

✓ Pearls and ✗ Pitfalls

- ✓ A diagnostic criterion for TM commonly used on CT and bronchoscopy is > 50% tracheal narrowing (cross-sectional area) during expiration.
- ✓ In most cases, the tracheal wall is normal or thin, although it can be thickened in cases of TM associated with relapsing polychondritis.
- ✗ In patients with TM/TBM, images obtained on inspiration may be completely normal or reveal only a lunate configuration and mild tracheomegaly. Because tracheal collapse is most prominent when intrathoracic pressure exceeds intraluminal pressure (expiration, cough, Valsalva), images on expiration are usually required to make this diagnosis.

Case 36

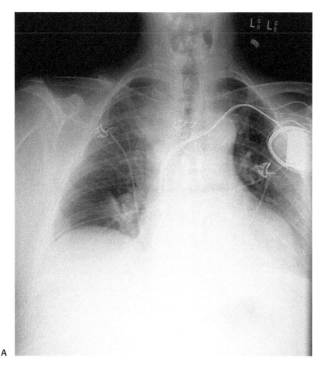

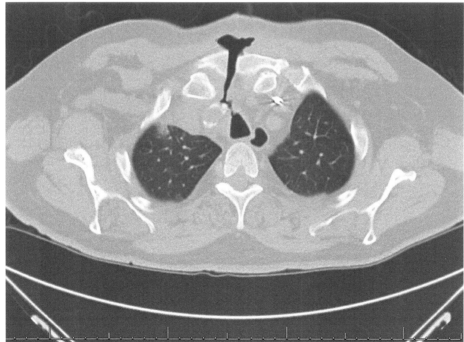

■ Clinical Presentation

A 62-year-old man after a motor vehicle crash.

■ Imaging Findings

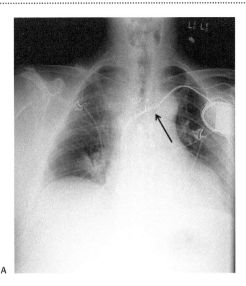 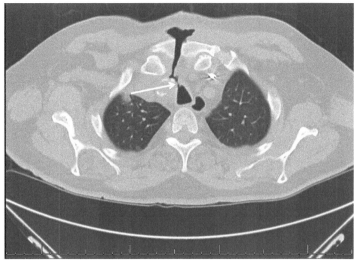

(A) Chest radiograph demonstrates pneumomediastinum (*arrow*). **(B)** Chest CT image (lung windows) shows a defect in the tracheal wall (*arrow*) with air extending into the mediastinum. In this case, the larger air pocket is somewhat unusual and is related to prior sternotomy. Typically, pneumomediastinum manifests as multiple small foci of air running along the fascial planes.

■ Differential Diagnosis

- **Tracheal rupture:** Discontinuity of the tracheal wall with associated pneumomediastinum is consistent with tracheal rupture.
- *Pneumomediastinum without tracheal rupture:* In severe blunt thoracic trauma, pneumomediastinum may develop without associated tracheobronchial or esophageal rupture.
- *Tracheal diverticulum:* A tracheal diverticulum may be seen as an abnormal collection of air in the right paratracheal region. It is usually posterolaterally located and should not be associated with pneumomediastinum or subcutaneous emphysema.

■ Essential Facts

- Major tracheobronchial injuries are two times more commonly seen secondary to penetrating trauma than after blunt trauma.
- Tracheobronchial injuries resulting from blunt thoracic trauma are relatively uncommon and found in < 2% of trauma patients.
- Tracheal ruptures comprise one fourth of all tracheobronchial injuries.
- Tracheal rupture is commonly associated with severe blunt trauma and has a high mortality rate (80%).
- Tracheal injury may result either from compression of the sternum against the thoracic spine or from a sudden increase of intraluminal pressure against a closed glottis.
- The most common site of tracheal laceration is at the junction of the cartilaginous and membranous portion of the posterolateral wall.

- The typical morphology of tracheal rupture is longitudinal/vertical, occurring more commonly in the distal third, close to the carina.
- The most common imaging findings are pneumomediastinum and subcutaneous emphysema (100%), often extending into the neck.
- Pneumothorax is relatively uncommon in isolated tracheal rupture (33%).
- On CT imaging, the tracheal rupture is directly visualized in 70% of cases.
- Esophageal rupture is another uncommon mechanism of pneumomediastinum in patients with blunt trauma.
- The fallen lung sign describes the appearance of a collapsed lung away from the mediastinum encountered with tracheobronchial injury.

✓ Pearls and ✗ Pitfalls

- ✓ In patients following trauma, the Macklin effect (alveolar rupture and air dissection along bronchovascular sheaths with mediastinal extension) is found to be the mechanism responsible for pneumomediastinum four times more often than is tracheobronchial injury.
- ✓ In patients with an endotracheal tube, an overly distended endotracheal balloon cuff can indicate tracheal rupture. The site of the tracheal laceration may be seen as herniation of the endotracheal balloon.
- ✗ A delay in diagnosis is the most important factor adversely influencing outcome. Patients with a delayed diagnosis (> 24 hours) sustain more complications and have a higher mortality rate.

Case 37

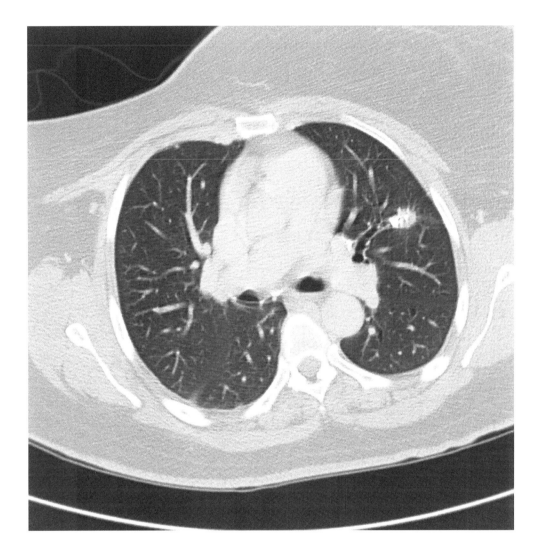

■ Clinical Presentation

A 60-year-old woman with chronic cough.

■ Imaging Findings

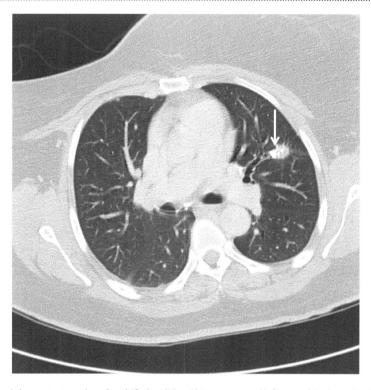

(A) Chest CT image (lung windows) demonstrates a densely calcified nodule within a segmental left upper lobe bronchus (*arrow*). There is postobstructive atelectasis.

■ Differential Diagnosis

- ***Broncholithiasis:*** Calcified material within the bronchial lumen represents broncholithiasis. In this case, it likely formed by erosion of a calcified lymph node into the bronchial lumen.
- *Carcinoid tumor:* When carcinoid tumor is totally ossified and within the bronchus, it simulates broncholithiasis.
- *Tracheobronchopathia osteochondroplastica (TBO):* TBO is an idiopathic condition with submucosal osteocartilaginous growth along the bronchial wall. Protrusion of the nodules into the airway can mimic broncholithiasis.

■ Essential Facts

- Typically the result of erosion of a calcified lymph node into the bronchial lumen.
- Usually associated with long-standing foci of necrotizing granulomatous lymphadenitis.
- May also occur secondary to in situ calcification of aspirated foreign material.

- Much rarer causes include extrusion of calcified bronchial cartilage plates and bronchial migration of calcified material such as a pleural plaque or renal stone via a fistula.
- Most commonly presents with nonproductive cough. A history of lithoptysis may be elicited.
- The calcified nodule may not be visible on chest radiograph, but secondary signs such as atelectasis, mucoid impaction, bronchiectasis, or expiratory air trapping may be present.
- High-resolution CT is usually confirmatory. Volume averaging makes evaluation difficult in CT scans with conventional slice thickness.
- Other calcified lymph nodes are also usually seen.

✓ Pearls and ✗ Pitfalls

- ✓ The proximal right middle lobe bronchus and the origin of the anterior segmental bronchus of the upper lobes are preferential sites.
- ✗ Bronchoesophageal and bronchoaortic fistula are rare complications.

Case 38

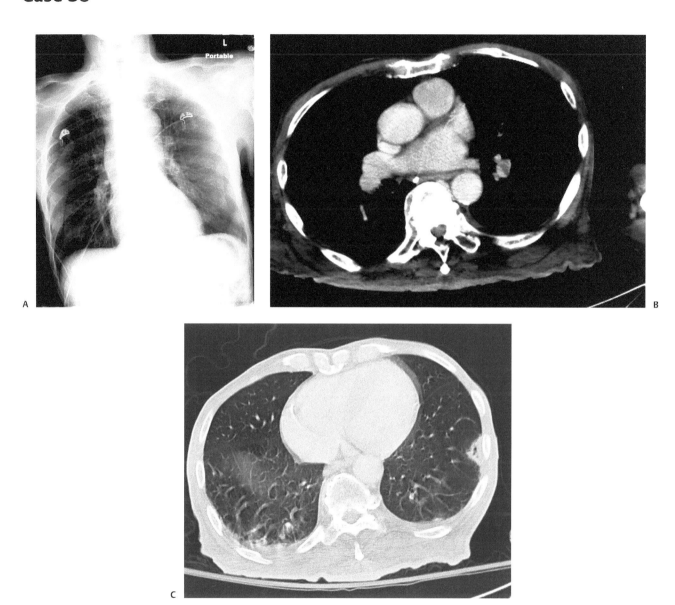

■ Clinical Presentation

A 40-year-old man with left-sided pleuritic chest pain.

■ **Imaging Findings**

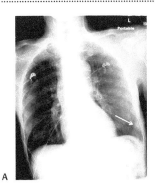 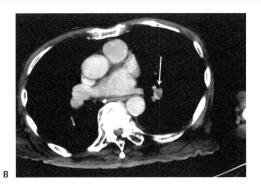 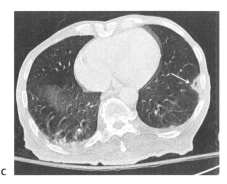

(A) Portable chest radiograph demonstrates a small peripheral opacity on the left (*arrow*). (B) Contrast-enhanced chest CT at the level of the pulmonary artery demonstrates a left lower lobe pulmonary embolus (*arrow*). (C) Contrast-enhanced chest CT (lung windows) shows a wedge-shaped peripheral opacity at the left base (*arrow*).

■ **Differential Diagnosis**

- ***Pulmonary infarct secondary to pulmonary embolism (PE):*** A peripheral wedge-shaped opacity in the setting of PE is highly suggestive of pulmonary infarct.
- *Septic emboli:* Septic emboli may manifest as diffuse bilateral nodular densities with a lower lobe predominance. A feeding vessel may be seen.
- *Tumor thrombus:* A tumor thrombus may demonstrate enhancement. It can manifest as a large central lesion or small nodules in the periphery.

■ **Essential Facts**

- Pulmonary infarction occurs in 10 to 15% of patients with PE.
- Patients are more likely to have pleuritic chest pain and hemoptysis.
- Pulmonary infarct is more likely in patients with coexisting cardiovascular disease and a large embolic burden.

- Pulmonary infarct is rare due to anastomoses between the pulmonary and bronchial vascular systems.
- Hemorrhage can coexist due to higher pressure in the bronchial arterial system, increased vascular permeability, and capillary endothelial injury.
- A wedge-shaped juxtapleural opacity has been referred to as a "Hampton hump."
- Infarcts are usually in the periphery and lower lobes.

✓ **Pearls and ✗ Pitfalls**

✓ Pulmonary infarction is very likely if peripheral consolidation contains central lucencies.
✓ Radiographic resolution may require weeks to months. A residual scar is often present.
✗ Cavitation can also be present in septic emboli and superinfection of a bland infarct.
✗ Wedge-shaped opacity can also be seen in a variety of other conditions such as organizing pneumonia, tumors, and Wegener granulomatosis.

Case 39

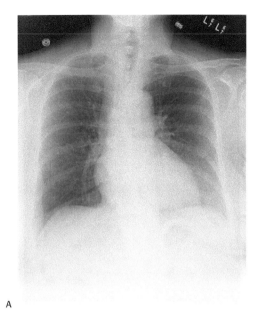

A

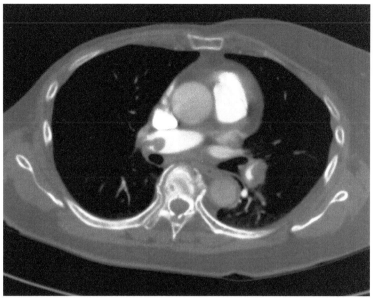

B

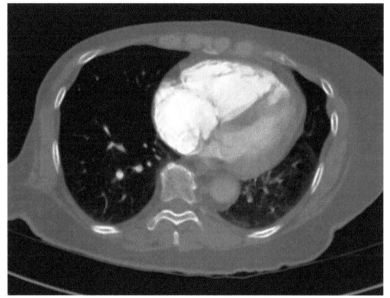

C

■ **Clinical Presentation**

A 52-year-old woman with pleuritic chest pain and hypotension.

■ **Imaging Findings**

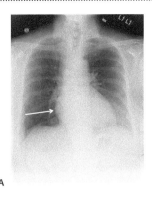
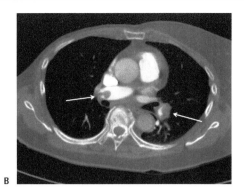
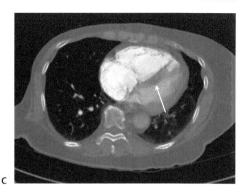

A   B   C

(A) Posteroanterior chest radiograph demonstrates borderline right atrial enlargement (*arrow*). The lungs are clear. **(B)** Contrast-enhanced chest CT image at the level of the pulmonary artery demonstrates bilateral pulmonary emboli (*arrows*). **(C)** Contrast-enhanced chest CT image demonstrates right atrial and ventricular enlargement with bowing of the interventricular septum (*arrow*) toward the left ventricle. Note the size discrepancy between the right and left ventricles.

■ **Differential Diagnosis**

- ***Pulmonary embolism (PE) with right heart strain***: Right-sided cardiac enlargement in the setting of large bilateral central PE is suggestive of right heart strain.
- *Primary pulmonary hypertension:* Can result in right-sided cardiac enlargement and right heart failure; however, there is typically central pulmonary artery enlargement.
- *Pulmonary valve stenosis:* Results in pulmonary artery enlargement typically isolated to the main and left pulmonary artery.
- *Tumor thrombus:* May demonstrate enhancement. Can manifest as a large central lesion or small nodules in the periphery.

■ **Essential Facts**

- PE can induce acute right heart failure.
- Signs of right ventricular strain on CT imaging include right ventricle/left ventricle ratio > 1 and leftward septal bowing.
- The superior vena cava and azygos vein may also be distended.
- Reflux into the hepatic veins and inferior vena cava can been seen in patients with right heart strain and tricuspid regurgitation.

- Total pulmonary artery embolic burden has also been investigated as a prognostic factor in patients with PE, although results have been equivocal.
- Radiography has poor sensitivity and specificity for the diagnosis of PE.
- The left ventricular cavity may be "D shaped" when there is right heart strain.

✓ **Pearls and** ✗ **Pitfalls**

- ✓ When a diagnosis of PE has been made, evaluate the heart for evidence of right heart strain.
- ✓ Westermark sign (regional oligemia), Hampton hump (peripheral wedge-shaped infarct), and Fleischner sign (enlarged pulmonary artery) are commonly described chest radiographic findings but have a low sensitivity.
- ✗ Pulmonary angiography is less sensitive for small subsegmental emboli and has poor interobserver agreement.
- ✗ Other embolic sources include air, fat, talc, and cement embolism.
- ✗ Webs and bands, nonocclusive or eccentric filling defects, and pouching/concave defects suggest chronic pulmonary embolism.

Case 40

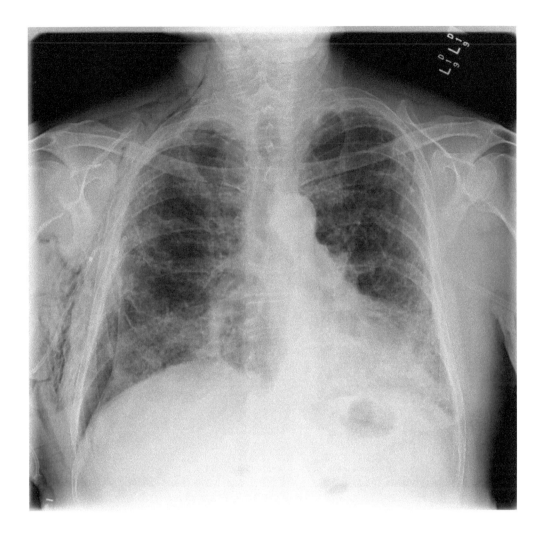

■ Clinical Presentation

A 40-year-old status post lung biopsy on the right.

■ Imaging Findings

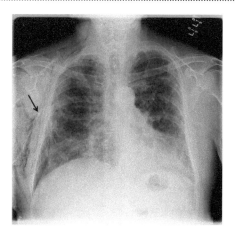

(A) Portable chest radiograph demonstrates a persistent right pneumothorax. Note that the pigtail drain is not fully in the pleural space. The side holes extend to the radiopaque marker, which is within the soft tissues (*arrow*).

■ Differential Diagnosis

- ***Malposition of a thoracostomy tube:*** Thoracostomy tubes placed for the evacuation of a pneumothorax or pleural fluid should be fully within the pleural space for adequate function.
- *Surgical drain in the soft tissues:* Pigtail drains can be placed into subcutaneous fluid collections at the time of surgery or percutaneously by interventional radiology. Review of the history and prior imaging findings in these complex patients is imperative to understand the type of support devices present.
- *Normally positioned thoracostomy tube:* The ideal position of a thoracostomy tube for the evacuation of a pneumothorax is in the upper anterior pleural space.

■ Essential Facts

- Closed thoracostomy tubes are commonly placed for the evacuation of air or fluid in the pleural cavity.
- Tubes range in size from 6 to 40F depending on purpose.
- Tube position is commonly monitored with chest radiographs.
- When adhesions of loculated pleural effusions are present, imaging guidance, usually with CT or ultrasound, may be needed for placement.
- Although the decision to place a chest tube depends on many factors, most importantly the clinical condition of the patient, tube placement is considered when a pneumothorax exceeds 25%.
- Other common indications for the placement of thoracostomy tubes include drainage of empyema, large recurrent pleural effusions, hemothorax, and malignant effusions.
- Tubes are commonly placed in an intercostal space between the fourth and ninth ribs, in the anterior chest wall, or in the midclavicular or anterior axillary line.

- For the drainage of a pneumothorax, an anterior location of the tube is preferred, whereas for the drainage of fluid, a posterior/dependent position is preferred.
- Malposition of tubes in extrathoracic (in the soft tissues of the chest wall or intra-abdominally), intramediastinal, intrafissural, or intraparenchymal locations can occur.
- Chest tube malposition is associated with increased morbidity and mortality.
- Hepatic and splenic lacerations are the two most common visceral injuries resulting from chest tube malposition.
- A persistent pneumothorax constitutes ongoing bubbling of air from a chest drain 48 hours after its insertion.
- Intrabronchial valves are now sometimes used for persistent air leaks following lung surgery.

✓ Pearls and ✗ Pitfalls

- ✓ Emergency placement of a thoracostomy tube is associated with a relatively high incidence of tube malposition and complications, the diagnosis of which is more limited with conventional radiography than with CT.
- ✓ When the side holes span the pleural space and soft tissues, extensive subcutaneous emphysema can result.
- ✓ Failure of the fluid column to move within a water seal drainage system during coughing or respiration is a cardinal sign of an occluded tube.
- ✗ The tube position relative to air or fluid can be misleading in a single anteroposterior view and can be better defined in a lateral projection.
- ✗ Kinked or clogged tubes or tubes that are occluded because the side holes are against the lung or mediastinum may result in a persistent pneumothorax.
- ✗ Despite proper positioning of a thoracostomy tube, the lung may not fully reexpand in cases of ex vacuo pneumothorax, a persistent air leak, or a bronchopleural fistula.

Case 41

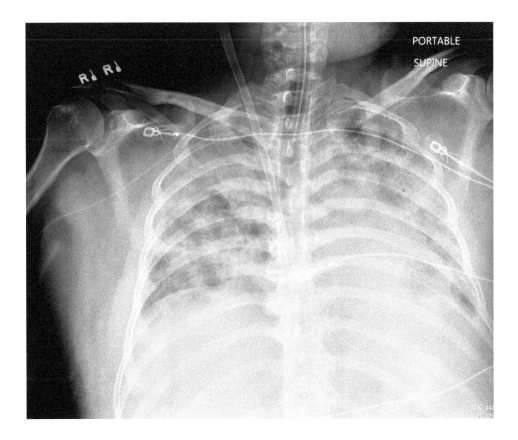

■ Clinical Presentation

A 40-year-old woman with pancreatitis and respiratory failure.

◼ Imaging Findings

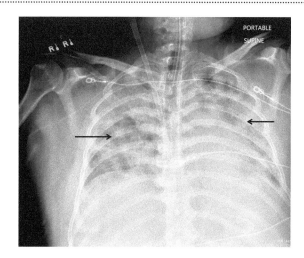

(A) Portable chest radiograph demonstrates dense bilateral upper lobe–predominant air-space and interstitial opacity (*arrows*). An endotracheal tube, nasogastric tube, and extracorporeal membrane oxygenation cannulas are present.

◼ Differential Diagnosis

- **Acute respiratory distress syndrome (ARDS):** Diffuse bilateral lung opacities in this patient are suggestive of ARDS in this critically ill patient.
- *Hydrostatic pulmonary edema:* The imaging features of hydrostatic pulmonary edema and ARDS overlap, and differentiation can be difficult without adequate clinical history and knowledge of the arterial blood gas or pulmonary artery wedge pressure. However, hydrostatic pulmonary edema is classically associated with pleural effusions and cardiomegaly. The opacity found in cardiogenic edema is classically more centrally located.
- *Desquamative interstitial pneumonia (DIP):* A smoking-related idiopathic interstitial pneumonia characterized by diffuse lower lung zone predominant ground-glass opacity. Although symptoms such as cough and dyspnea can be severe, respiratory distress requiring mechanical ventilation is not expected. Most patients improve with smoking cessation and steroid treatment.
- *Pneumocystis jirovecii pneumonia:* On CT, *Pneumocystis* pneumonia demonstrates patchy ground-glass opacity on a background of interlobular septal thickening. Pleural effusions, however, are uncommon. *Pneumocystis* pneumonia is most commonly seen in patients with AIDS.

◼ Essential Facts

- Diffuse pulmonary parenchymal injury associated with noncardiogenic pulmonary edema.
- Results in severe respiratory distress and hypoxemic respiratory failure.
- Associated with a wide variety of clinical disorders resulting in direct or indirect lung injury.

- Pneumonia, aspiration, trauma, fat and amniotic fluid embolism, inhalational injury, sepsis, drug overdose, and pancreatitis are among the best documented causes.
- Diagnosis is made on clinical grounds: acute onset, bilateral lung opacity, pulmonary artery wedge pressure ≤ 18 (or no clinical signs of congestive heart failure), and $Pao_2:Fio_2 \leq 200$ mm Hg.
- With severe ARDS, $Pao_2:Fio_2$ may be < 100 mm Hg.
- The pathologic hallmark is diffuse alveolar damage (DAD).
- Progresses through exudative, fibroproliferative, and fibrotic phases.
- Mortality approaches 60%.
- Nearly all patients have ground-glass opacity.
- Lung opacity is typically bilateral and dependent.
- Lung opacity evolves rapidly with maximal severity in the first 3 days; might progress to frank consolidation.
- Pneumothorax occurs in ~10% of cases and is not necessarily related to positive pressure ventilation.
- In patients who survive, the ground-glass opacity and consolidation clears although a reticular interstitial abnormality with architectural distortion and traction bronchiectasis may persist. Cysts and bullae may develop.

✓ Pearls and ✗ Pitfalls

- ✓ The most common risk factor for ARDS is sepsis.
- ✓ The presence of a pleural effusion is atypical and may suggest complicating pneumonia.
- ✓ The lack of cardiomegaly, septal lines, vascular redistribution, and peribronchial cuffing favor ARDS over cardiogenic edema.
- ✗ The term *acute interstitial pneumonia* is reserved for idiopathic cases of DAD.
- ✗ The correlation between the imaging findings and the degree of hypoxemia is variable.

Case 42

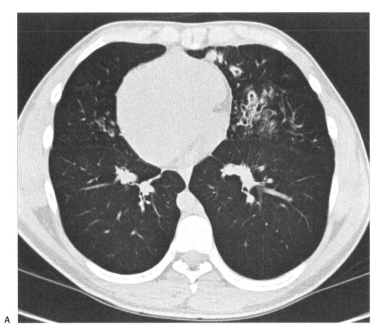

A

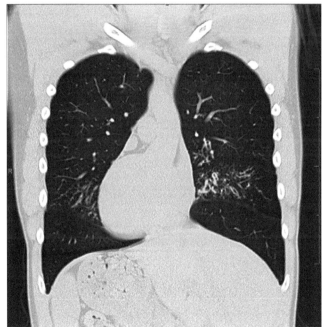

B

■ Clinical Presentation

....

A 25-year-old man with chronic cough undergoing workup with spouse for infertility.

■ **Imaging Findings**

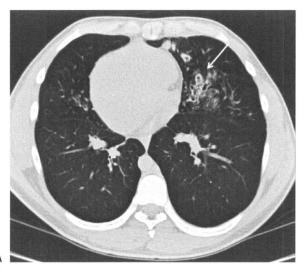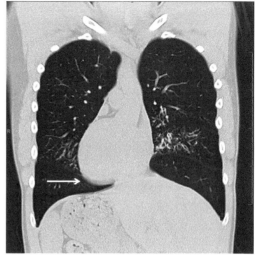

(A) Noncontrast chest CT image (lung windows) demonstrates bronchiectasis and bronchial wall thickening. There are multiple centrilobular nodules and areas of tree-in-bud opacity (*arrow*). There is consolidation in the "left middle lobe" in this patient with situs inversus. **(B)** Noncontrast chest CT, coronal reformat image (lung windows) confirms the dextrocardia (*arrow*) and bronchiectasis.

■ **Differential Diagnosis**

- ***Primary ciliary dyskinesia/Kartagener syndrome:***
  Lower lobe–predominant bronchiectasis is seen in primary ciliary dyskinesia. Fifty percent of these patients have situs inversus.
- *Cystic fibrosis:* Bronchiectasis is usually upper lobe predominant. Infertility is also present. Cystic fibrosis is typically more severe and progressive, and patients present earlier in life. No association with situs inversus.
- *Williams–Campbell syndrome:* A congenital disorder of defective cartilage in fourth to sixth bronchial generations, either diffusely or in one focal area of lung. The lung distal to the bronchiectasis may be emphysematous. There are no extrathoracic manifestations, and situs inversus is not expected.

■ **Essential Facts**

- Immotile cilia syndrome includes patients with a spectrum of ciliary abnormalities, including ciliary akinesia, dyskinesia, and aplasia.
- Kartagener syndrome is a subgroup of primary ciliary dyskinesia in which situs inversus, sinusitis, and bronchiectasis occur together.
- Typical clinical manifestations include chronic cough, rhinitis, and sinusitis. Cilia dysfunction results in impaired mucociliary clearance.
- The inheritance pattern of primary ciliary dyskinesia is autosomal recessive. Most men are infertile because of immotile spermatozoa.

- Patients can be screened by measuring exhaled nasal nitric oxide (low or absent); however, definitive diagnosis requires electron microscopy to confirm specific defects. Genetic testing is available for specific mutations.
- Situs inversus occurs in approximately half of patients (body asymmetry is randomized) with immotile cilia syndrome and is not an essential part of the disorder.
- Moderate hyperinflation, bronchial thickening, and bronchiectasis are the most common imaging findings.
- Small centrilobular nodules are often seen on high-resolution (HR) CT.
- Bronchiectasis is classified into three categories: cylindrical, varicose, and cystic. Patients with primary ciliary dyskinesia typically have varicose bronchiectasis.
- Nasal polyps and aplasia of the frontal sinuses can also be seen.
- Associated with congenital cardiac abnormalities such as transposition of great vessels. Pyloric stenosis and epispadias are other associations.

✓ **Pearls and ✗ Pitfalls**

✓ The "signet ring sign" refers to visualization of a dilated bronchus adjacent to the pulmonary artery in cross section.
✓ Lack of bronchial tapering or visualization of bronchi within 1 cm of the pleura may be early findings of bronchiectasis on HRCT.
✗ Bronchiectasis may not manifest until adulthood.
✗ Often results in recurrent pneumonia and scarring. Mycetoma formation and hemorrhage may ensue.

Case 43

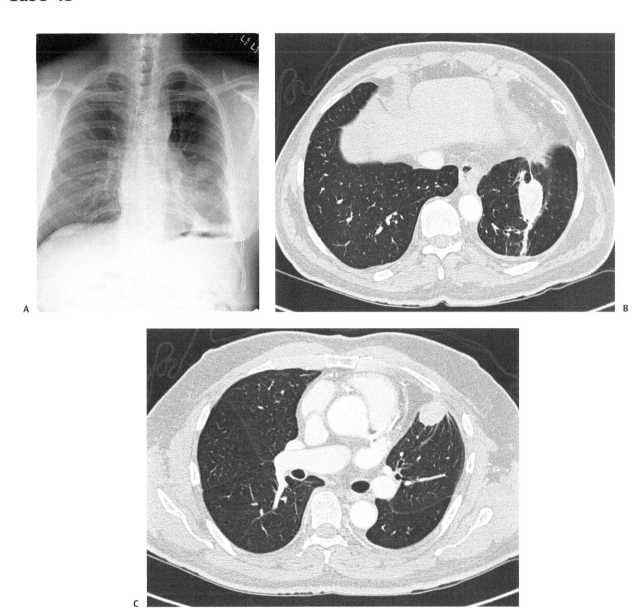

■ Clinical Presentation

A 52-year-old woman with remote history of infection and chronic cough.

■ Imaging Findings

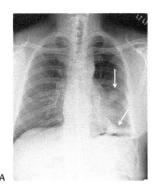 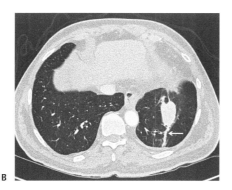 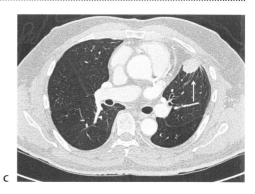

(A) Posteroanterior chest radiograph demonstrates left pleural thickening, volume loss, and two well-defined masses (*arrows*). **(B)** Contrast-enhanced chest CT (lung windows) at the level of the left base demonstrates pleural thickening, a dense mass, and long curvilinear opacities extending posteriorly (*arrow*). **(C)** Contrast-enhanced chest CT (lung windows) slightly superiorly shows similar findings involving the second mass (*arrow*).

■ Differential Diagnosis

- ***Rounded atelectasis:*** The presence of curvilinear opacities, the "comet tail sign," and association with pleural thickening make this the top consideration.
- *Bronchogenic carcinoma:* Although this should be considered, the association with pleural thickening and presence of the "comet tail sign" favor rounded atelectasis.
- *Metastases:* Multiple pulmonary nodules in a patient of this age make pulmonary metastatic disease a top consideration. However, the association with the "comet tail sign" and absence of known malignancy make this less likely.

■ Essential Facts

- Unusual form of atelectasis associated with extensive pleural folding and invagination.
- Abuts pleural effusion or thickening.
- Interlobular septa are thickened and fibrotic.

- Most commonly associated with asbestos-related pleural disease but may occur with any cause of pleural fibrosis.
- Typically found in the posterior aspect of the lower lobes.
- The swirling bronchovascular bundle is thought to resemble a comet's tail.
- Atelectatic lung may show homogeneous contrast enhancement.
- Air bronchograms are present in 60%.

✓ Pearls and ✗ Pitfalls

- ✓ The presence of the "comet tail sign" helps differentiate rounded atelectasis from other pleural-based masses.
- ✗ May enlarge over time.
- ✗ Contrast enhancement may mimic neoplastic lesions.
- ✗ Fine needle aspiration or biopsy is necessary if imaging findings are equivocal.

Case 44

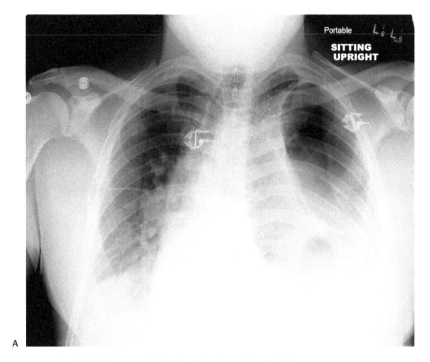

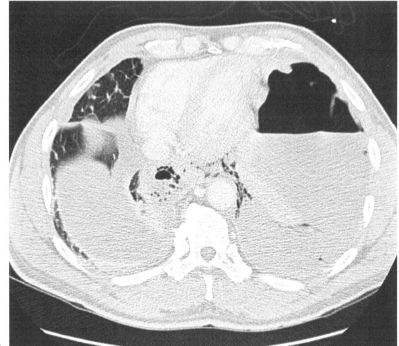

■ Clinical Presentation

A 50-year-old man with chest pain after alcohol binge.

■ Imaging Findings

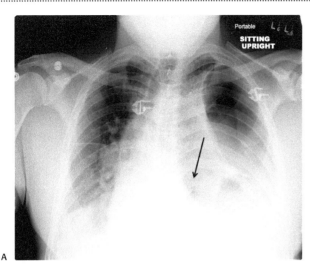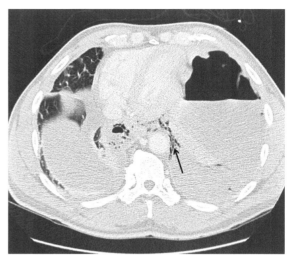

(A) Portable chest radiograph demonstrates a left hydropneumothorax, a right pleural effusion, and pneumomediastinum (*arrow*). (B) Contrast-enhanced chest CT image (lung windows) shows the pneumomediastinum with air tracking in the fascial planes to advantage (*arrow*). A left pleural effusion is present. The air and fluid seen on this CT image is the stomach, although the hydropneumothorax seen on chest X-ray is visible on more cranial images.

■ Differential Diagnosis

- **Boerhaave syndrome:** The development of pneumomediastinum, pleural effusion, and hydropneumothorax after an episode of forceful vomiting suggests esophageal rupture.
- *Tracheobronchial injury:* Pneumomediastinum is always concerning for the presence of tracheobronchial injury, which in trauma patients can be associated with pleural air and fluid.
- *Acute mediastinitis:* Mediastinal air and fluid can be seen in infectious mediastinitis resulting from a variety of conditions such as posterior mediastinal extension of a retropharyngeal abscess, postsurgical complications, and esophageal and airway injuries, among others.

■ Essential Facts

- Boerhaave syndrome refers to the "spontaneous" perforation of the esophagus during instrumentation or external trauma. It is typically associated with forceful vomiting and/or retching; it has also been described as "effort rupture" of the esophagus.
- Rupture is likely related to the sudden increase in intraluminal pressure.
- Pain is the presenting symptom in the majority of patients (85%), followed by vomiting (71%).
- The diagnosis should be suspected in the presence of the Mackler triad: vomiting, strong and sudden chest pain, and subcutaneous emphysema.
- Other presenting symptoms include shock, fever, jaundice, dyspnea, and back pain.

- The most common site of perforation is the left side of the distal esophagus.
- Imaging manifestations include pneumomediastinum with periesophageal air, pleural effusion (bilaterally or on the left side), pneumothorax, and pneumopericardium.
- A delayed diagnosis is associated with a high rate of mortality from polymicrobial mediastinitis and sepsis.
- Contrast esophagography or CT imaging after the oral administration of contrast demonstrates extravasation of the contrast medium at a supradiaphragmatic or subdiaphragmatic level.

✓ Pearls and ✗ Pitfalls

- ✓ "Spontaneous" rupture of the esophagus has also been described in other situations and conditions in which the intraluminal pressure increases suddenly, such as weightlifting, coughing, hiccups, childbirth, and seizures.
- ✓ On chest radiography, pneumomediastinum may be associated with the "V sign of Naclerio," a focal, sharply marginated V-shaped air lucency in the left lower mediastinum.
- ✗ Boerhaave syndrome is commonly misdiagnosed as myocardial infarction, aortic dissection, pulmonary embolism, pancreatitis, or perforated peptic ulcer.
- ✗ Boerhaave syndrome should not be confused with a Mallory–Weiss tear, which is a longitudinal mucosal laceration near the gastroesophageal junction (also often postemetic) resulting in upper gastrointestinal hemorrhages.

Case 45

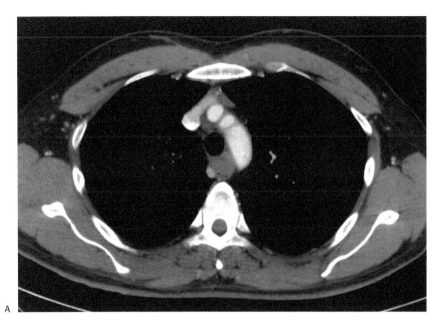

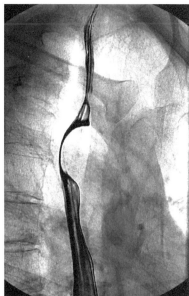

A

B

■ Clinical Presentation

A 50-year-old man with dysphagia.

■ Imaging Findings

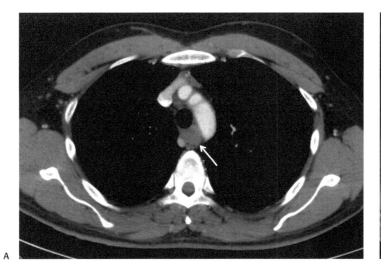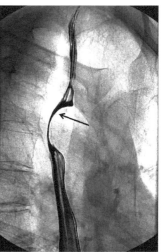

(A) Contrast-enhanced chest CT scan demonstrates a smoothly marginated soft tissue mass in the anterior esophagus (*arrow*). (B) Esophagram shows that the mass has smooth margins (*arrow*) and nearly completely obstructs the esophageal lumen.

■ Differential Diagnosis

- *Esophageal leiomyoma:* A well-defined soft tissue density mass may represent an esophageal leiomyoma.
- *Esophageal fibroma/schwannoma:* Other benign esophageal tumors (e.g., fibromas, schwannomas) have identical imaging appearances, presenting as a noninfiltrative soft tissue mass.
- *Esophageal carcinoma:* A mass arising from the esophageal wall should raise concern for the possibility of an esophageal carcinoma. Typically, the margins are more irregular.

■ Essential Facts

- Leiomyoma is the most common benign esophageal tumor, accounting for > 60% of benign neoplasms arising from the esophagus.
- Leiomyomas are well-encapsulated tumors composed of a mixture of benign smooth muscle and fibrous tissue.
- They may be multiple in 5% of patients.
- The most common location of esophageal leiomyomas is in the distal esophagus (> 60%), followed by the middle third (30%). Involvement of the upper esophagus is uncommon (10%).
- These slow-growing submucosal lesions are commonly asymptomatic but may result in epigastric discomfort and dysphagia.
- Symptomatic patients are on average 45 years old, and men are more commonly affected (2:1).

- Ulceration and bleeding are less common with esophageal than with gastric leiomyomas.
- On CT, they appear as round or lobulated soft tissue masses that are homogeneous in density, with a well-defined interface separating them from adjacent mediastinal structures.
- Large esophageal leiomyomas appear on chest radiographs as mediastinal masses, typically in the retrocardiac region.
- These tumors are generally enucleated and do not need esophageal resection (97%).
- MRI allows a better determination of the submucosal location of these tumors so that they can be differentiated from mucosal lesions such as carcinomas.

✓ Pearls and ✗ Pitfalls

✓ Esophageal leiomyomatosis may be associated with Alport syndrome, an X-linked genetic condition affecting biosynthesis of type IV collagen. Diffuse leiomyomatosis of the esophagus, female genitalia, or both may be present. Other findings include nephritis, hematuria, sensorineural hearing loss, and cataracts.

✓ The presence of calcification is highly suggestive of esophageal leiomyoma.

✗ CT cannot differentiate between leiomyomas and noninvasive esophageal carcinoma, sarcoma, or gastrointestinal stromal tumor. Soft tissue density masses detected on CT imaging should be further evaluated with upper gastrointestinal endoscopy.

Case 46

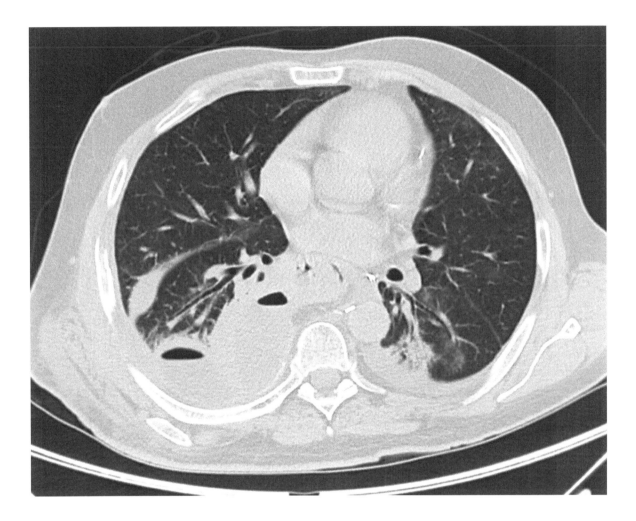

■ Clinical Presentation

A 50-year-old man with fever and weight loss.

■ **Imaging Findings**

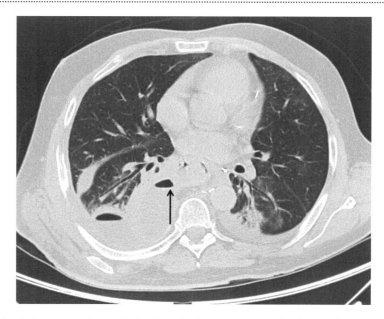

(A) Chest CT image (lung windows) demonstrates irregularity involving the distal esophagus with right lower lobe consolidation and a loculated hydro-pneumothorax (*arrow*).

■ **Differential Diagnosis**

- ***Esophagopulmonary fistula:*** Distal esophageal perforation, due to trauma, increased pressure, or cancer, which results in a fistula with the pleural space and pulmonary parenchyma.
- *Aspiration:* Aspiration can result in pneumonia and empyema. In some cases, empyema has an air-fluid level due to a gas-forming organism.
- *Hiatal hernia:* The air and fluid collection can be due to a diaphragmatic or hiatal hernia, although these are usually on the left.

■ **Essential Facts**

- The esophagus abuts the posterior surface of the left mainstem bronchus, the left lung, aorta, and heart. Because there is direct contact with the pleura on the right, without interposed aorta as is found on the left, pathology involving the midesophagus involves the right pleura more easily than the left.
- The majority of esophageal fistulas seen in adult patients result from acquired diseases such as intrathoracic malignancies (> 60%), in particular esophageal cancer (77%) and lung cancer (16%).
- Esophagorespiratory fistulas occur in 5 to 10% of patients with advanced esophageal cancer.
- Trauma, endoscopy, chemical injury, prolonged intubation, and infections such as tuberculosis can also result in esophageal fistulas.

- Based on the site of the tract, a fistula may develop between the esophagus and the trachea, lungs, and/or bronchi.
- Advanced esophageal carcinomas (T4) result in fistulas between the esophagus and respiratory tract or pleural space in up to 15% of cases.
- The incidence of fistula formation increases with concomitant radiation therapy.
- The initial clinical presentation is recurrent pneumonia with a variable degree of parenchymal consolidation secondary to aspiration and sepsis.
- CT after the oral administration of contrast reveals an abnormal collection of contrast in the airways or lung parenchyma.
- If necrotizing pneumonia develops, oral contrast may accumulate within the cavity.

✓ **Pearls and ✗ Pitfalls**

✓ The prognosis of patients with esophageal cancer and a fistula between the esophagus and respiratory tract is extremely poor, with an approximately 1-month overall survival. Palliative measures such as esophageal stenting can be considered.

✗ Cross-sectional imaging is limited in defining the exact morphology of the fistula. Esophagography is usually required to confirm the diagnosis and define the location and anatomy of the fistulous tract.

Case 47

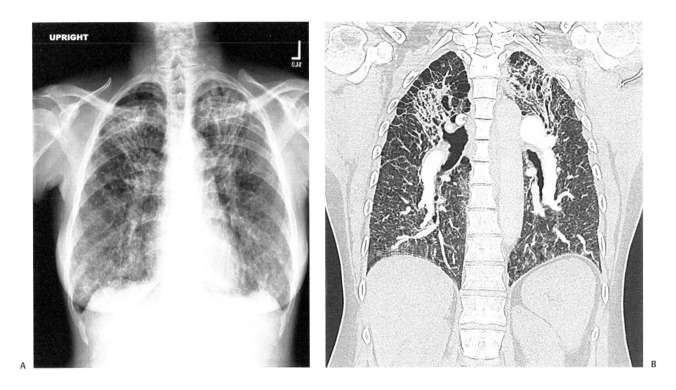

A

B

■ Clinical Presentation

A 45-year-old woman with erythema nodosum and severe dyspnea.

■ Imaging Findings

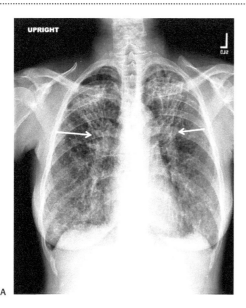
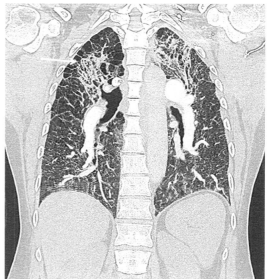

(A) Chest radiograph demonstrates an upper lobe–predominant interstitial abnormality with upper lobe retraction (*arrows*). There is mild enlargement of the central pulmonary arteries. **(B)** Chest CT (lung windows) coronal reformat demonstrates severe upper lobe fibrosis and traction bronchiectasis (*arrow*).

■ Differential Diagnosis

- ***Sarcoidosis with pulmonary hypertension:*** The upper lobe predominance and clinical history make sarcoidosis the best choice. End-stage sarcoidosis can result in pulmonary hypertension.
- *Idiopathic pulmonary fibrosis:* Typically, lower lobe–dependent subpleural reticulation, traction bronchiectasis, and honeycombing.
- *Pulmonary Langerhans cell histiocytosis (PLCH):* Although upper lobe–predominant lung disease is seen with PLCH, this typically demonstrates large lung volumes with cysts and nodules. Lymphadenopathy is uncommon. It is almost exclusively seen in smokers.

■ Essential Facts

- Sarcoidosis is an immunologically mediated multiorgan granulomatous disease of unknown etiology.
- Sarcoidosis typically manifests in young adults and people of middle age.
- It has a highly variable clinical course and prognosis; 50% of patients are asymptomatic.
- Although almost any organ can be affected, intrathoracic involvement is seen in 90% of cases.
- HRCT shows bilateral small perivascular nodules with irregular "beaded" thickening of the bronchovascular bundles and interlobular septa.
- Pulmonary involvement is typically upper lobe predominant.
- End-stage disease results in architectural distortion with upper lobe retraction, traction bronchiectasis, honeycombing, and cysts.

- Chronic alveolar hypoxia due to interstitial lung disease can result in pulmonary hypertension.
- Hypoxic vasoconstriction results in increased resistance in the pulmonary arterial bed.
- On CT, a transverse diameter of the main pulmonary artery > 29 mm is suggestive of pulmonary hypertension.
- Dilation of the right atrium and ventricle, thickening of the anterior RV wall, and flattening of the interventricular septum are manifestations of cor pulmonale on CT.
- The right interlobar artery is enlarged (> 16 mm in men, > 14 mm in women).

✓ Pearls and ✗ Pitfalls

- ✓ End-stage sarcoidosis can result in pulmonary hypertension.
- ✓ Primary pulmonary hypertension is a rare disorder occurring primarily in middle-aged females. There is likely a genetic component and the disorder has been associated with HIV infection, appetite suppressants, cocaine use, and portal hypertension.
- ✓ Scleroderma is the most common collagen vascular disease to cause pulmonary hypertension.
- ✗ The major complications of sarcoidosis are fibrosis, cor pulmonale, and mycetoma formation.
- ✗ Imaging findings of cor pulmonale include right-sided cardiac dilation, dilation of the azygous vein, and reflux of contrast into the hepatic veins.

Case 48

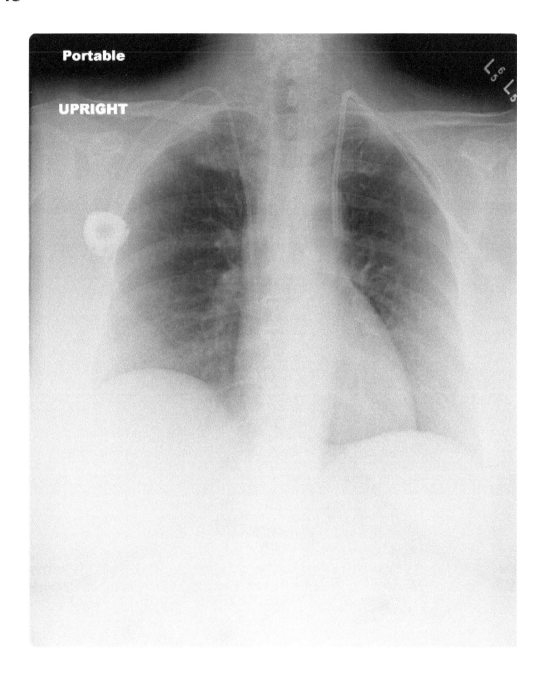

■ Clinical Presentation

A 40-year-old woman with leukemia status left post central line placement.

■ Imaging Findings

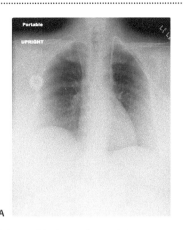
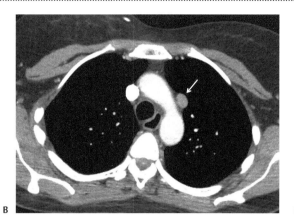
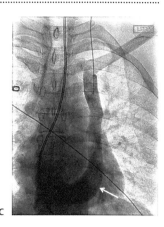

(A) Portable chest radiograph demonstrates a right jugular single lumen port catheter with the tip at the right atrial–superior vena cava junction. The new left venous catheter overlies the left mediastinum in a vertical course. **(B)** Contrast-enhanced chest CT image (soft tissue windows) in a different patient shows an oval vascular structure in the left mediastinum (*arrow*). **(C)** Left jugular venogram (soft tissue windows) in a different patient shows a left superior vena cava with drainage into the coronary sinus (*arrow*) and right atrium.

■ Differential Diagnosis

- ***Persistent left superior vena cava (PLSVC):*** PLSVC is typically found incidentally on a chest radiograph obtained after placement of a left-sided central venous catheter or on CT imaging.
- *Partial anomalous pulmonary venous return (PAPVR):* A large venous structure can also be seen to the left of the aortic arch in patients with PAPVR of the left upper lobe, but it will typically connect to the brachiocephalic vein, not to the coronary sinus, and the venous drainage is from the lung parenchyma.
- *Malpositioned catheter:* Catheters can be malpositioned in mammary or mediastinal veins, arteries, the mediastinum, or the pleural space.

■ Essential Facts

- PLSVC is the most common congenital thoracic venous anomaly.
- The prevalence is < 0.5% in the general population but up to 10% in patients with congenital heart disease.
- The left superior vena cava (SVC) represents persistence of the left anterior and common cardinal veins and left horn of the sinus venosus.
- The right SVC may be normal, small, or absent.
- A bridging left brachiocephalic vein is variably present.

- Drainage is usually into the right atrium via a dilated coronary sinus.
- Another configuration results in a left azygos arch; in such cases, the left superior intercostal vein connects the left SVC and the accessory hemiazygos vein.
- Chest radiographs may show mild mediastinal widening with a soft tissue density to the left of the aortic knob.
- On cross-sectional images, the PLSVC is seen as a vascular structure connecting the confluence of the left subclavian vein and the internal jugular vein with the coronary sinus.

✓ Pearls and ✗ Pitfalls

- ✓ Congenital cardiac anomalies are more common with absence of the right SVC.
- ✓ Other causes of a dilated coronary sinus include elevated right heart pressures and a coronary arteriovenous fistula to the sinus.
- ✗ Rarely, there is abnormal communication with the left atrium at the level of the left atrial appendage or coronary sinus. This results in a small right-to-left shunt (Raghib syndrome).
- ✗ A single anteroposterior view of the chest is limited for evaluating the course of a venous catheter.
- ✗ During cardiac surgery, a PLSVC is a relative contraindication to retrograde cardioplegia.

Case 49

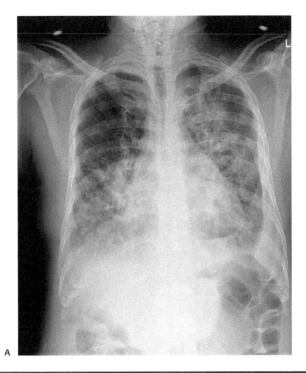

A

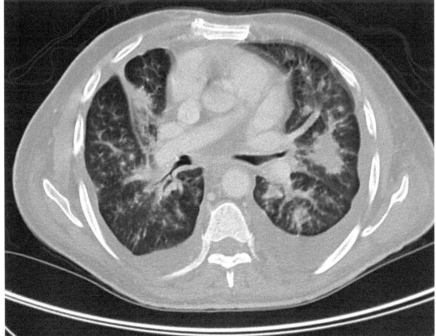

B

■ **Clinical Presentation**

A 40-year-old immunocompromised man with progressive shortness of breath and cough.

■ Imaging Findings

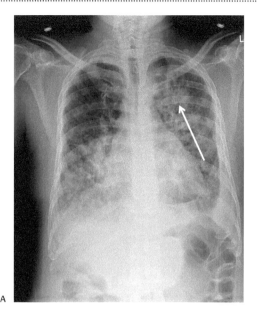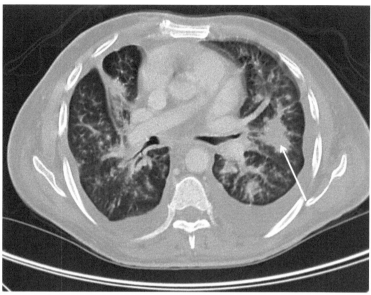

(A) Portable chest radiograph demonstrates bilateral pleural effusions and patchy multifocal irregular opacities (*arrow*). **(B)** Contrast-enhanced chest CT image (soft tissue windows) demonstrates irregular nodular coalescent opacities (*arrow*). Bilateral pleural effusions are seen.

■ Differential Diagnosis

- ***Kaposi sarcoma (KS):*** Bilateral pulmonary nodules in a peribronchovascular distribution, especially in an HIV-positive patient, are suggestive of lung involvement of KS.
- *Lymphoma:* Multicentric non-Hodgkin lymphoma may also manifest as enlarged peribronchovascular nodules and pleural effusion.
- *Opportunistic infection:* Tuberculosis, as well as atypical mycobacterial and other opportunistic infections, should also be considered in the differential diagnosis of multiple pulmonary nodules in an immunocompromised host.

■ Essential Facts

- AIDS-related KS occurs principally in men who have sex with men infected with human herpesvirus type 8.
- AIDS-related KS is a multicentric disease that may involve lymph nodes, the gastrointestinal tract, and the lung parenchyma in the presence of extensive mucocutaneous disease.
- Pulmonary KS is found in ~10% of patients with AIDS and in 50% of patients with cutaneous KS.
- The prevalence of pulmonary KS at postmortem examination in patients with AIDS is also high (30 to 50%).
- Affected patients typically have a low CD4 lymphocyte count ($< 100/mm^3$).

- Thoracic involvement from KS includes bilateral pulmonary nodules in a peribronchovascular distribution, coalescent nodular and irregular opacities with a "flame shape" appearance, and hilar-mediastinal lymphadenopathy.
- Enhancing neck, axillary, abdominal, and pelvic lymph nodes are also common.
- Bilateral pleural effusions are common, and their presence has been associated with a poor outcome.
- Cavitary pulmonary lesions have also been reported.
- Osteolytic lesions in the sternum and thoracic spine as well as soft tissue masses with skin and subcutaneous fat involvement are other imaging findings.
- Nuclear medicine studies with sequential thallium and gallium scanning have been used to help differentiate between KS and other pulmonary disease in AIDS. Gallium uptake is usually negative in KS and positive in infection or lymphoma. Thallium uptake is typically positive in lymphoma and KS. Indium-111–labeled polyclonal human immunoglobulin scanning is negative in KS.

✓ Pearls and ✗ Pitfalls

- ✓ The incidence of KS has declined significantly since the introduction of highly active antiretroviral therapy.
- ✗ The imaging manifestations of thoracic KS can be misleading because it can be seen as an isolated event or associated with opportunistic infection.

Case 50

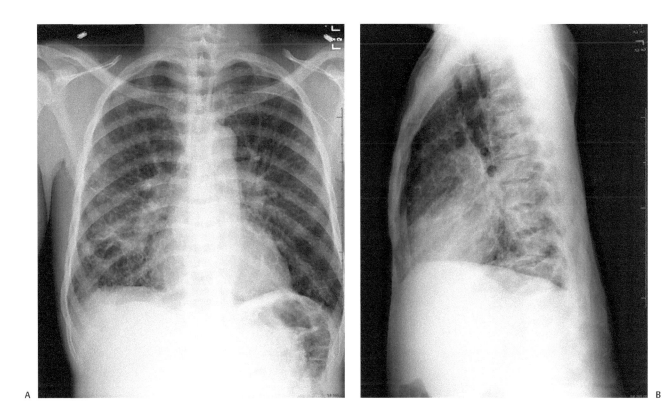

A   B

■ Clinical Presentation

A 25-year-old man with acute chest pain.

■ Imaging Findings

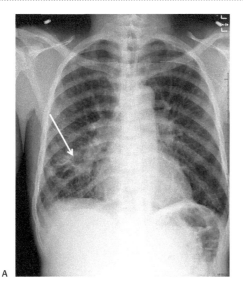 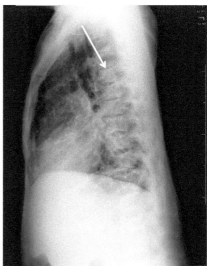

(A) Frontal chest radiograph demonstrates a patchy right-sided opacity (*arrow*). The spleen is not seen. **(B)** Lateral chest radiograph shows the H-type vertebral bodies to advantage (*arrow*).

■ Differential Diagnosis

- ***Sickle cell disease (SCD) with acute chest syndrome (ACS):*** ACS in patients with SCD presents with a variable degree of parenchymal opacities, which may be unilateral or bilateral.
- *SCD with pneumonia:* Patients with SCD have a high incidence of pneumonia, which presents with a variable degree of parenchymal opacities.
- *SCD with pulmonary edema:* Pulmonary edema may develop in patients with SCD due to severe anemia, aggressive volume resuscitation, renal insufficiency, dilated cardiomyopathy, and pulmonary hypertension.

■ Essential Facts

- ACS is an acute pulmonary disease that develops in patients with SCD. It is one of the most common causes of hospitalization in these patients and is responsible for 25% of deaths among them.
- ACS occurs in 15 to 40% of patients with SCD and is more prevalent in children and in patients with homozygous disease.
- ACS is defined as the presence of a new pulmonary opacity on chest radiograph in conjunction with at least one other new symptom or sign: chest pain, wheezing, cough, tachypnea, and/or fever higher than 38°C (100.4°F).
- ACS can be caused by different mechanisms in both infectious and noninfectious conditions. Infection, fat embolism, and rib infarction are the most common.
- Pulmonary embolism and in situ thrombosis in the pulmonary vasculature are other, less common causes of ACS.

- The most common infectious agents in patients with ACS/SCD are *Chlamydia pneumoniae* and *Mycoplasma pneumoniae*. Other, less common infectious agents are *Streptococcus pneumoniae* and *Haemophilus influenzae*.
- Fat emboli originate in bone marrow that becomes infarcted during acute crises. Necrotic fragments break loose and are trapped in the pulmonary vascular bed.
- Chronic lung disease develops in 4% of patients with SCD, presumably secondary to recurrent episodes of infarction and infection. Interstitial pulmonary fibrosis, parenchymal irregular scars, pleural thickening, and bronchiectasis develop and involve predominantly the lower lobes.
- Pulmonary arteriolar intimal hyperplasia develops, resulting in pulmonary arterial hypertension.
- Bone infarcts affecting the ribs and humeral heads are also common imaging findings.
- Chronic and recurrent episodes of splenic infarction are common. The replacement of the tissue of the spleen by scar and calcification leads to a small, densely calcified, nonfunctional organ (autosplenectomy).

✓ Pearls and ✗ Pitfalls

- ✓ Infarction affecting the vertebral body end plate creates a step-off deformity known as the Reynolds sign, which is associated with concurrent overgrowth of the adjacent secondary ossification center and results in H-shaped deformity, considered pathognomonic for SCD.
- ✗ Paraspinal masses resulting from extramedullary hematopoiesis are additional imaging findings on thoracic imaging examinations and should not be confused with neoplasm or lymphadenopathy. Their nature can be confirmed by imaging with technetium-99m sulfur colloid.

Case 51

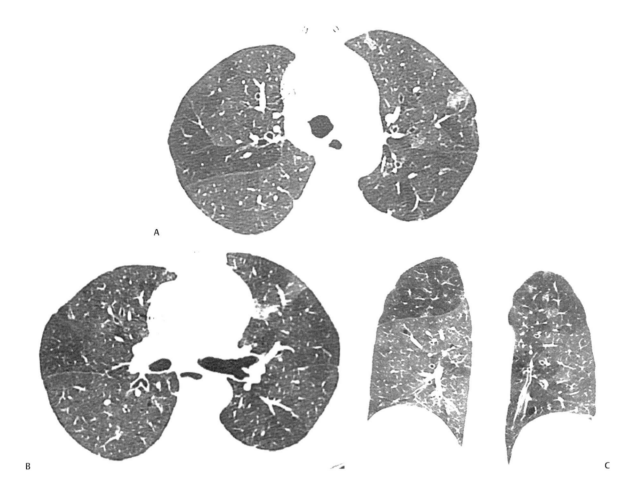

A

B

C

■ Clinical Presentation
....

A 58-year-old man, 2 years post bilateral lung transplantation for idiopathic pulmonary fibrosis, presents with progressive shortness of breath and declining pulmonary function on expirometry.

■ Imaging Findings

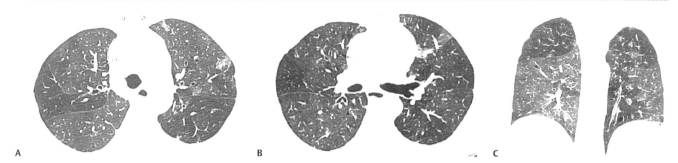

A   B   C

(A–C) CT chest axial (A, B) and coronal (C) images demonstrate mosaic pattern of lung attenuation with diminished vascularity within the areas with air trapping. Patchy ground-glass opacities are also appreciated.

■ Differential Diagnosis

- **Bronchiolitis obliterans syndrome**.
- *Bronchiolitis obliterans organizing pneumonia.*
- *Follicular bronchiolitis.*
- *Opportunistic infection.*

■ Essential Facts

- Bronchiolitis obliterans syndrome (BOS) is a major complication of lung transplantation that is associated with poor prognosis and poor survival.
- BOS may also develop as a complication of allogenic hematopoietic stem cell transplantation and bone marrow transplantation.
- BOS is caused by inflammation, destruction, and fibrosis of small airways in the lung that lead to obliterative bronchiolitis (OB).
- Bronchiolitis obliterans (BO) or OB is the histologic hallmark of chronic lung allograft dysfunction and is characterized by patchy submucosal peribronchiolar fibrosis and cicatrization involving the respiratory bronchioles, resulting in total or near-total occlusion of the noncartilaginous airway.
- The characteristic clinical manifestation is a gradual decline in lung function with sudden or gradual decline in forced expiratory volume in 1 second (FEV_1).
- BOS affects 50% or more of lung transplant recipients who survive beyond 5 years, and it accounts for a significant proportion of lung allograft loss and recipient mortality.
- No effective treatment exits for BOS. Immunosuppression remains the mainstay of therapy but intensified pharmacological immunosuppression has little effect on established BOS.

■ Other Imaging Findings

- Routine thoracic radiographs lack sensitivity and specificity for the diagnosis of BOS.
- High-resolution CT (HRCT) is the best imaging modality for the diagnosis of BOS. The presence of air trapping on expiratory views or mosaic pattern of lung attenuation on HRCT supports the possibility of BOS in a lung transplant recipient or bone marrow transplant patient who develops a decline in lung function.
- HRCT with inspiratory and expiratory images should be considered in the evaluation of transplant recipients with FEV_1 decline when BOS is a possibility.
- Expiratory CT may reveal air trapping that is not evident on inspiratory scans.

✓ Pearls and ✗ Pitfalls

- ✓ BOS is the most common long-term noninfectious pulmonary complication of allogenic hematopoietic stem cell transplantation.
- ✗ Because of the patchy distribution of OB and small sample size, the yield of transbronchial biopsy is poor (< 20%).

Case 52

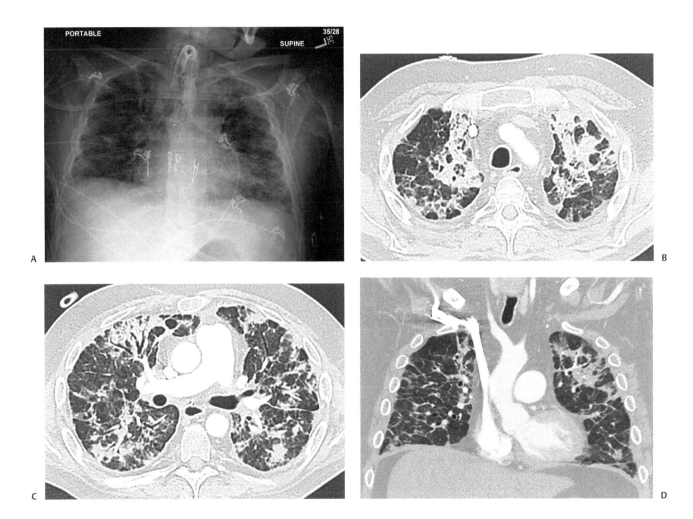

■ Clinical Presentation

A 33-year-old man with a history of bilateral lung transplant for cystic fibrosis 3 years earlier has worsening respiratory function and progressive shortness of breath. Pulmonary function test reveals severe restriction with mild obstruction.

■ Imaging Findings

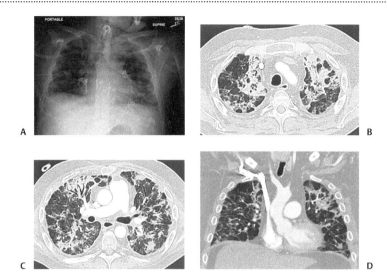

(A–D) Conventional radiograph, anteroposterior view **(A)**, shows diminished lung volumes with diffuse reticulation throughout the bilateral lungs. CT images, axial **(B, C)** and coronal **(D)** reconstruction, demonstrate increased reticulation and interlobular septal thickening with patchy areas of denser opacity and consolidation.

■ Differential Diagnosis

- ***Restrictive allograft syndrome.***
- *Bronchiolitis obliterans syndrome.*
- *Recurrent pretransplant underlying condition.*

■ Essential Facts

- Survival after lung transplantation (5-year survival ~55%) remains shorter than survival after transplantation of other solid organs.
- This has been mainly attributed to the development of chronic rejection.
- Rejection is responsible for 30% mortality after lung transplantation.
- Chronic lung allograft dysfunction (CLAD) is an umbrella term that embraces all forms of chronic lung dysfunction (≥ 3 weeks) after transplant.
- Currently, two principal phenotypes of CLAD dysfunction are recognized: obstructive CLAD and restrictive CLAD.
- Obstructive CLAD is the typical, which from a histopathology standpoint is characterized by obliterative bronchiolitis.
- Restrictive CLAD has been termed restrictive allograft syndrome (RAS), which from a histopathology standpoint is characterized by pleuroparenchymal fibroelastosis (100%) and interstitial fibrosis (> 90%) predominantly in a biapical subpleural distribution, which are seen in nearly all patients with RAS.
- RAS is characterized by restrictive pulmonary function decline with decreased forced vital capacity and total lung capacity in addition to decline in forced expiratory volume in 1 second.

- No effective treatment exists for CLAD. Immunosuppression remains the mainstay of therapy, but intensified pharmacologic immunosuppression has little effect on established bronchiolitis obliterans syndrome or RAS.
- Retransplantation is not considered a good option for RAS. Affected patients seem to redevelop CLAD earlier, and they have a low 3-year survival rate after retransplantation.

■ Other Imaging Findings

- On CT imaging, RAS manifests as increased reticulation, interlobular septal thickening, scarring, and pleural thickening more significantly affecting the mid and upper lung zones.
- Architectural distortion with traction bronchiectasis is also common.
- The progressive pulmonary restriction manifests as diminished lung volumes.

✓ Pearls and ✗ Pitfalls

- ✓ Progressive restriction, with diminished lung volume, associated with increased reticulation and pleural thickening in a lung transplant patient suggest RAS, the restrictive form of CLAD.
- ✗ Roughly 50% of cases of pleuroparenchymal fibroelastosis are secondary to CLAD after lung transplantation or bone marrow transplantation. The other 50% are idiopathic, familial, or associated with drug toxicity from chemotherapy agents.

Case 53

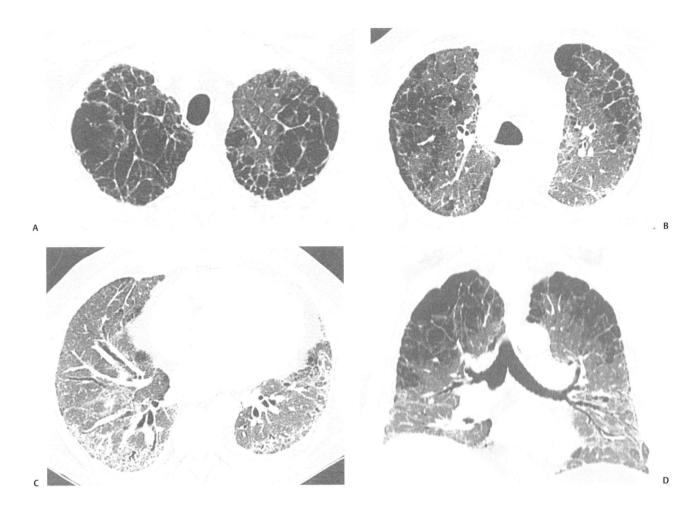

A

B

C

D

■ Clinical Presentation

A 69-year-old man with progressive shortness of breath and hypoxemia.

■ Imaging Findings

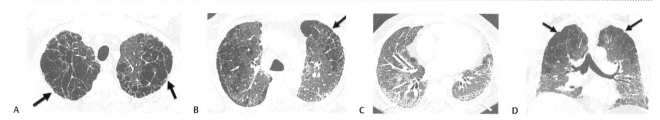

(A–D) CT images of the chest: axial images **(A–C)** and coronal reconstruction image **(D)** show advanced changes of centrilobular emphysema, more pronounced in the upper lobes (*black arrows*), with changes of interstitial pulmonary fibrosis with traction bronchiectasis and increased reticulation in the bilateral lower lobes (*white arrows*).

■ Differential Diagnosis

- ***Combined pulmonary fibrosis and emphysema.***
- *Hypersensitivity pneumonitis.*
- *Centrilobular emphysema.*
- *Usual interstitial pneumonia.*
- *Asbestosis.*

■ Essential Facts

- Coexistence of upper lobe emphysema and lower lobe pulmonary fibrosis in the same patient, resulting in a clinical syndrome known as combined pulmonary fibrosis and emphysema (CPFE), which is clinically characterized by dyspnea and abnormalities in gas exchange.
- Histologic analysis demonstrates predominantly centrilobular emphysema in the upper lobes and interstitial pulmonary fibrosis in the lower lobes.
- The coexistence of emphysema (obstruction) and fibrosis (restriction) leads to a characteristic functional profile. Affected patients commonly have a relatively normal spirometry (normal forced vital capacity, forced expiratory volume in 1 second, and total lung capacity), in the setting of a severely impaired gas exchange with decreased diffusing capacity of lung for carbon monoxide.
- CPFE is associated with high mortality, with a median survival between 2 and 8 years and a 5-year survival rate between 35 and 80%.
- Pulmonary hypertension is a common complication (50%), and appears to be more frequent and more severe than in population with idiopathic pulmonary fibrosis or emphysema alone.
- Patients with CPFE also have an increased risk for the development of lung cancer (> 40%).
- There is no specific treatment. In current smokers, smoking cessation is encouraged. Lung transplantation should be considered given the significant mortality.

■ Other Imaging Findings

- The radiographic characteristics include the presence of upper lobe emphysema and lower-lobe interstitial pulmonary fibrosis.
- Conventional chest radiograph may demonstrate reticulonodular opacities in the lung bases and subpleural regions, with hyperlucency and diminished vascular marking in the upper lung zones.
- High-resolution CT demonstrates well demarcated areas of centrilobular emphysema in the upper lobes, with the characteristic decreased attenuation with or without bullae, and areas of interstitial pulmonary fibrosis with increase reticulation and interlobular septal thickening with peripheral and basal predominance, with honeycombing, architectural distortion and /or traction bronchiectasis or bronchiolectasis.

✓ Pearls and ✗ Pitfalls

- ✓ Strong male predominance (90%).
- ✓ Strong association with cigarette smoking. Nearly all affected patients (98%) are either current or former smokers.
- ✗ Emphysema can occur in patients with asbestosis (10–36%) and other mineral dust exposures (e.g., silicosis, coal workers' pneumoconiosis, talcosis) with or without cigarette smoking.

Case 54

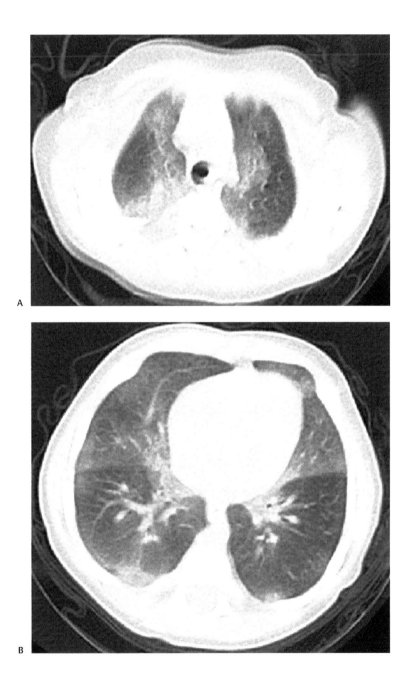

A

B

■ Clinical Presentation

A 6-month-old boy with persistent cough and wheezing who has had hypoxemia, digital clubbing, failure to thrive, and respiratory symptoms since birth.

■ **Imaging Findings**

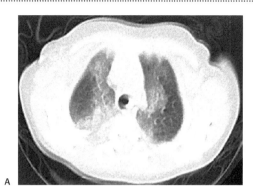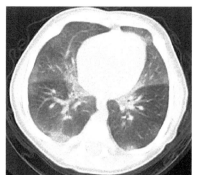

(A, B) CT images of the chest. Axial images in the upper lung zone **(A)** and lower lung zone **(B)** reveal a mosaic pattern of lung attenuation with focal areas of ground-glass opacity and air trapping.

■ **Differential Diagnosis**

- ***chILD syndrome.***
- *Immunodeficiency.*
- *Chronic aspiration.*

■ **Essential Facts**

- chILD (childhood interstitial lung disease) syndrome is a rare complex and heterogeneous disorder with an estimated prevalence between 0.13 and 16.2 per 100,000 children/year.
- chILD syndrome is considered present when an infant (< 2 years old) with diffuse lung disease (DLD) has the common causes of DLD excluded as the primary diagnosis and has at least three of the following four criteria: (1) respiratory symptoms (e.g., cough), (2) respiratory signs (e.g., retractions, digital clubbing), (3) hypoxemia, and (4) diffuse abnormalities on chest X-ray or CT scan.
- chILD syndrome represents a heterogeneous group of disorders that have been classified into four major categories: (1) diffuse developmental disorders (e.g., acinar dysplasia, congenital alveolar dysplasia), (2) alveolar growth abnormalities (e.g., pulmonary hypoplasia, pulmonary changes from chromosomal abnormalities like trisomy 21), (3) specific conditions of undefined etiology (e.g., pulmonary glycogenosis, neuroendocrine cell hyperplasia of infancy), (4) surfactant dysfunction genetic mutations.
- Some chILD entities are associated with very high mortality, whereas others have a more favorable outcome. Overall mortality rate is high (13–30%), with 50% of patients experiencing ongoing mortality.
- Corticosteroids and hydroxychloroquine are the most common treatment medications, but there have been no controlled trials of any therapeutic intervention.
- Lung transplantation is an option for infants and children with life-threatening chILD diseases with end-stage lung disease, with a 5-year survival rate ~50%.

■ **Other Imaging Findings**

- Conventional chest radiographs are usually the first imaging study performed; they are frequently abnormal but rarely provide a specific diagnosis.
- High-resolution (HR) CT is recommended in the evaluation to better characterize the nature and distribution of the lung disease. The imaging manifestation varies significantly depending on the underlying condition and may include diffuse ground-glass opacities, interlobular septal thickening, cystic changes, mosaic attenuation, and air trapping.
- Controlled ventilation HRCT (CVHRCT), which requires mask ventilation and general anesthesia, has been proposed as the best technique to assess for air trapping and ground-glass opacities and to eliminate motion artifacts in infants and children with diffuse lung disease.
- No studies have compared CVHRCT with conventional HRCT in chILD syndrome or DLD, and there is some question whether the increased risk of anesthesia is justified.

✓ **Pearls and ✗ Pitfalls**

✓ Tachypnea is consistently the most common clinical sign (75–90%), followed by hypoxemia, crackles, wheezing, and cough. Failure to thrive is also an additional common clinical manifestation.

✗ The diagnosis of chILD syndrome requires that the more common causes of DLD (cystic fibrosis, immunodeficiency syndromes, congenital heart disease, bronchopulmonary dysplasia, pulmonary infection, primary ciliary dyskinesia, and recurrent aspiration) have been excluded.

Case 55

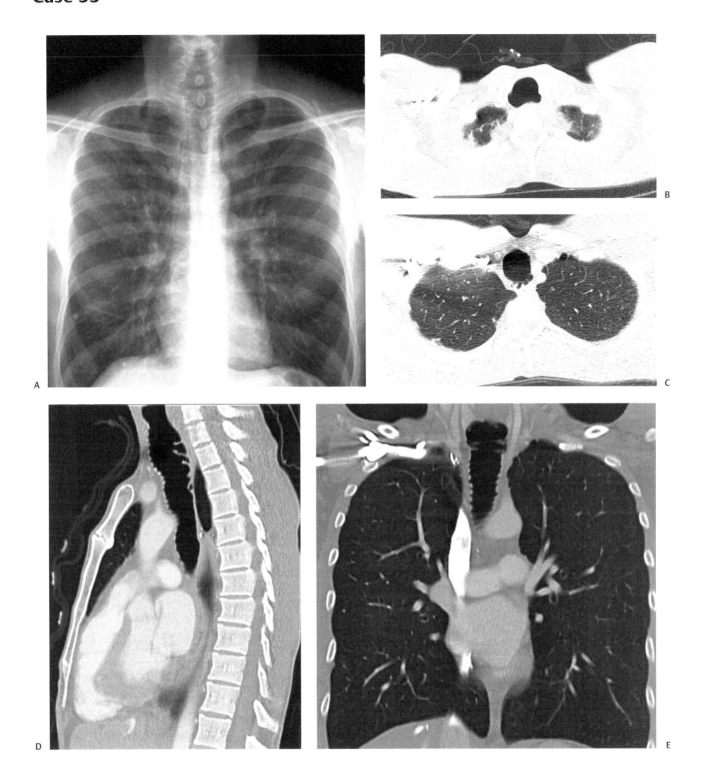

Clinical Presentation

A 44-year-old man (never a smoker) with chronic cough and nail-clubbing deformity.

▪ Imaging Findings

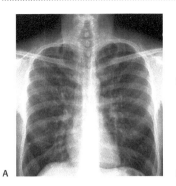
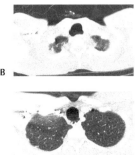
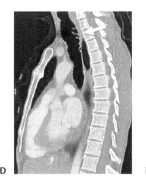
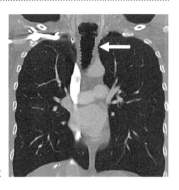

(A) Conventional radiograph, anteroposterior view, shows increased lung volumes with a dilated trachea. (B–E) Chest CT images. Axial images (B, C), sagittal view (D), and coronal reconstruction (E) show abnormally dilated trachea with posterior and lateral wall diverticulosis (*arrows*).

▪ Differential Diagnosis

- ***Mounier–Kuhn syndrome.***
- *Williams–Campbell syndrome.*
- *Secondary tracheobronchomegaly associated with different chronic pulmonary conditions:* Typically manifests with chronic cough (i.e., pulmonary fibrosis, chronic infection, chronic obstructive pulmonary disease [COPD]/emphysema).

▪ Essential Facts

- Mounier–Kuhn syndrome (MKS) is a rare disorder of uncertain etiology likely secondary to a congenital defect or atrophy of the elastic and smooth muscle tissues of the trachea and main bronchi, resulting in significant tracheobronchial dilation.
- There is thinning of the muscular mucosa as well as atrophy of longitudinal muscle and elastic fibers.
- The loss of elastic fibers around the respiratory tract may be partial or complete and may be patchy in distribution.
- There are numerous saccular diverticula between cartilages with bulging dilations on the posterior wall.
- There is also absence of myenteric plexus in the tracheal wall.
- The exact etiology of MKS is not known, but it seems to be congenital.
- No clear hereditary pattern has been recognized.
- Many adult affected patients have a history of cigarette smoking.
- Cough is the most common clinical complaint (> 70%), followed by recurrent respiratory infections (50%) and dyspnea (> 40%).
- Patients with MKS commonly show obstructive physiology on pulmonary function test.
- Finger clubbing is common.
- No definitive data are available regarding disease progression. Anecdotal data suggest that once certain enlargement has taken place, the anatomical changes do not progress over time.

- There is no definitive treatment for this condition. Mucolytic therapy, physical therapy, and postural drainage are recommended to facilitate expectoration.

▪ Other Imaging Findings

- Tracheobronchomegaly is commonly missed on plain chest X-rays.
- On CT image, the normal diameter of the trachea, measured 2 cm above the aortic arch, is 27 mm (sagittal) and 25 mm (coronal) for males and 23 mm and 21 mm, respectively, for females. For an adult, an increased diameter of the trachea > 3 cm, or of the right mainstem bronchus > 2.4 cm or for the left mainstem bronchus > 2.3 cm.
- Tracheobronchial diverticulosis, which is found in ~50% of patients with MKS, is better appreciated on CT with multiplanar reconstruction.
- Bronchiectasis is identified with CT in a significant number of affected patients (30–45%).
- Tracheobronchomalacia is found in at least 28% of affected subjects.

✓ Pearls and ✗ Pitfalls

- ✓ The sporadic association of this condition with Ehlers–Danlos syndrome, Marfan syndrome, and cutis laxa syndrome suggest a smooth muscle and connective tissue disorder.
- ✓ Tracheobronchomegaly is manifest not only by abnormal dilation of the trachea and bronchi but also by the protrusion of the redundant musculomembranous tissue between the cartilaginous rings with the formation of tracheal diverticulosis, resulting in scalloped or lobulated appearance of the air column.
- ✗ COPD is commonly diagnosed (> 25%) in patients with congenital tracheobronchomegaly.

Case 56

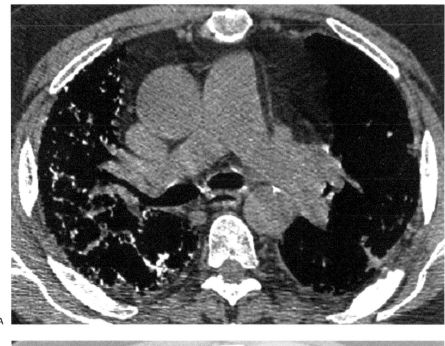

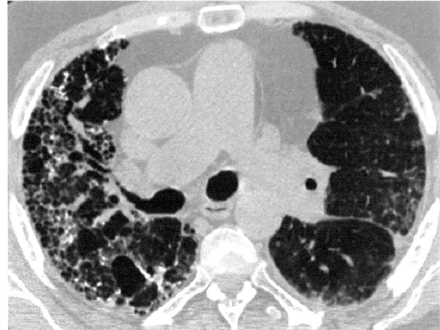

■ Clinical Presentation
....

A 63-year-old man with progressive shortness of breath and known pulmonary fibrosis.

▪ Imaging Findings

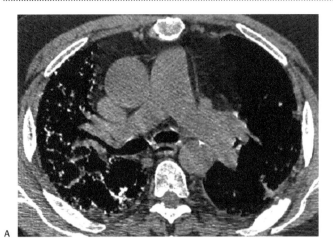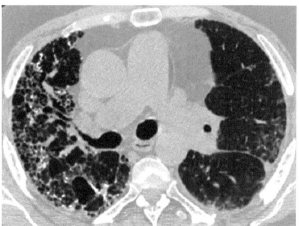

(A, B) CT images of the chest: axial images with mediastinal (A) and bone window (B) show dense punctate and branching calcifications in the lung parenchyma with more significant fibrosis.

▪ Differential Diagnosis

- ***Dendriform pulmonary ossification.***
- *Metastatic pulmonary calcification.*
- *Talc granulomas.*

▪ Essential Facts

- Dendriform pulmonary ossification (DPO) is a chronic process characterized by progressive metaplastic ossification and formation of mature bone in the lung parenchyma, affecting the pulmonary interstitium or alveolar spaces.
- There are two morphologic forms of pulmonary ossification: DPO and nodular pulmonary ossification (NPO).
- In DPO, the heterotopic bone has a delicate dendritic branching pattern that typically affects the alveolar interstitium.
- In NPO, the more rounded nodular ossification predominantly affects the alveolar spaces.
- Patients can be asymptomatic or have symptoms from the underlying pulmonary or cardiac disease. More commonly found in the elderly, affecting males more than females (M:F = 7:1).
- Although considered an uncommon disease, it is probably underrecognized, and the exact prevalence is not known. Reported in as much as 9% of patients with idiopathic pulmonary fibrosis.
- No known treatment is available.

▪ Other Imaging Findings

- Because of the very small size of the calcifications, diffuse pulmonary ossification is typically not recognized on conventional chest radiographs.
- On CT imaging, because of the small size of the parenchymal calcification, the abnormality may be more easily recognized with window settings appropriate for calcium, as fine nodular or branching calcifications in the periphery of the lungs, commonly associated with increased reticulation and predominantly in the mid and lower lung zones.

✓ Pearls and ✗ Pitfalls

- ✓ DPO is more commonly seen associated with interstitial pulmonary fibrosis, chronic obstructive pulmonary disease, organizing pneumonia, Hamman–Rich syndrome, adult respiratory distress syndrome, fibrosing alveolitis, pneumoconiosis, and other diffuse pulmonary disorders. Sometimes, it is truly idiopathic.
- ✓ NPO is more commonly associated with preexisting heart disease including mitral valve stenosis, chronic left ventricular heart failure, and aortic or subaortic stenosis.
- ✗ Laboratory exams such a serum chemistry have no value. Calcium and phosphorus levels are normal.

Case 57

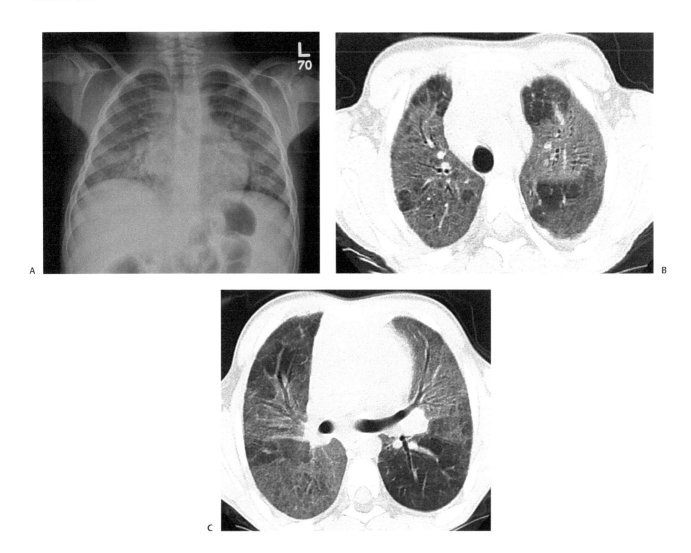

■ Clinical Presentation

A 7-year-old boy with history of oculocutaneous albinism, epistaxis, melena, and easy bruising presents with progressive respiratory symptoms.

■ Imaging Findings

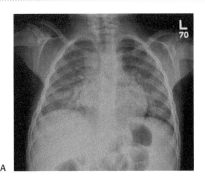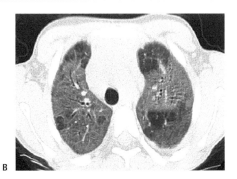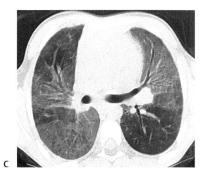

(A) Chest radiograph shows ground-glass opacities in the bilateral lungs. **(B, C)** Noncontrast CT images of the chest. Axial images in the upper and middle lung zones demonstrate diffuse reticulation and ground-glass opacity in a patchy distribution (mosaic pattern of lung attenuation) affecting the bilateral lungs.

■ Differential Diagnosis

- ***Hermansky–Pudlak syndrome.***
- *Idiopathic pulmonary fibrosis.*
- *Familial idiopathic pulmonary fibrosis.*
- *Nonspecific interstitial pneumonia.*

■ Essential Facts

- Hermansky–Pudlak syndrome (HPS) is an autosomal-recessive genetic disorder characterized by oculocutaneous albinism, platelet dysfunction, and accumulation of ceroid-lipofuscin in lysosomes of cells of multiple organs and reticuloendothelial system.
- Clinical findings include oculocutaneous albinism with skin and hair hypopigmentation. Later in life, patients manifest with hemorrhagic diathesis, epistaxis, melena, and easy bruising.
- Pulmonary fibrosis develops in 50 to 70% of affected patients, usually late in life.
- Nine types of the syndrome have been described, most of which are associated with mutation in the *HPS* gene, located in the long arm of chromosome 10. Type 1 is the most common and is more severe, with a strong association with pulmonary disease.
- The clinical manifestations of HPS are related to several defects in protein trafficking resulting in dysfunction of lysosome-related organelles, including melanosomes (oculocutaneous albinism), platelet-dense granules (bleeding disorder), and lamellar bodies of type II alveolar cells (pulmonary fibrosis).
- In the lungs, HPS is characterized by diffuse extensive fibrosis of the interalveolar septa and peribronchial stroma, likely secondary to the accumulation of ceroid-lipofuscin in alveolar macrophages. Abnormal accumulation of surfactant has also been reported.

- Usual interstitial pneumonia, like interstitial pneumonia with advanced pulmonary fibrosis and honeycombing, occurs in the advanced stage of the disease. Type II pneumocytes display characteristic foamy swelling and degeneration with desquamation into alveolar space.
- There is no effective available treatment for pulmonary fibrosis due to HPS. The only definitive treatment for pulmonary fibrosis is lung transplantation, which has been performed in several cases.

■ Other Imaging Findings

- Imaging manifestations consist of diffuse interstitial lung disease, with predominant peripheral distribution, which may affect the upper, middle, or lower lung zones.
- In the early stages, there is interlobular septal thickening, reticulation, perihilar fibrosis, and patchy ground-glass opacities.
- In older patients with more advanced disease, imaging manifestation of advanced fibrosis with traction bronchiectasis, honeycombing, and subpleural cysts is common.

✓ Pearls and ✗ Pitfalls

- ✓ In North America, most patients with HPS are from Puerto Rico, but sporadic cases have been reported in other countries, affecting both females and males and all races and ethnicities.
- ✗ Clinical correlation is essential for the diagnosis, because the imaging manifestations are nonspecific and are similar to those of several diffuse/interstitial diseases of the lung.

Case 58

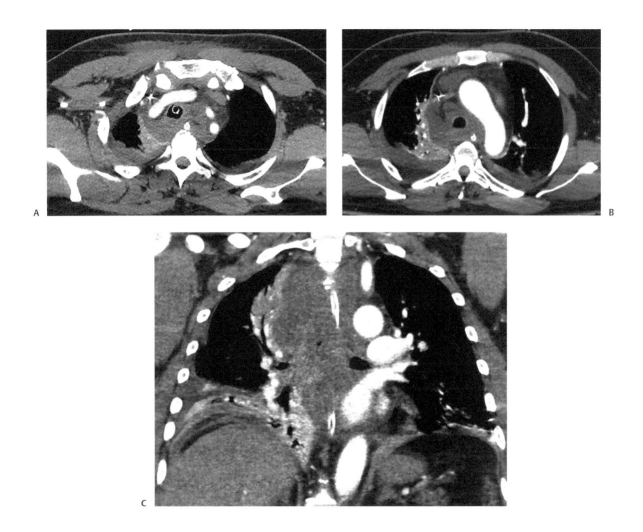

■ Clinical Presentation

A 42-year-old man with severe odynophagia, and right peritonsillar abscess on a CT of the neck. Two days later, the patient develops severe chest pain and shortness of breath.

■ Imaging Findings

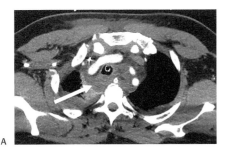 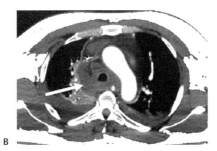 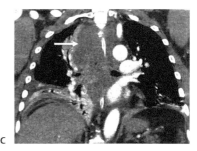

(A–C) Contrast-enhanced CT images. Axial image at the level of the thoracic inlet **(A)**, axial image at the level of the aortic arch **(B)**, and coronal reconstruction though the middle mediastinum **(C)** demonstrate a very large mediastinal fluid collection in the middle mediastinum (*arrows*) associated with bilateral pleural effusions and bibasilar atelectasis.

■ Differential Diagnosis

- ***Descending necrotizing mediastinitis.***
- *Mediastinal hematoma.*
- *Mediastinal lymphangioma.*

■ Essential Facts

- Descending necrotizing mediastinitis (DNM) is a rare acute polymicrobial infection of the mediastinum, caused by direct spread of head and neck infections. It is a lethal condition carrying a high mortality of ~30 to 50%.
- Early diagnosis plays a crucial role in the management of this life-threatening condition. CT is the imaging modality of choice, first to identify the source of infection in head and neck and then to establish the contiguity of this infectious process to the mediastinum.
- There are three pathways for head and neck infection to extend to the mediastinum: from the pretracheal space to the anterior mediastinum, through the lateral pharyngeal space to the middle mediastinum, and the most common route through the retropharyngeal and "danger space" to the posterior mediastinum.
- The sources of infection include odontogenic, oropharyngeal epiglottitis, cervical lymphadenitis, parotitis, thyroiditis, and jugular intravenous drug abuse.
- Several hypotheses for the pathophysiology of DNM have been proposed. Suggested mechanism of downward spread of neck infection include the effect of gravity,

the negative intrathoracic pressure, the relatively poor vascularity of these anatomic spaces with tissue hypoxia, and paucity of cellular immune response.
- Type 1 mediastinal infection (localized above the carina) is generally treated medically with antibiotics, whereas type 2A infection (lower anterior mediastinum) and type 2B mediastinal infection (anterior and posterior mediastinum) require more aggressive treatment with a surgical approach.

■ Other Imaging Findings

- Other imaging findings in acute mediastinitis include mediastinal widening, mediastinal gas bubbles, focal fluid collections, mediastinal fat stranding, and increased attenuation, with enlarged lymph nodes occasionally associated with pleural effusion/empyema.

✓ Pearls and ✗ Pitfalls

- ✓ Increased attenuation of the mediastinal fat on CT imaging is the most sensitive imaging sign of acute mediastinitis (> 90% sensitivity).
- ✗ Mediastinal fluid collection on CT imaging is only seen in ~50% of patients with acute mediastinitis.

Case 59

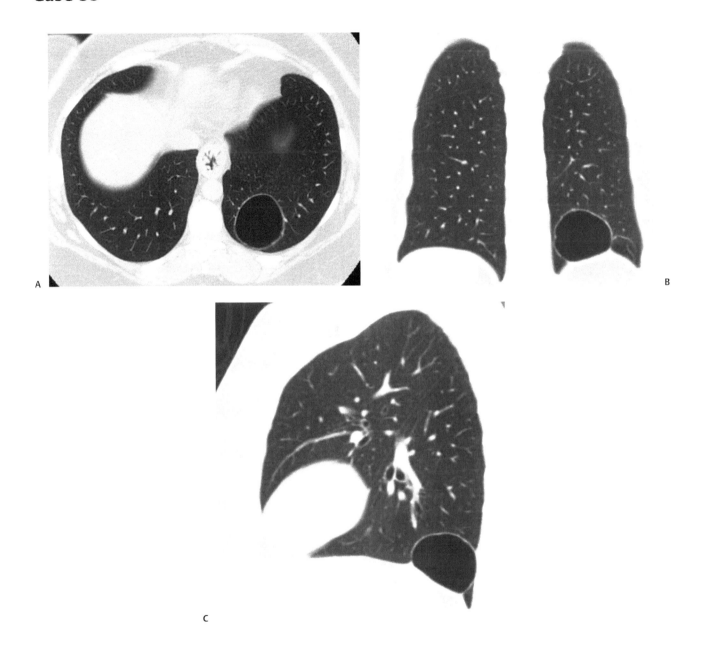

A

B

C

■ Clinical Presentation

A 35-year-old woman with past medical history of pneumonia; follow-up CT image.

■ Imaging Findings

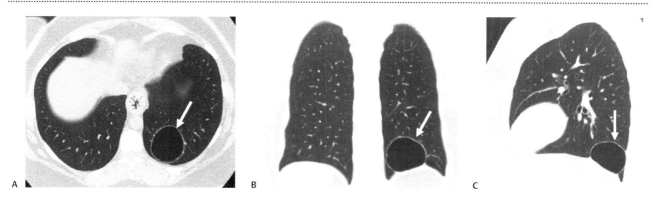

(A–C) Noncontrast CT images of the chest: axial **(A)**, coronal **(B)**, and sagittal **(C)** images. A thin-walled, relatively large air-containing cyst is identified in the inferior aspect of the left lower lobe (*arrows*). No septation, mural nodule, or soft tissue component is appreciated in this unilocular lesion.

■ Differential Diagnosis

- ***Pneumatocele.***
- *Lung abscess.*
- *Pulmonary sequestration.*
- *Congenital cystic adenomatoid malformation.*
- *Malignancy.*

■ Essential Facts

- Pneumatocele is defined as a thin-walled, air-filled cyst in the lung parenchyma, which most often results from previous pulmonary infection or trauma. Other less common causes include mechanical ventilation (positive pressure) and hydrocarbon ingestion.
- The most common infectious agent associated with pneumatocele formation is *Staphylococcus aureus*, followed by *Streptococcus* and *Haemophilus influenzae*. Tuberculosis and *Escherichia coli* pulmonary infection have also been reported.
- Posttraumatic pneumatoceles, which are commonly described as traumatic pulmonary pseudocysts, are usually surrounded by an area of pulmonary hemorrhage or contusion, and they can result from penetrating and nonpenetrating trauma.
- Postinfectious pneumatoceles occur in as much as 8% of pneumonias in children typically under 3 years of age. Tend to be transient and may entirely resolve in about 6 weeks.

- Exact mechanism for the formation of postinfectious pneumatocele is not entirely clear, but the two most likely mechanisms include bronchial obstruction with ball-valve mechanism, tissue necrosis, or a combination.
- Pneumatoceles are usually asymptomatic, tend to resolve spontaneously, and do not require invasive procedures or surgical intervention.

■ Other Imaging Findings

- On both radiographs and CT images, pneumatocele appears as a round, thin-walled, air-filled unilocular lesion without significant tissue on its wall.

✓ Pearls and ✗ Pitfalls

✓ Posttraumatic pneumatoceles, which are commonly described as traumatic pulmonary pseudocysts, are usually surrounded by an area of pulmonary hemorrhage or contusion, and can result from penetrating and nonpenetrating trauma.

✗ Posttraumatic pneumatoceles occur after blunt chest trauma in 1 to 8% of cases and can be single or multiple.

Case 60

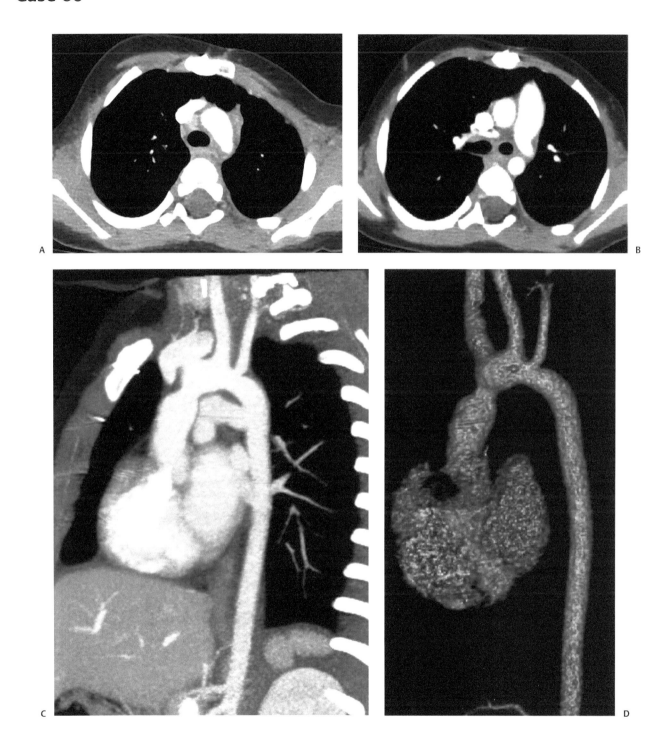

Clinical Presentation

An 11-month-old boy with past medical history of surgical repair of congenital heart disease (interrupted aortic arch, atrial septal defect, and ventricular septal defect), cleft palate, respiratory symptoms, and mouth, arm, and hand spasms.

■ Imaging Findings

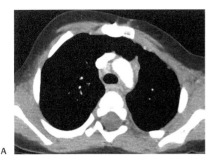 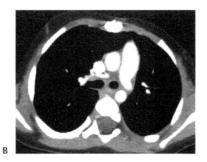 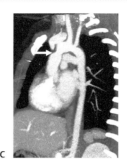 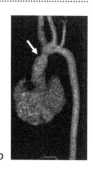

A   B   C   D

(A–D) Contrast-enhanced CT images: axial image at the level of the aortic arch **(A)**, axial image at the level of the pulmonary artery **(B)**, sagittal oblique reconstruction **(C)**, and volume rendered three-dimensional reconstruction **(D)**. These CT images show the absence of thymic tissue in the anterior mediastinum as well as mild residual narrowing of the proximal aortic arch (*arrows*).

■ Differential Diagnosis

- *DiGeorge syndrome.*

■ Essential Facts

- DiGeorge syndrome, also called 22q11.2 deletion syndrome, is a common genetic disorder caused by a defect in chromosome 22. It results in the poor development of several organs and systems and is currently considered to be the most common microdeletion syndrome. Inheritance pattern is autosomal dominant.
- Medical problems commonly associated with DiGeorge syndrome include congenital heart disease (conotruncal malformations including interrupted aortic arch, tetralogy of Fallot, truncus arteriosus), T-cell–mediated immunodeficiency with absent or hypoplastic thymus, a cleft palate, hypocalcemia/hypoparathyroidism, learning difficulties, and delayed development with behavioral and emotional problems.
- Before the discovery of the chromosome 22 defect, the disorder was known by several names: DiGeorge syndrome, velocardiofacial (velo-cardio-facial) syndrome, Shprintzen syndrome, CATCH22 (**C**ardiac abnormalities, **A**bnormal facies, **T**hymic aplasia, **C**left palate, **H**ypocalcemia/**H**ypothyroidism), and others. The term *22q11.2 deletion syndrome* is preferred today and is generally considered a more accurate description of the underlying abnormality.
- 22q11.2 deletion syndrome is present in 7% of patients with complex congenital heart disease and in > 30% of those with conotruncal abnormalities (50% of interrupted aortic arch, 34% of truncus arteriosus, 16% of tetralogy of Fallot).

- After surgical correction for their congenital heart disease, patients with 22q11.2 deletion syndrome experience more significant heart and respiratory failure, pneumonia, sepsis, hypocalcemia, and postintubation laryngeal stridor and require prolonged mechanical ventilation and longer postoperative hospitalization.
- No specific treatment or cure is available. Cardiac surgery is performed according to the underlying congenital heart disease as well as surgical correction of cleft palate when present. Additional therapies include pharmacologic intervention for hypoparathyroidism, and thymic transplant in case of severe thymus dysfunction.

■ Other Imaging Findings

- Involution of the thymus may occur in response to intrauterine stress. However, depleted thymic tissue in the larger term neonate should raise the question of an immunodeficiency syndrome. In a patient with known congenital heart disease, and in particular those patients with conotruncal anomalies, a small or absent thymic silhouette on chest radiograph suggests 22q11.2 deletion syndrome.

✓ Pearls and ✗ Pitfalls

- ✓ Absent or hypoplastic fetal thymus on prenatal ultrasound allows identification of a group at high risk for chromosome 22q11.2 deletion syndrome, particularly when in association with prenatal diagnosis of congenital heart disease.
- ✗ Premature infants normally have little thymic tissue visible on early chest radiographs.

Case 61

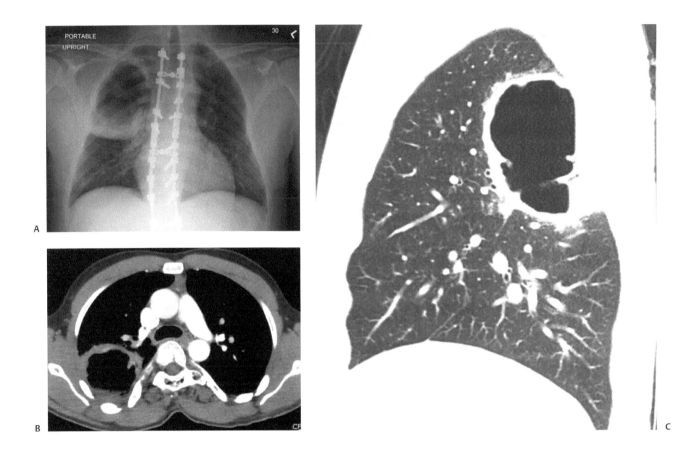

■ Clinical Presentation

Cough and fever in a 24-year-old man with past medical history of scoliosis and recurrent cutaneous abscesses and pulmonary infections.

■ Imaging Findings

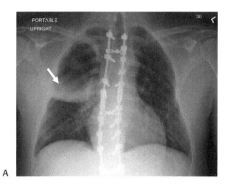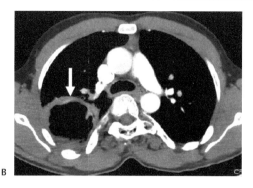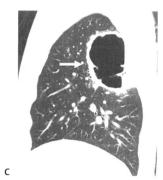

(A) Anteroposterior chest radiograph. A large cavitary lesion is noted in the right upper lobe (*arrow*). Postoperative changes from previous spinal instrumentation is also identified along the thoracic spine. **(B)** Contrast-enhanced CT axial image through the upper thoracic region confirms a thick-walled cavity with an intraluminal air-fluid level in the right upper lobe (*arrow*). **(C)** Sagittal reconstruction through the right lung shows the intrapulmonary abscess in the posterior aspect of the upper lobe (*arrow*).

■ Differential Diagnosis

- ***Hyperimmunoglobulin E syndrome (Job syndrome).***
- *Common variable immune deficiency.*
- *Severe combined immunodeficiency.*
- *Chronic granulomatous disease.*
- *AIDS.*

■ Essential Facts

- The hyperimmunoglobulin E syndrome (HIES) was first described in patients with severe chronic dermatitis, furunculosis, and multiple skin abscesses, which the authors perceived to be similar to the diseases attributed to the biblical prophet Job, and hence designated it Job syndrome.
- The clinical triad of symptoms found in the majority of patients (> 75%) include recurrent staphylococcal abscesses, recurrent airway infection, and increased serologic levels of immunoglobulin E (IgE).
- HIES is a complex immune deficiency that affects several body organs/systems, particularly the immune system, with particular susceptibility to staphylococcal and mycotic infections.
- HIES is a condition with a heterogeneous genetic mechanism.
- The autosomal-dominant form is associated with facial, dental, skeletal, and connective tissue abnormalities in addition to the immune deficiency.
- The autosomal-recessive form is not associated with facial, dental, or skeletal abnormalities, but affected patients suffer recurrent otitis media, mastoiditis, sinusitis, pneumonias, and sepsis and have increased risk for malignancy as well as aortic and cerebral aneurysms.

- Affected individuals present with recurrent pneumonias; formation of pneumatoceles; eczema and skin infection with multiple abscesses; and musculoskeletal abnormalities including scoliosis, osteopenia, and increased risk for bone fracture.
- Males and females are affected with the same frequency.
- Elevated IgE level is a cardinal feature of this condition.
- Eosinophilia is an additional common serologic abnormality.
- Most patients with HIES are treated with long-term antibiotic therapy to prevent staphylococcal infections.

■ Other Imaging Findings

- Common pulmonary imaging presentation of HIES includes alveolar air-space disease and consolidation, pneumatoceles, and occasionally spontaneous pneumothorax when subpleural pneumatoceles rupture into the pleural space.

✓ Pearls and ✗ Pitfalls

✓ The combination of recurrent cutaneous and sinopulmonary infection that begins in infancy with frequent development of pneumatoceles following pneumonia, despite adequate therapy, suggests HIES.

✗ Staphylococcal pulmonary infection not associated with HIES are more common cause of pneumatocele formation.

Case 62

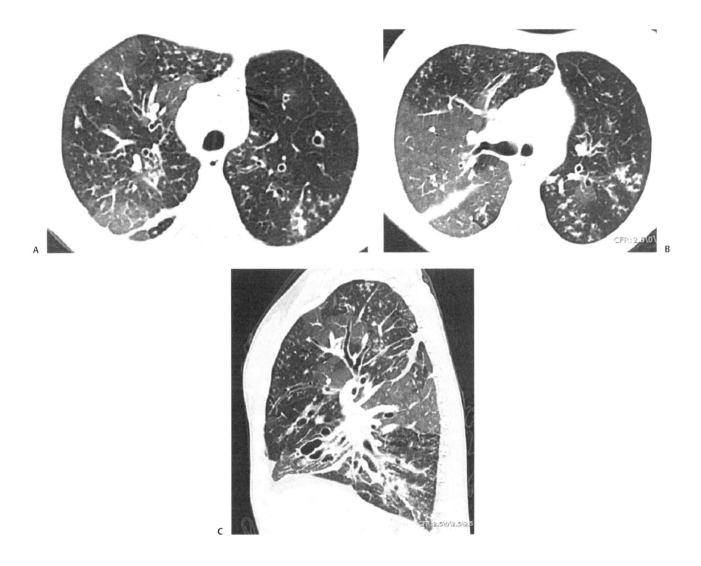

■ Clinical Presentation

A 17-year-old girl with history of chronic cough and recurrent otitis, sinusitis, and pulmonary infections.

■ Imaging Findings

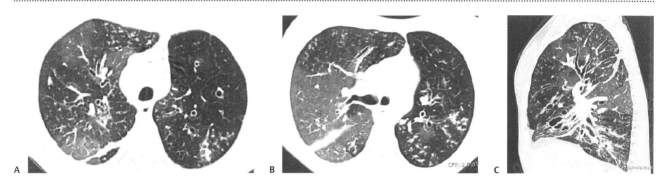

(A–C) Contrast-enhanced CT images of the chest with lung windows. (A) Axial image above the aortic arch. (B) Axial image through the carina. (C) Sagittal reconstruction image. Extensive abnormalities are noted throughout the bilateral lungs; ground-glass opacities in a patchy distribution alternating with areas of air trapping produce a pattern of mosaic attenuation. In addition, tree-in-bud nodularity and cylindrical bronchiectasis are identified.

■ Differential Diagnosis

- **Common variable immune deficiency.**
- *Cystic fibrosis.*
- *Primary ciliary dyskinesia.*
- *Allergic bronchopulmonary aspergillosis.*
- *Sarcoidosis.*

■ Essential Facts

- Common variable immune deficiency (or common variable immunodeficiency [CVID]) is a disorder that involves a combination of low serum levels of most or all immunoglobulins (immunoglobulin [Ig] G, IgA, and/or IgM) and antibodies, abnormal B and T lymphocytes, and lack of plasma cells in bone marrow that are capable of producing antibodies, which results in increased susceptibility to the development of recurrent bacterial infection.
- CVID is one of the most common primary immunodeficiencies in adults. CVID should not be diagnosed in children younger than age 4, because physiologic immaturity of the immune system can mimic the clinical manifestations of CVID.
- Males and females are affected, and the diagnosis is not made in the majority of cases until the 3rd or 4th decade of life.
- Most commonly affected organs are the lungs and bronchi, sinuses, and ears.
- Recurrent pulmonary infections commonly produce permanent damage to the airways with formation of bronchiectasis and bronchiolectasis.
- Association with autoimmune disorders such as autoimmune thrombocytopenic purpura, autoimmune hemolytic anemia, autoimmune neutropenia, and pernicious anemia is common (25–50%).

- Affected individuals also have increased risk for malignancy, in particular non-Hodgkin lymphoma and gastric carcinoma.
- Treatments include immunoglobulin replacement therapy and long-term broad-spectrum antibiotic use.
- Patients with bronchiectasis may need daily respiratory therapy to mobilize bronchopulmonary secretions.

■ Other Imaging Findings

- Other imaging findings in CVID include air trapping, bronchial wall thickening, bronchiectasis (50–65%), emphysema, ground-glass opacities (37%), air-space consolidation, pulmonary nodules that are typically multiple (38–67%), and mediastinal lymphadenopathy.
- Pulmonary function test is a weak predictor of chronic pulmonary abnormalities in patients with CVID. Repetitive (biannual) CT seems to better monitor the progression of structural airway disease (bronchial wall thickening, bronchiectasis, and air trapping) and interstitial lung disease in these patients.
- Splenomegaly is also a common finding (70%).

✓ Pearls and ✗ Pitfalls

- ✓ Lymphadenopathy, usually cervical, mediastinal, and abdominal, is a common finding in CVID.
- ✗ Lymphoid tissue may contain sarcoidlike changes, with noncaseating granulomas that are very similar to those seen in sarcoidosis, in up to 20% of patients.

Case 63

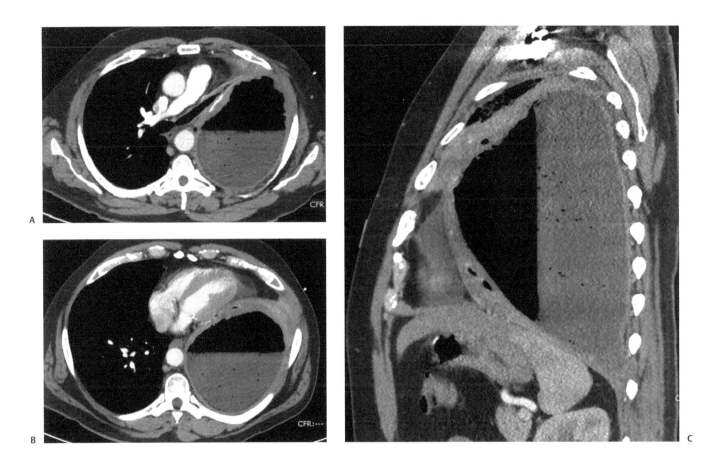

■ Clinical Presentation

....

A 49-year-old man with fever, cough, and left-sided chest pain.

■ **Imaging Findings**

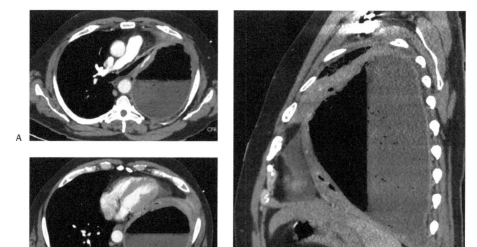

(A–C) Contrast-enhanced CT images: axial image at the level of the pulmonary artery **(A)**; axial image above the diaphragm **(B)**; and left sagittal reconstruction image **(C)**. CT images reveal a large air-fluid level in the left hemithorax with collapsed lung parenchyma seen anteriorly, consistent with a large hydropneumothorax.

■ **Differential Diagnosis**

- ***Empyema with bronchopleural fistula.***
- *Empyema from a gas-forming organism.*
- *Lung abscess.*
- *Empyema necessitans.*

■ **Essential Facts**

- Bronchopleural fistula (BPF) consists of an abnormal sinus tract and communication between a bronchus and the pleural space, which can result from a necrotizing pneumonia and empyema, tuberculosis, lung neoplasm, surgery, mechanical ventilation, trauma, or radiation therapy.
- Regardless of the underlying disease, BPF is a serious complication with increased morbidity and mortality, requiring prolonged hospital stay, operative or interventional approach, and increased health care cost.
- BPF is a relatively common complication after lung resection surgery; there is higher incidence after pneumonectomy (5–20%) than after lobectomy (0.5%).
- In a patient with pneumonia the presence of an air-fluid level on chest radiograph or CT image suggests either the formation of a lung abscess or of an empyema with BPF.
- A lung abscess, due to its spherical shape, typically presents a similar anteroposterior and transverse diameter. Conversely, in an empyema with BPF, which has an elongated or lenticular nonspherical shape, there is a disparity in these two diameters.
- Treatment of BPF includes various surgical and medical procedures as well as the use of bronchoscopy and endobronchial therapy with different glues, coils,

and sealants. In BPF secondary to infection, pleural space drainage tubes and appropriate use of antibiotics are also critical.

■ **Other Imaging Findings**

- Imaging findings that suggest BPF include a progressively enlarging pneumothorax, development of a new air-fluid level in a patient with preexisting pleural fluid collection, and development of a tension pneumothorax.
- In the case of an empyema with BPF, the intrathoracic air-fluid level characteristically extends to the chest wall. In some cases, CT image may directly demonstrate the lung or airway sinus tract and the pleural space.

✓ **Pearls and ✗ Pitfalls**

✓ In the presence of a hydropneumothorax, careful evaluation of the lung parenchyma for the detection of a sinus tract between the airways or lung parenchyma and the pleural cavity is essential for the diagnosis of BPF.

✗ The presence of intrapleural air or air-fluid level in a preexisting pleural fluid collection suggests recent clinical instrumentation (e.g., thoracentesis), complicating BPF, and/or rarely, infection from gas-forming organisms.

✗ Intrapleural gas secondary to infection from a gas-forming organism (e.g., anaerobic bacteria) typically presents as multiple small gas bubbles. In the absence of previous instrumentation, a large amount of intrapleural air in a patient with pneumonia or empyema suggests BPF.

Case 64

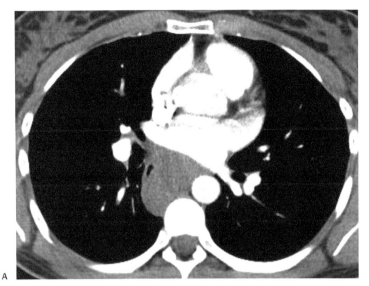

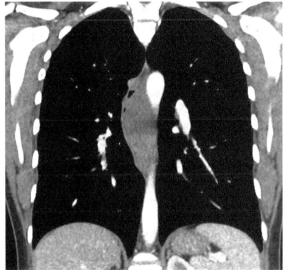

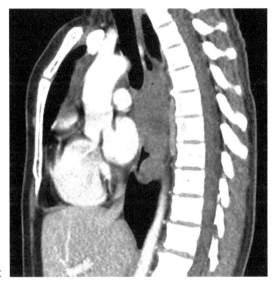

■ Clinical Presentation

A 50-year-old woman with dysphagia.

■ **Imaging Findings**

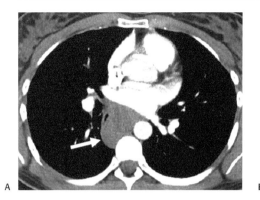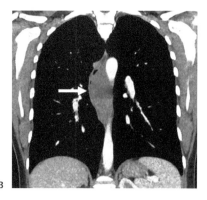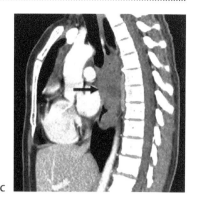

(A–C) Contrast-enhanced CT of the chest: axial image **(A)**; coronal reconstruction image **(B)**; and sagittal reconstruction image **(C)**. All CT images demonstrate an elongated large soft tissue density mediastinal mass in the retrocardiac region (*arrows*) with right lateral displacement of the esophageal lumen with no obvious invasion of adjacent structures.

■ **Differential Diagnosis**

- ***Gastrointestinal stromal tumor of the esophagus.***
- *Leiomyoma/leiomyosarcoma of the esophagus.*
- *Esophageal cancer.*
- *Foregut duplication cyst.*

■ **Essential Facts**

- Gastrointestinal stromal tumors (GISTs) are the most common mesenchymal neoplasms of the gastrointestinal tract but represent < 1% of all gastrointestinal tumors. About 25% of mesenchymal esophageal tumors are GISTs, of which 90% are localized in the distal esophagus.
- GISTs are usually found in the stomach or small intestine but can occur anywhere along the gastrointestinal tract. GISTs differentiate from the interstitial cell of Cajal (gut pacemaker cells) found in the muscularis propria and around the myenteric plexus.
- The majority of these tumors are located in the stomach (70%) and the small intestine (25%), whereas GISTs of the colorectum (4%) and esophagus (1%) are less common.
- With average size about 8 cm at the time of diagnosis, esophageal GISTs tend to be larger than their counterparts in the stomach and small bowel, and they also tend to have a higher mitotic rate and hence worse prognosis.
- In comparison to gastric GIST, esophageal GIST occurs more frequently in men as well as in patients younger than 60 at diagnosis. GISTs have been reported in all age groups including infants, but it is most common in patients older than 40 years and is extremely rare in patients younger than 30 years.
- Approximately 4500 new cases of GIST are diagnosed annually in the United States.
- Dysphagia is the most common clinical manifestation (50%), followed by weight loss (20%) and bleeding (10%). Roughly one quarter (25%) represent an incidental finding in asymptomatic individuals.

- Complete surgical resection of the tumor is the only curative therapeutic option in the management of nonmetastatic, resectable esophageal GIST neoplasms.

■ **Other Imaging Findings**

- On barium study, GISTs are smooth submucosal lesions, which most frequently grow endophytically parallel to the lumen of the esophagus.
- Esophageal GISTs appear on CT images as well-marginated lesions predominantly in the distal esophagus, isoattenuating to muscle after contrast injection.
- All esophageal GISTs show marked metabolic activity and avid uptake on positron emission tomography scans.

✓ **Pearls and ✗ Pitfalls**

✓ A small minority of GISTs are associated with hereditary syndromes such as neurofibromatosis type 1 and the Carney triad (epithelioid gastric stromal tumors, pulmonary chondromas, and extra-adrenal paragangliomas), observed predominantly in young women, and considered to be a specific form of multiple endocrine neoplasia.

✗ In the past, such lesions were classified as leiomyomas or leiomyosarcomas because they possessed smooth muscle features when examined under light microscopy, but electron microscopy studies found little evidence of the smooth muscle origin of these tumors. Immunohistochemistry analysis shows that these tumors do not have immunophenotypic features of smooth muscle cells but rather express antigens related to neural crest cells.

Case 65

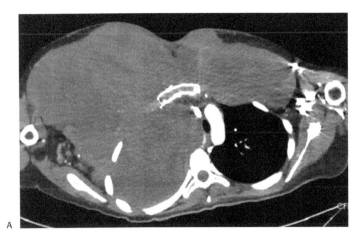

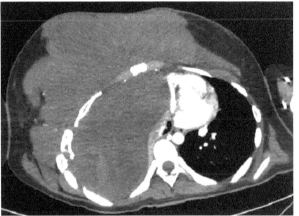

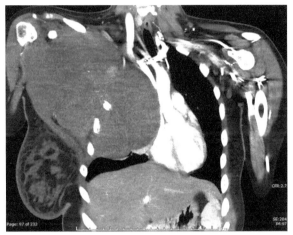

■ **Clinical Presentation**

A 19-year-old woman with past medical history of multiple bone osteomas and colonic polyposis presenting with a large right-sided chest wall mass.

■ Imaging Findings

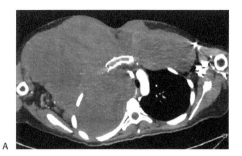 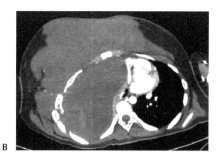 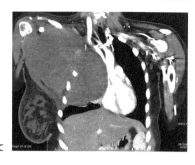

A   B   C

(A–C) Contrast-enhanced CT images. **(A)** Axial image at the level of the aortic arch. **(B)** Axial image at the level of the right atrium. **(C)** Coronal reconstruction image. CT images show a very large infiltrative, slightly heterogeneous in density, enhancing soft tissue mass involving the anterior chest wall with a very large intrathoracic component and significant mass effect on the right lung and mediastinum.

■ Differential Diagnosis

- ***Desmoid tumor.***
- *Fibrosarcoma.*
- *Rhabdomyosarcoma.*
- *Lymphoma.*

■ Essential Facts

- Desmoid tumors (also known as aggressive fibromatosis) are fibrous neoplasms originating from the myofibroblast, the mesenchymal stem cells of fascial or musculoaponeurotic structures. Despite their benign histologic appearance with no significant mitotic activity and extremely rare metastatic potential, they tend to be locally aggressive and produce large exuberant masses with local invasion.
- Most cases are sporadic, but there is a clear association with familial adenomatoid polyposis (FAP), an autosomal inherited condition. Overall, desmoid tumors are rare in the general population (0.03% of all tumors), but the incidence is much higher in patients with colorectal FAP. Approximately 10 to 15% of patients with FAP develop desmoid tumor.
- Gardner syndrome is characterized by FAP, colon cancer, gastric polyps, soft tissue tumors (fibromas, desmoid tumors), epidermoid cysts of the skin, dental and retinal abnormalities, and bone tumors (osteomas). Several other tumors known to be associated with Gardner syndrome include small bowel carcinoma, pancreatic cancer, papillary thyroid carcinoma, hepatoblastoma, adrenal gland carcinoma, cholangiocarcinoma, and medulloblastoma.
- The sporadic form may affect both men and women, but desmoid tumor associated with FAP most commonly occurs in young women.
- Desmoid tumors may arise from any muscle, but the most common location is in the rectus abdominis muscle of the abdominal wall. Chest wall desmoids account for about 20 to 40% of desmoid tumors.

- Desmoid tumors are classified as abdominal wall, extra-abdominal, and intra-abdominal.
- When possible, complete surgical resection is the treatment of choice. Given the often large size at the time of presentation, complete resection is commonly challenging and requires chest wall reconstruction with prosthetic material.
- Neither adjuvant radiation therapy nor chemotherapy has been shown to reduce the rate of local recurrence.

■ Other Imaging Findings

- Desmoid tumors present as large, homogeneous, not significantly enhancing soft tissue density masses on CT images, similar to normal muscle. Similarly, on MR images, the signal intensity of these tumors follows that of normal muscle on T1-weighted images but presents high signal intensity on T2-weighted sequences.
- On fluorodeoxyglucose–positron emission tomography, desmoid tumors exhibit only mild metabolic activity.

✓ Pearls and ✕ Pitfalls

- ✓ Local desmoid tumor recurrence after surgery is very high (70%), even after complete resection, and is particularly high in patients with positive surgical margins.
- ✕ Gardner syndrome and FAP were considered separate entities until the identification of the *APC* (adenomatous polyposis coli) gene, which is a tumor suppressor gene. Mutations in this gene are currently recognized as responsible for both conditions. Currently, Gardner syndrome is considered a subtype of FAP.

Case 66

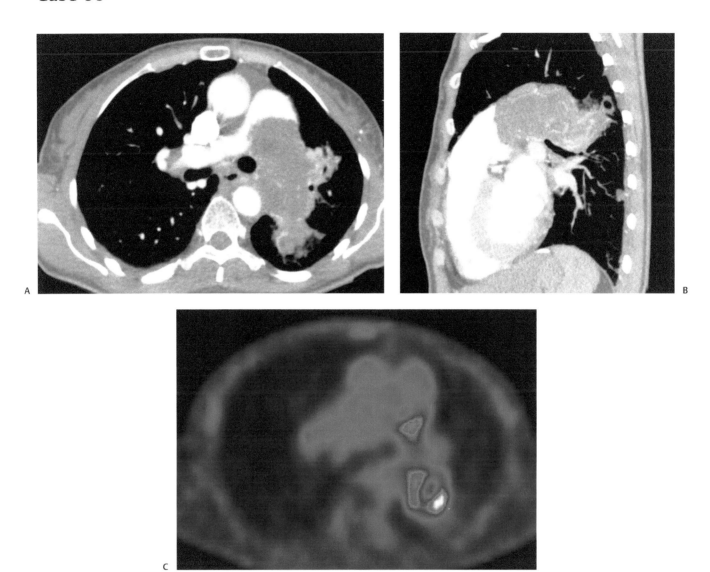

■ Clinical Presentation

A 67-year-old female patient with chest pain and exertional dyspnea.

■ Imaging Findings

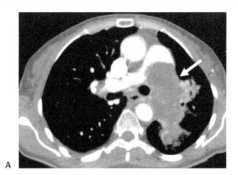
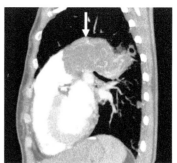
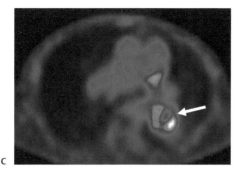

(A, B) Contrast-enhanced CT images. (A) Axial image at the level of the pulmonary artery. (B) Sagittal reconstruction image depicting a large soft tissue density mass (*arrows*) expanding the pulmonary trunk and left pulmonary artery with internal neovascularity and complete luminal obstruction. (C) Positron emission tomography–CT reveals increased uptake and metabolic activity with the mass.

■ Differential Diagnosis

- ***Pulmonary artery sarcoma.***
- *Pulmonary artery thrombus.*
- *Lung cancer.*
- *Lymphoma.*

■ Essential Facts

- Primary pulmonary artery sarcomas are rare, aggressive tumors with poor prognosis.
- Median overall survival after diagnosis is < 2 years, and in many cases is just a few weeks or months.
- Pulmonary artery sarcomas arise from the vascular endothelium from pluripotent intimal cells and can present with bilateral pulmonary artery involvement.
- Typically, these are poorly differentiated malignant mesenchymal tumors with fibroblastic or myofibroblastic differentiation.
- Some cases demonstrate distinct histologic features that allow subclassification as rhabdomyosarcoma, leiomyosarcoma, angiosarcoma, malignant fibrous histiocytoma, osteogenic sarcoma, and so forth.
- Mean age at diagnosis is 50 years, with no gender predilection.
- Symptoms almost always include dyspnea, hemoptysis, and chest pain, and in some cases pulmonary hypertension, mimicking pulmonary embolism. Some patients also report systemic symptoms like weight loss and fever.

- When possible, surgical radical resection is the preferred treatment option. Tumors respond to chemotherapy alone; response to radiation therapy is often poor.

■ Other Imaging Findings

- Most common imaging finding is an area that is variable in size and of low density within the pulmonary vasculature. The affected vessel may appear enlarged, reflecting the expansile nature of the lesion. The tumoral lesion may present with areas of internal calcification. Contrast enhancement of the tumor may be appreciated.
- Increased metabolic activity on fluorodeoxyglucose–positron emission tomography in case of pulmonary artery sarcoma is helpful in differentiating the endovascular tumoral mass from pulmonary thromboembolism.

✓ Pearls and ✗ Pitfalls

- ✓ A pulmonary artery endovascular mass that continues growing despite anticoagulation therapy should rise the possibility of pulmonary artery sarcoma.
- ✗ Most common initial misdiagnosis of pulmonary artery sarcoma is with pulmonary embolism. When the tumoral mass extends to the lung and mediastinum, they can also be confused with lung cancer, mediastinal tumors, and fibrosing mediastinitis.

Case 67

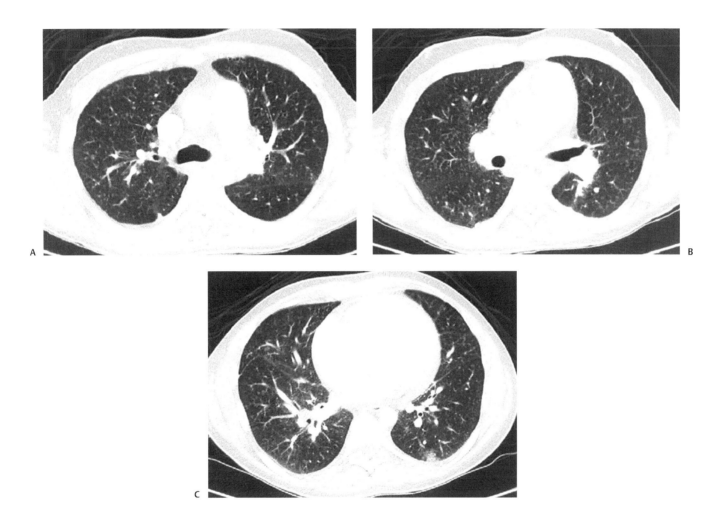

■ Clinical Presentation

A 38-year-old man with pulmonary hypertension and worsening shortness of breath.

■ **Imaging Findings**

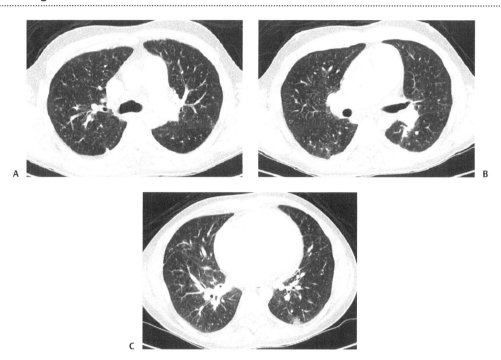

(**A–C**) Contrast-enhanced CT images of the chest. Axial images at the level of the left pulmonary artery (**A**), right pulmonary artery (**B**), and right atrium (**C**) demonstrate abnormal dilation of the central pulmonary arteries, right atrial and right ventricular enlargement, and innumerable small pulmonary nodules with interlobular septal thickening.

■ **Differential Diagnosis**

- ***Pulmonary capillary hemangiomatosis.***
- *Pulmonary veno-occlusive disease.*
- *Interstitial pulmonary edema.*
- *Lymphangitic carcinomatosis.*

■ **Essential Facts**

- Pulmonary capillary hemangiomatosis (PCH) is an uncommon cause of pulmonary hypertension characterized by extensive abnormal proliferation of pulmonary capillaries within alveolar septae.
- The pathologic hallmark of PCH is abnormal proliferation of thin-walled capillaries at least two layers thick, with infiltration and expansion of interlobular septae, centered around bronchovascular bundles with extension to the wall of small pulmonary arteries, veins, and bronchi. The proliferative process may even extend to the pleura, pericardium, and mediastinal lymph nodes.
- Men and women of all ages can be equally affected, but the most common presentation age is between 20 and 40 years.
- The most common clinical manifestations include progressive dyspnea, cough, and chest pain. Arterial blood gases demonstrate arterial hypoxemia.
- Hemodynamic examination demonstrates normal or even low pulmonary capillary wedge pressure, with increased mean pulmonary artery pressure.

- In the most common classification system of pulmonary hypertension (Dana Point, 2008), PCH and pulmonary veno-occlusive disease (PVOD) were put together in their own category.
- Prognosis is poor, with 3- to 5-year survival after symptom onset.
- Lung transplantation is the preferred treatment option because no effective pharmacologic therapy exists.

■ **Other Imaging Findings**

- In addition to the imaging signs of arterial pulmonary hypertension, PCH manifests with diffuse centrilobular ground-glass nodules in the bilateral lungs as well as interlobular septal thickening.
- Hilar and mediastinal lymphadenopathy and pleural effusion may also be present.

✓ **Pearls and ✗ Pitfalls**

- ✓ The definitive diagnosis of PCH and PVOD requires histopathologic evaluation of lung tissue.
- ✗ PCH is closely related with PVOD, with striking clinical, hemodynamic, radiologic, genetic, and histopathologic overlap. Recently, a common genetic mutation (*EIF2AK4*) has been described in both entities, raising the question of whether they actually represent different diseases or are merely variations of the same condition.

Case 68

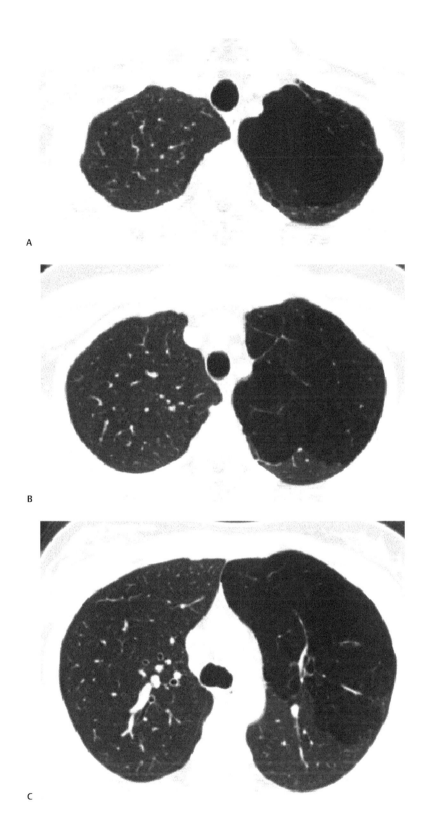

A

B

C

■ Clinical Presentation

A 30-year-old woman with chronic cough and shortness of breath.

■ Imaging Findings

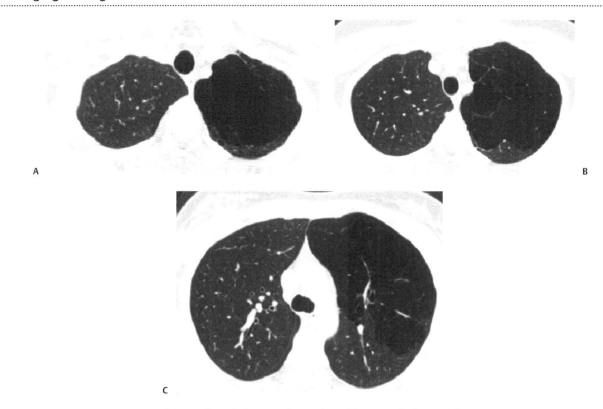

(A–C) Noncontrast chest CT images. Axial images through the upper lung at three different levels show significant reduction in lung parenchyma and vascularity in the left upper lobe with formation of large thin-walled blebs.

■ Differential Diagnosis

- ***Congenital lobar emphysema.***
- *Swyer–James syndrome.*
- *Congenital interruption of a pulmonary artery.*
- *α_1-Antitrypsin deficiency.*
- *Centrilobular emphysema.*

■ Essential Facts

- Congenital lobar emphysema (CLE), or congenital lobar overinflation, is characterized by pulmonary lobar overinflation with compression of the adjacent normal lung tissue. Airway obstruction is believed to be the cause, but actual obstruction is only demonstrated in 25% of the cases.
- CLE commonly manifests early in life with progressive dyspnea and tachypnea. In > 95% of cases, the disease manifests in the first 6 months of life, with only few rare cases diagnosed in adults. The left upper lobe is more commonly affected (50%), followed by the right middle lobe (35%).
- The disease is more commonly seen in males than in females (3:1 ratio).
- CLE typically has a unilateral distribution with involvement of one single lobe.

- Surgical resection is recommended in patients with respiratory symptoms or recurrent infection; conservative management is recommended for asymptomatic cases.

■ Other Imaging Findings

- The most significant imaging finding of CLE is single lobe overinflation and air trapping, with diminished vascularity and compression of the surrounding lung parenchyma.
- Displacement of the mediastinum and ipsilateral diaphragm may be observed.

✓ Pearls and ✗ Pitfalls

- ✓ Association between CLE and congenital heart disease is reported in 15% of cases, including left-to-right shunts (atrial septal defect, ventricular septal defect), tetralogy of Fallot, right-sided aortic arch, and patent ductus arteriosus.
- ✗ Ventilation perfusion scan will demonstrate minimal or no perfusion in the affected lobe.

Case 69

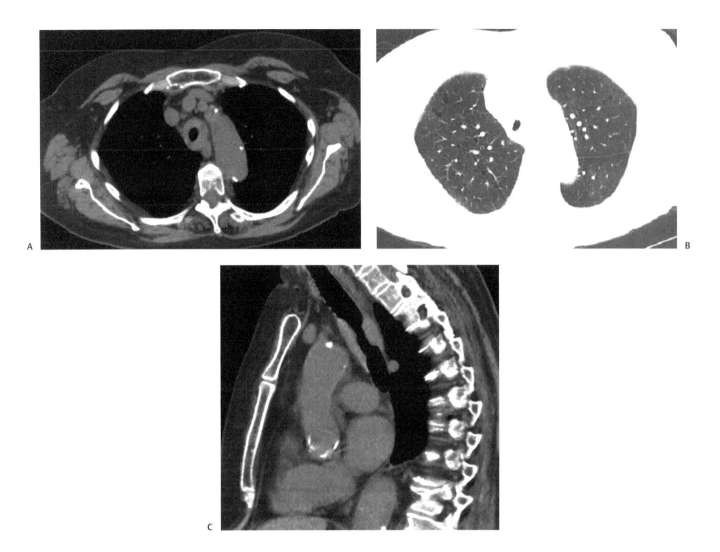

■ Clinical Presentation

A 68-year-old man with a history of cigarette smoking presents with cough, hemoptysis, and chest pain.

■ **Imaging Findings**

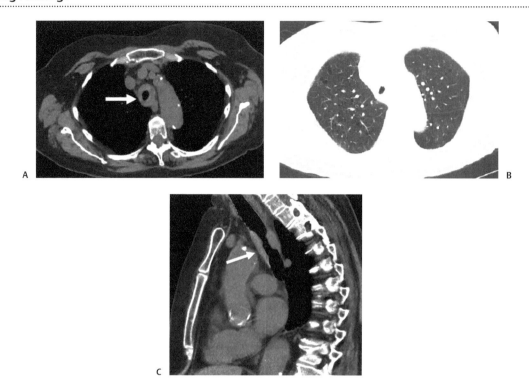

(A) Noncontrast CT image of the chest. Axial image at the level of the aortic arch demonstrates concentric soft tissue thickening of the tracheal wall with moderate luminal narrowing (*arrow*). (B) Lung window image at the same level shows pulmonary emphysema in the bilateral lungs. (C) Sagittal reconstruction image through the trachea depicts the concentric soft tissue tracheal wall mass (*arrow*) with nodular contour of the tracheal lumen.

■ **Differential Diagnosis**

- ***Tracheal carcinoma.***
- *Sarcoidosis.*
- *Amyloidosis.*
- *Granulomatous infection (e.g., tuberculosis, histoplasmosis).*
- *Vasculitis.*

■ **Essential Facts**

- Primary tracheal cancers are rare, with an estimate of 0.1 per 100,000 per year.
- Primary tracheal tumors in adults are usually malignant (90%) and are more commonly benign in children.
- Average age at the time of diagnosis is ~60 years, with a slightly higher incidence in males than females. Patients with adenoid cystic carcinomas tend to be younger.
- Around half of all primary tracheal cancers are squamous cell carcinomas, followed by adenoid cystic carcinomas (25%).
- Primary malignant tracheal tumors may arise from the respiratory epithelium, salivary glands, or mesenchymal elements of the tracheal wall.
- Most commonly, presenting symptoms are dyspnea, hemoptysis, cough, and hoarseness.
- Most patients with tracheal squamous cell carcinomas are smokers or former smokers.

- Adenoid cystic carcinoma is not associated with cigarette smoking.
- Squamous cell carcinoma may be multicentric in origin and can also be associated with synchronous or metachronous carcinomas of the oropharynx, larynx, or lung.
- Whenever possible, surgical resection is the treatment of choice for malignant primary tracheal tumors. Overall survival and prognosis depends on whether or not the tumor is resectable.

■ **Other Imaging Findings**

- CT is the best imaging modality to evaluate tracheal tumors, assess tumoral extension, and visualize possible infiltration of the mediastinum and adjacent structures.
- Malignant tracheal tumors may present as a focal sessile endoluminal mass or polypoid soft tissue density, or as a focal circumferential mass or thickening of the tracheal wall.

✓ **Pearls and ✗ Pitfalls**

✓ Conventional chest radiographs are rarely diagnostic of tracheal tumors.
✗ Most patients with primary malignant tracheal tumors present with an advanced local disease, and diagnosis is usually delayed.

Case 70

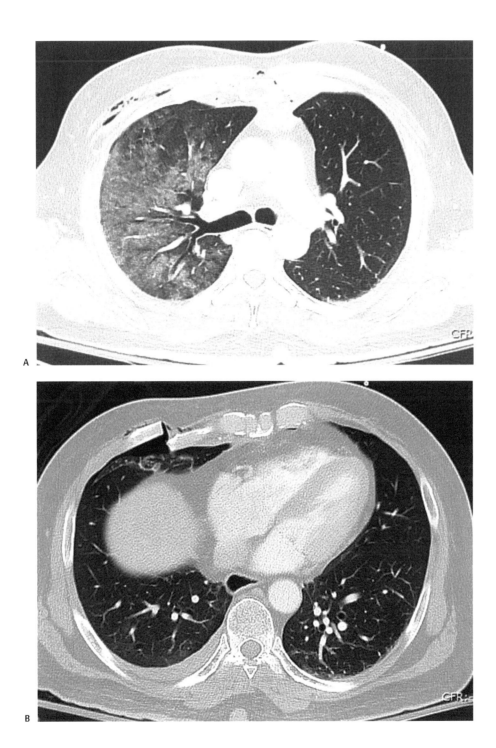

■ Clinical Presentation

Restrained driver with chest pain after motor vehicle accident.

■ Imaging Findings

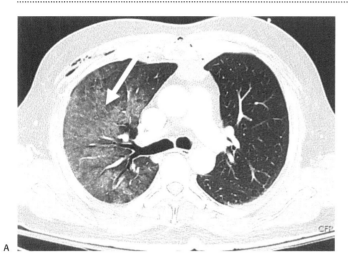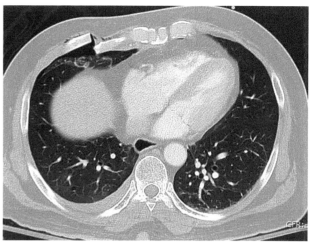

A

B

(A) Contrast-enhanced CT image of the chest. Lung window axial image shows extensive ground-glass opacities in the right lung (*arrow*). (B) Bone window axial image at a lower level in the same patient shows rib fracture, pneumothorax, and hemothorax ipsilateral to the upper lung zone ground-glass pulmonary opacities.

■ Differential Diagnosis

- ***Pulmonary contusion.***
- *Pulmonary edema.*
- *Fat embolism.*

■ Essential Facts

- Pulmonary contusion is a common consequence of thoracic trauma seen in 25 to 50% of patients with multiple traumatic injuries that impart substantial amounts of kinetic energy to the thorax.
- Falls and rapid deceleration after motor vehicle accidents are the most common mechanism in civilians, whereas in military confrontations, the shock wave produced by explosion and high-velocity projectiles is also common.
- Trauma patients with pulmonary contusion have a higher incidence of pneumonia, acute respiratory distress syndrome (ARDS), and long-term respiratory disability, and they have a significant mortality rate (10–25%).
- From a histopathologic standpoint, pulmonary contusion is characterized by interstitial and alveolar hemorrhage and edema, without cut or tear in the lung tissue.
- Pulmonary contusion interferes with gas exchange, leading to hypoxemia (decreased O_2) and hypercarbia (increased CO_2).
- The traumatic lung injury in pulmonary contusion generally resolves entirely 7 to 10 days after the traumatic event.

- Patients with pulmonary contusion that is evident on chest radiographs have a longer hospital stay and are more likely to require mechanical ventilation.
- There is no specific treatment. Management is mainly supportive, with optimization of oxygenation and ventilation as required, as well as pain control and restoration of pulmonary mechanics.

■ Other Imaging Findings

- Hemorrhage and edema into the lung parenchyma is responsible for the radiologic changes that are usually evident in the first 6 hours and may worsen for 24 to 48 hours; they generally resolve between 7 and 10 days after injury.
- Imaging presentation of pulmonary contusion consists of variable-sized patchy areas of consolidation and ground-glass opacities, with a nonsegmental distribution.

✓ Pearls and ✗ Pitfalls

- ✓ Pulmonary contusion may evolve and progress in the early hours after the traumatic event, with a much higher incidence of radiographic pulmonary abnormalities 24 hours after injury than on the initial radiographs.
- ✗ Conventional chest radiographs have poor sensitivity for the detection of pulmonary contusion, in comparison to chest CT, with a false-negative rate between 20 and 66%.

Case 71

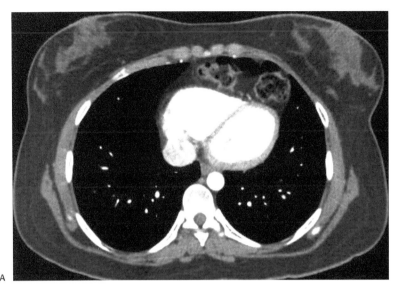

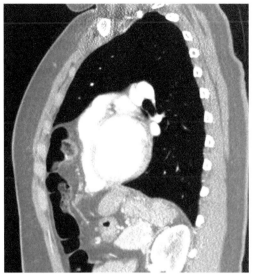

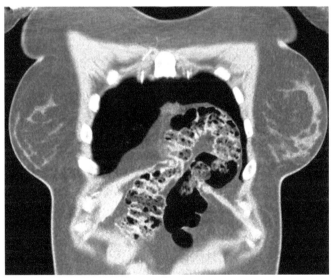

▪ Clinical Presentation

A 20-year-old woman with atypical chest pain.

■ **Imaging Findings**

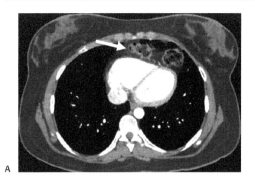 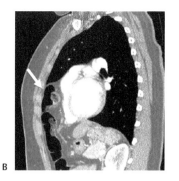 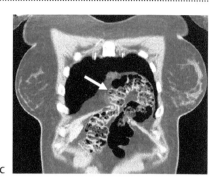

(A–C) Contrast-enhanced CT images of the chest. **(A)** Axial image at the level of the interventricular septum depicts a bowel loop (transverse colon) in the anterior mediastinum, between the heart and the sternum (*arrow*). **(B)** Sagittal reconstruction image. **(C)** Coronal reconstruction image. The multiplanar images show the continuity between the intrathoracic bowel loop in the anterior mediastinum (*arrows*) and the rest of the transverse colon. A mild degree of mass effect is noted on the anterior surface of the heart. The coronal reconstruction image nicely demonstrates the presence of an anterior diaphragmatic defect.

■ **Differential Diagnosis**

- ***Morgagni hernia.***
- *Colonic interposition.*
- *Eventration of the diaphragm.*

■ **Essential Facts**

- Morgagni hernias are a relatively rare type of congenital retrosternal hernias that originate from a defective closure of the anterior and medial septum tranversus (the ventral component of the diaphragm) during early embryogenesis.
- Morgagni hernias are < 5% of all congenital diaphragmatic hernias.
- Diagnosis is commonly delayed, with most cases diagnosed during adult life.
- The anatomic defect is known as the foramen of Morgagni in the right and as the Larrey space or hiatus in the left side. Herniation of abdominal content on either side is considered a Morgagni hernia, but left-sided hernias are sometimes also known as Larrey hernias.
- Morgagni hernia typically has a covering, or sac, that herniates into the anterior mediastinum and most commonly contains omentum, transverse colon, or small bowel.
- These hernias are commonly asymptomatic but may manifest with chest pain, dyspnea, or gastrointestinal symptoms. Strangulation and bowel necrosis are extremely rare but have been described.
- Most common location of a Morgagni hernia is to the right (90%), but occasionally left-sided and bilateral hernias may occur. Protection by the pericardium on the left side has been suggested for the predominant right-sided location of these hernias.

- Several different congenital anomalies are associated with congenital diaphragmatic hernias, including intestinal malrotation.
- Surgical repair is commonly recommended for symptomatic cases in particular, and in bowel-containing hernias to prevent complications.

■ **Other Imaging Findings**

- Morgagni hernias appear as an abnormal density in the anterior right cardiophrenic angle.
- Depending on the content of the hernia, sac density and morphology will vary. Omentum-containing hernias have fat density, whereas bowel-containing hernias will show characteristic appearance of the intestinal content.

✓ **Pearls and ✗ Pitfalls**

✓ Fetal diaphragmatic hernias usually occur through the Bochdalek space on the left side and not through the foramen of Morgagni.

✗ Omental fat–containing Morgagni hernias on the right side may be difficult to differentiate from epicardial fat pad or fat-containing tumors (lipoma, thymolipoma). The detection of curvilinear vessels within the mass extending to the abdomen through the diaphragmatic defect is characteristic of an omental hernia. This can be better demonstrated with multidetector CT with sagittal and coronal reconstructions.

Case 72

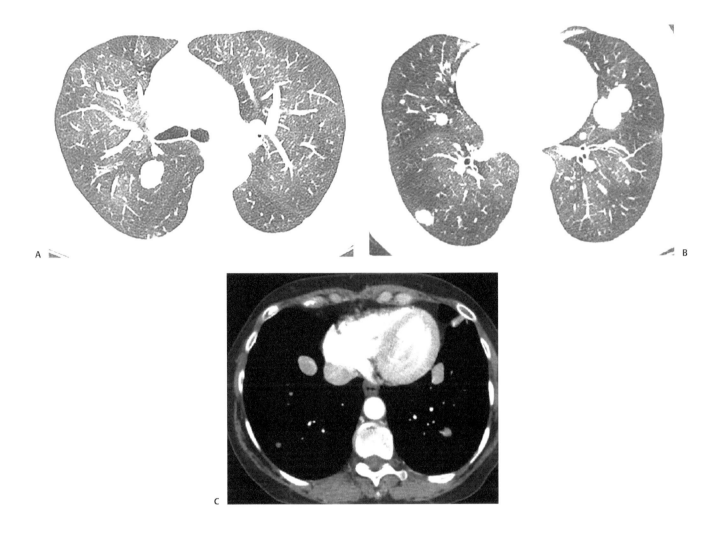

■ Clinical Presentation

A 55-year-old woman with chronic cough and dyspnea.

■ Imaging Findings

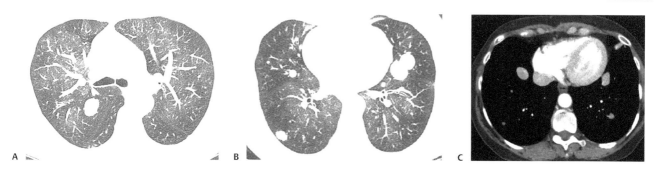

(A, B) Contrast-enhanced CT images of the chest. Lung window images at two different levels show mosaic pattern and lung attenuation in the bilateral lungs with multiple pulmonary nodules. **(C)** Mediastinal window, axial image above the diaphragm demonstrates the soft tissue density of the multiple pulmonary nodules.

■ Differential Diagnosis

- ***Diffuse idiopathic pulmonary neuroendocrine cell hyperplasia (DIPNECH).***
- *Pulmonary metastasis.*
- *Cellular bronchiolitis.*

■ Essential Facts

- DIPNECH is a rare condition that is part of the spectrum of pulmonary neuroendocrine cell proliferation and neoplasms, which also includes carcinoid tumorlets and carcinoid tumors.
- Tumorlets and carcinoids reflect a continuum in a proliferative process that evolves from neuroendocrine cell hyperplasia; the tumors are arbitrarily classified as tumorlet (lesions < 5 mm) or as carcinoid (lesions > 5 mm), based on lesion size.
- There is a significant association between DIPNECH and pulmonary carcinoid tumors. More than 50% of patients with proven DIPNECH will have pulmonary carcinoid tumors, whereas 5% of patients with pulmonary carcinoid tumors have DIPNECH in the lung parenchyma.
- Pulmonary carcinoid tumors in the context of DIPNECH are usually multiple and bilateral, measuring up to 2 cm in diameter.
- Pulmonary neuroendocrine cells (Kulchitsky cells) are mucosal epithelial cells of the tracheobronchial tree that extend from the trachea to the terminal bronchioles, which act as chemoreceptors to hypoxemia.
- Pulmonary neuroendocrine cell hyperplasia has been described in association with numerous conditions, including cigarette smoking, high-altitude hypoxemia, bronchiectasis, asthma, bronchiolitis, cystic fibrosis, pulmonary fibrosis, and many more.
- Since 1999, DIPNECH has been recognized by the World Health Organization classification of lung tumors as a preneoplastic condition.

- The vast majority of affected patients are adult females (> 90%), with an age range between 36 and 84 years (average, 66 years).
- Most patients are symptomatic, with cough and dyspnea being the most common clinical manifestation, but ~20% are asymptomatic.
- There are no guidelines for treatment or management of DIPNECH. Some patients are treated with steroids and octreotide, a somatostatin analogue, but no evidence-based recommendations are available.

■ Other Imaging Findings

- Mosaic pattern of lung attenuation is the most common imaging finding, and it results from abnormal neuroendocrine cell proliferation in the bronchial wall. Mucoid impaction and bronchiectasis secondary to bronchial stenosis may also occur.
- Pulmonary nodules of variable size may also be present. These tend to be spherical in shape, and depending on their size may represent tumorlets (< 5 mm) or carcinoid tumors (> 5 mm).
- DIPNECH-associated carcinoid tumors are soft tissue in density and do not calcify as do carcinoids unrelated to DIPNECH.

✓ Pearls and ✗ Pitfalls

✓ Almost all carcinoid tumors observed in patients with DIPNECH are typical carcinoids (95%), and only small percentages are atypical carcinoids (5%).

✗ Despite being classified as a preneoplastic condition, DIPNECH is commonly indolent and has good prognosis. No case of evolution into a high-grade neuroendocrine carcinoma has been reported.

Case 73

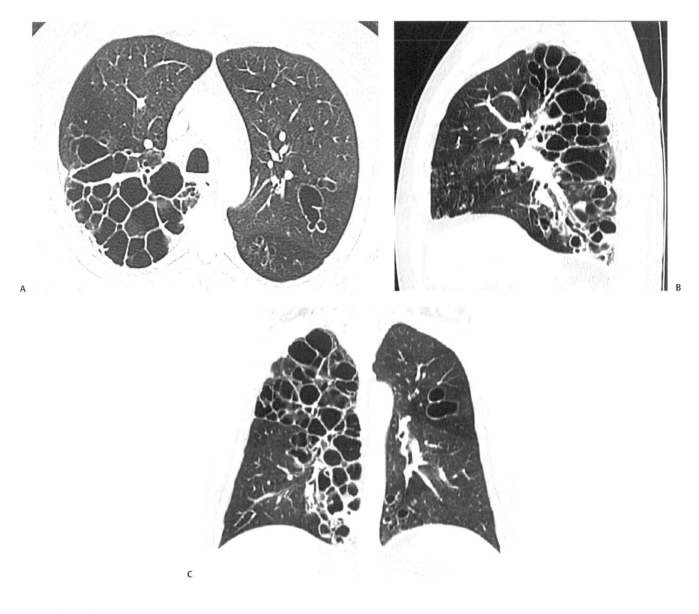

A

B

C

■ Clinical Presentation

A 25-year-old man with chronic cough and recurrent pulmonary infections.

■ Imaging Findings

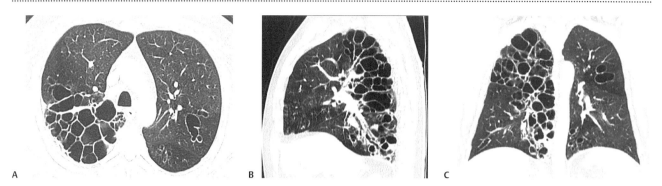

(A–C) Contrast-enhanced CT images of the chest: lung window axial **(A)**, sagittal **(B)**, and coronal **(C)** images. These different images demonstrate cystic bronchiectasis throughout the bilateral lungs, more extensively affecting the right upper and right lower lobes.

■ Differential Diagnosis

- ***Williams–Campbell syndrome.***
- *Cystic fibrosis.*
- *Idiopathic bronchiectasis.*
- *Ciliary dyskinesia.*
- *Allergic bronchopulmonary aspergillosis.*

■ Essential Facts

- Williams–Campbell syndrome is a rare congenital syndrome in which complete or partial deficiency of bronchial wall cartilage results in the formation of cystic and cylindrical bronchiectasis in the bilateral lungs.
- The defect can affect from the first to the eighth bronchial divisions, but it is most commonly seen involving the fourth, fifth, and sixth bronchial generations without affecting the trachea or central bronchi.
- The majority of cases manifest with respiratory symptoms in childhood (cough, wheezing, recurrent pulmonary infection), but several adult cases have been reported, suggesting that less severe cartilage deficiency may manifest late or remain underdiagnosed for years.
- The exact mechanism is not clear, and both a genetic mechanism (autosomal recessive) as well as a postinfectious etiology (adenovirus) have been proposed.

- Pathology examination of the affected bronchi show deficient cartilaginous plates in the bronchial wall.
- Because there is no specific treatment, prophylaxis for preventing recurrent infection with antibiotics and respiratory therapy is the most common approach. Some cases of bilateral lung transplantation have been reported.

■ Other Imaging Findings

- CT demonstrates diffuse bilateral cystic and cylindrical bronchiectasis, with normal trachea and mainstem bronchi.
- Dynamic CT images in inspiration and expiration may show cystic bronchiectasis "ballooning" in inspiration with expiratory collapse.

✓ Pearls and ✗ Pitfalls

- ✓ The diagnosis of Williams–Campbell syndrome requires exclusion of other conditions that may produce congenital and acquired bilateral cystic and cylindrical bronchiectasis.
- ✗ Different from Mounier–Kuhn syndrome, which can also present with bronchiectasis, in Williams–Campbell syndrome, the trachea and mainstem bronchi are normal.

Case 74

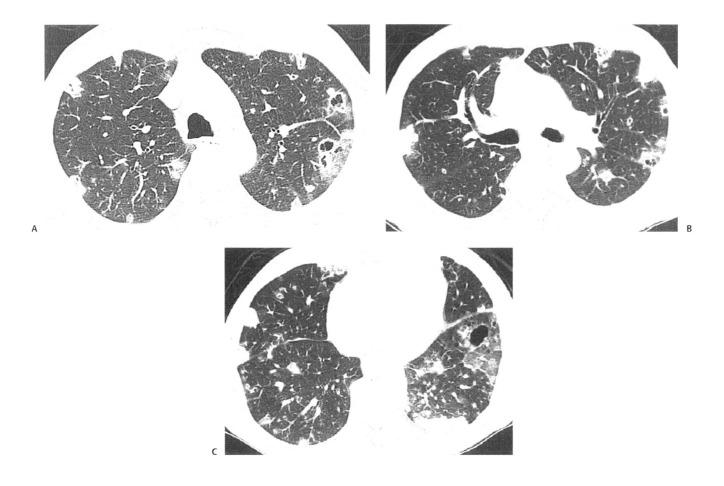

A

B

C

■ Clinical Presentation

A 50-year-old man with a history of intravenous drug abuse has fever and cough.

■ Imaging Findings

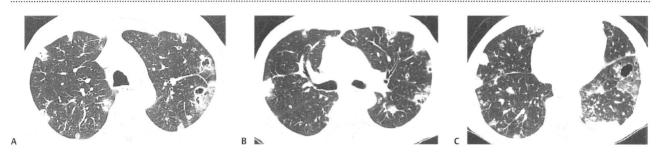

A   B   C

(A–C) Contrast-enhanced CT images: lung window axial images at three different levels. Numerous nodular and patchy opacities, some of which present with cavitation, are noted predominantly in the periphery and subpleural region of the bilateral lungs. In several of the nodular opacities, pulmonary vessels can be tracked extending into the focal abnormality.

■ Differential Diagnosis

- ***Septic pulmonary embolism.***
- *Multilobar pneumonia.*
- *Metastatic disease.*
- *Granulomatosis with polyangiitis.*

■ Essential Facts

- Septic pulmonary embolism occurs when there is embolization of infected thrombi from an extrapulmonary infectious site into the pulmonary vasculature, resulting in lung parenchyma infection.
- The most common causes of septic pulmonary embolism are intravenous drug abuse (25–75%), right heart infective endocarditis (15–75%), septic thrombophlebitis, suppurative head and neck infection, skin infection, and infected intravascular catheters and other medical devices.
- In patients with infective endocarditis and septic pulmonary embolism, most common location of cardiac infection/vegetation is in the tricuspid valve (65–85%), resulting in valvular destruction and insufficiency.
- *Staphylococcus aureus* is the most common pathogen identified, follow by *Candida* infection.
- Clinical manifestations include fever, chest pain, cough, dyspnea, and septic shock.

- Rupture of subpleural cavitary lesions into the pleural space may result in pneumothorax and empyema.
- Treatments include antibiotic therapy and appropriate management of the primary site or source of the infection.

■ Other Imaging Findings

- Pulmonary nodules, often in the periphery of the lung, is the most common CT finding (60%). Wedge-shaped peripheral pulmonary opacities (23%), and a feeding vessel approaching or entering a nodule or opacity (the feeding vessel sign), are also commonly reported (25–50%).
- Cavitation of lung nodules or pulmonary opacity is also a common finding (25%).

✓ Pearls and ✗ Pitfalls

- ✓ Conventional chest radiographs have low sensitivity for the detection of septic pulmonary embolism and may even be normal. If the clinical suspicion is high, then a CT image of the chest should be obtained.
- ✗ The feeding vessel sign (a vessel entering a nodule or pulmonary opacity) is also commonly seen in pulmonary metastases and is not specific for pulmonary septic embolism.

Case 75

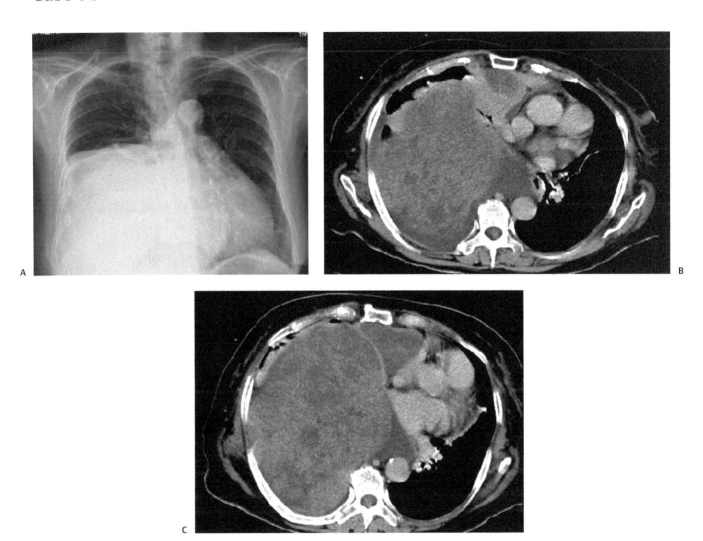

■ Clinical Presentation

A 75-year-old woman with chest pain, bilateral hand clubbing, and hypoglycemia.

▪ Imaging Findings

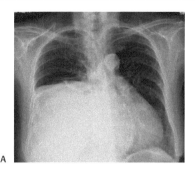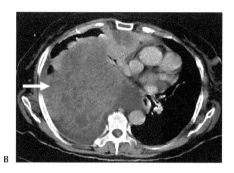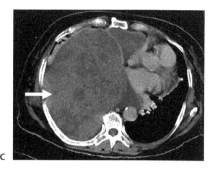

A   B   C

(A) Chest radiograph, frontal view. A very large masslike opacity is appreciated in the lower aspect of the right hemithorax with mass effect on the medi-astinum with shifting of the cardiac silhouette to the left. **(B, C)** Contrast-enhanced CT images of the chest. Axial images at two different levels confirm a large heterogeneous density solid mass in the right hemithorax (*arrows*) compressing the right lung and displacing the heart and mediastinum to the left.

▪ Differential Diagnosis

- ***Solitary fibrous tumor of the pleura.***
- *Mesothelioma.*
- *Thoracic sarcoma.*

▪ Essential Facts

- Solitary fibrous tumor of the pleura (SFTP) is a rare, primary, usually benign (90%) mesenchymal tumor that is now considered to be a soft tissue neoplasm of pluripotent fibroblastic or myofibroblastic origin.
- The tumor more commonly arises from the visceral (80%) than from the parietal pleura (20%) and can be sessile or pedunculated. Intrapulmonary and mediastinal origin are less common but may also occur.
- Pedunculated tumors attached to the visceral pleura are more easily removed, have a lower recurrence rate, and have better prognosis.
- Men and women between 30 and 70 years old are equally affected.
- There is no association between asbestos exposure and SFTP.
- Excellent prognosis after complete surgical resection. The sessile types have a higher recurrence rate, even after complete resection.

▪ Other Imaging Findings

- SFTP presents as a pleural-based soft tissue density mass with mild degree of enhancement after contrast injection. On CT imaging, tumors tend to be hyperdense and homogeneous, but large tumors may present internal areas of necrosis and hemorrhage as well as focal calcification.

✓ Pearls and ✗ Pitfalls

- ✓ Paraneoplastic syndromes such as refractory hypoglycemia (Doege–Potter syndrome), clubbing, and hypertrophic pulmonary osteoarthropathy (Pierre Marie–Bamberger syndrome) have been reported associated with this tumor (< 20%), in particular with large tumors > 7 cm in diameter.
- ✓ Hypoglycemia results from tumor production of insulinlike growth factor, and hypertrophic pulmonary osteoarthropathy results from tumor production of a growth hormone–like substance.
- ✗ These tumors were formerly considered to be mesothelial or submesothelial lesions of the pleura and were known as "benign mesotheliomas."

Case 76

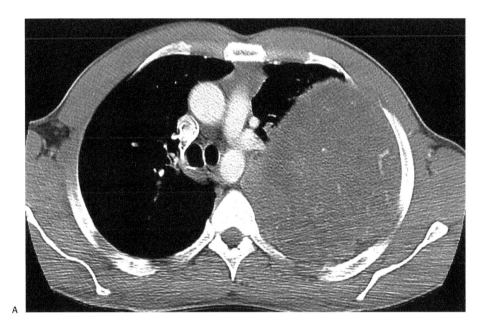

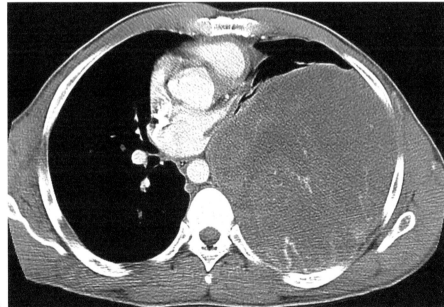

■ Clinical Presentation

A previously healthy 28-year-old man with chest pain.

■ Imaging Findings

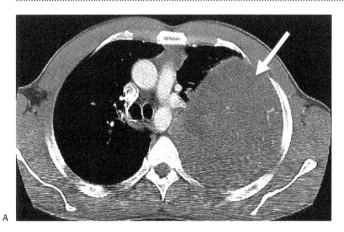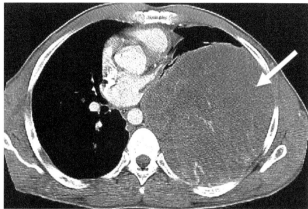

(A, B) Contrast-enhanced CT axial images at the level of the carina **(A)** and left atrium **(B)** display a large soft tissue mass in the left hemithorax (*arrows*) with irregular neovascularity and displacement of the heart and mediastinum to the right. No chest wall abnormality is appreciated.

■ Differential Diagnosis

- ***Sarcoma.***
- *Solitary fibrous tumor of the pleura.*
- *Lymphoma.*
- *Lung cancer.*

■ Essential Facts

- Sarcomas represent a diverse group of malignant mesenchymal tumors with different histopathology that can arise from several different structures within the thoracic cavity and chest wall.
- Overall, primary thoracic sarcomas are rare and less common than metastatic disease from extrathoracic sarcomas.
- Most common primary thoracic sarcomas arise from the chest wall from either bone (e.g., chondrosarcoma, Ewing sarcoma, osteosarcoma) or soft tissue (e.g., malignant fibrous histiocytoma, fibrosarcoma, leiomyosarcoma, rhabdomyosarcoma).
- The most frequent types of primary pulmonary sarcomas include leiomyosarcoma, fibrosarcoma, malignant fibrous histiocytoma, rhabdomyosarcoma, synovial sarcoma, and Kaposi sarcoma.
- Primary intrathoracic sarcomas may also arise in the mediastinum as well as from the heart and great vessels.

■ Other Imaging Findings

- Primary thoracic sarcomas have a wide range of imaging appearance and manifestation. A common imaging finding consists of a well-defined large mass, usually > 5 cm in diameter, often > 10 cm in size, with a smooth or lobulated margin.
- Associated pleural effusion is common, but associated mediastinal or hilar lymphadenopathy, cystic/cavitary changes, and internal calcifications are relatively rare.
- Significant amount of calcification when present, in a pleural-based mass, favors a chondrosarcoma or osteosarcoma.
- Contrast-enhanced CT image may reveal neovascularity with small irregular vessels.

✓ Pearls and ✗ Pitfalls

- ✓ The possibility of an intrathoracic sarcoma should be considered in the presence of a large intrathoracic mass, > 5 cm in diameter, with small and lobulated margins, and with internal neovascularity and no significant lymphadenopathy.
- ✗ The different histologic subtypes of thoracic sarcomas are commonly indistinguishable based on their imaging presentation.

Case 77

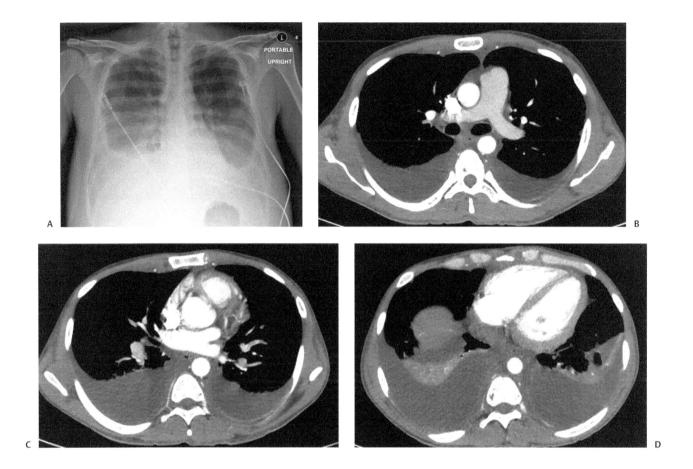

■ Clinical Presentation

Man who is HIV positive with Kaposi sarcoma and recurrent bilateral pleural effusion.

■ Imaging Findings

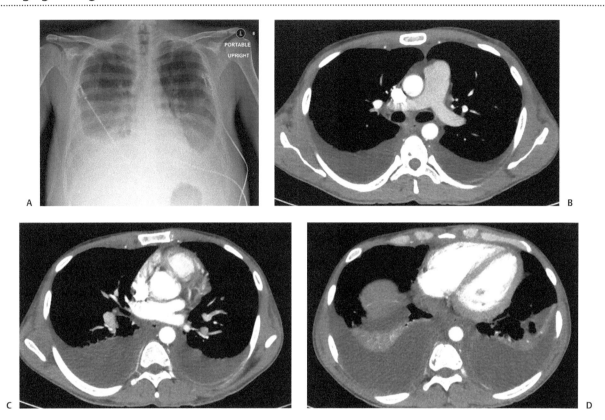

(A) Chest radiograph shows bilateral pleural effusions blunting the lateral costophrenic angles. **(B–D)** Contrast-enhanced CT axial images at three different levels confirm the presence of large bilateral pleural effusions. No mediastinal or pleural bases mass is identified.

■ Differential Diagnosis

- ***Primary effusion lymphoma.***
- *Pyothorax associated lymphoma.*
- *Pleural effusion.*

■ Essential Facts

- Primary effusion lymphoma (PEL) is a rare large-cell non-Hodgkin (B cell) lymphoma localized predominantly in body cavities.
- It was initially described in HIV-infected patients with Kaposi sarcoma.
- PEL accounts for ~4% of all HIV-associated non-Hodgkin lymphomas.
- Characteristic presentation of PEL consists of lymphomatous effusions in the absence of extracavitary solid tumor.
- Pleural, peritoneal, and pericardial spaces are commonly involved, but the disease usually involves only one body site.
- PEL is commonly associated with human herpesvirus type 8 (HHV-8) infection in HIV-positive individuals with AIDS, mostly men, with severe immunodeficiency or in organ-transplantation–related immunosuppression. Coinfection with Epstein–Barr virus is also very common (> 90%).

- Symptoms are due to the mass effect of the accumulation of malignant effusion: dyspnea results from pleural or pericardial effusion; abdominal distention results from intraperitoneal fluid.
- Management consists of a combination of chemotherapy and antiretroviral therapy (if patient is HIV positive), but no effective treatment is yet available. Response to chemotherapy is poor. Prognosis is poor, with median survival time of < 6 months.

■ Other Imaging Findings

- Moderate to large amount of low-density fluid, typically with no associated solid tumor component in the pleural space, pericardium, or peritoneal cavity.

✓ Pearls and ✗ Pitfalls

- ✓ Preexisting Kaposi sarcoma and multicenter Castleman disease are common and are additional manifestations of HHV-8 infection.
- ✗ Occasionally, PEL can also present in extracavitary regions with a component of solid mass.

Case 78

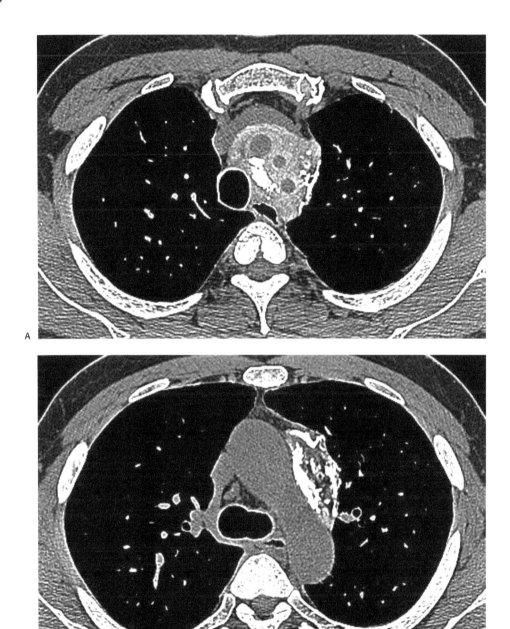

■ Clinical Presentation

A 37-year-old man with chest pain, cough, and dyspnea.

■ Imaging Findings

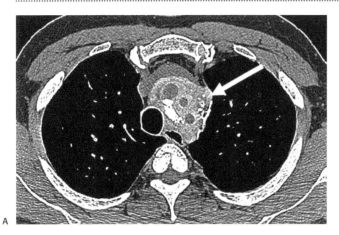
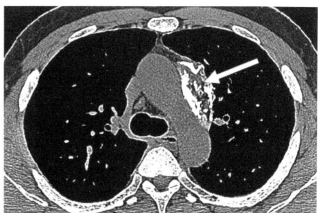

(A, B) Noncontrast CT image of the chest. Axial images through the upper chest at and above the aortic arch show an irregularly calcified mass in the middle mediastinum (*arrows*) surrounding the brachiocephalic vessels and extending to the prevascular space.

■ Differential Diagnosis

- ***Fibrosing mediastinitis.***
- *Treated lymphoma.*
- *Tuberculosis.*
- *Silicosis.*

■ Essential Facts

- Fibrosing mediastinitis, or mediastinal fibrosis, is characterized by abnormal accumulation of excessive amounts of dense fibrous tissue in the mediastinum.
- The prevalence of fibrosing mediastinitis is not well known but is generally considered to be a rare condition.
- Two major forms of the disease are recognized—the focal granulomatous form, commonly associated with histoplasmosis, and the diffuse nongranulomatous form, which is considered an idiopathic process that is known to be associated with other fibrosing conditions such as retroperitoneal fibrosis, primary sclerosing cholangitis, and orbital pseudotumor.
- The fibrotic tissue that gradually encases the mediastinal structures may produce pulmonary artery or pulmonary vein stenosis, superior vena cava obstruction, tracheobronchial stenosis, or esophageal obstruction.
- Less common complications include constrictive pericarditis, coronary artery or aortic stenosis, and nerve injury (recurrent laryngeal nerve or phrenic nerve).
- No curative treatment is available. Anecdotal reports have described some success with the administration of corticosteroids and tamoxifen. Surgical or percutaneous intervention (stenting) are additional therapeutic options to alleviate vascular obstruction or tracheobronchial stenosis.

■ Other Imaging Findings

- Conventional radiography is limited in the evaluation of fibrosing mediastinitis and is often normal. When abnormal, the most common findings include nonspecific mediastinal widening, with increased density in the paratracheal and subcarinal regions of the middle mediastinum.
- On CT imaging, abnormal soft tissue density, predominantly in the middle mediastinum, is the most constant imaging finding. The degree of calcification is quite variable, typically more extensive in the focal form than in the diffuse form.
- The diffuse form may manifest as an infiltrative process, with visceral encroachment producing vascular or airway luminal narrowing or stenosis.
- Contrast-enhanced multidetector CT with multiplanar reconstruction is the imaging modality of choice for the evaluation of fibrosing mediastinitis. Internal calcification, in particular the stipple pattern, is better appreciated with CT than with MRI.

✓ Pearls and ✗ Pitfalls

✓ In the United States, where *Histoplasma capsulatum* is endemic, the granulomatous form is the most common type of fibrosing mediastinitis (70%).

✗ On 18-fluorodeoxyglucose–positron emission tomography (FDG-PET), fibrosing mediastinitis may exhibit variable degrees of metabolic activity. Masslike mediastinal fibrosis with increased metabolic activity on FDG-PET may mimic a malignant mediastinal tumor.

Case 79

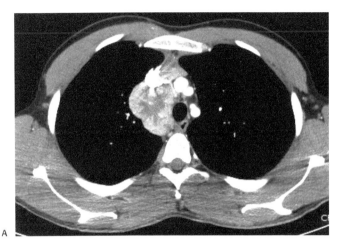

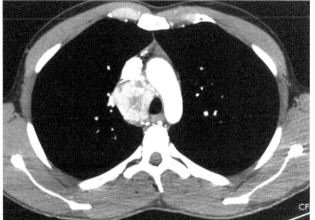

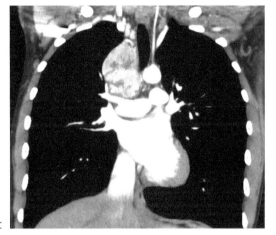

■ Clinical Presentation

....

A previously healthy 21-year-old man with chest pain and cough (CT of the neck and abdomen were normal).

■ Imaging Findings

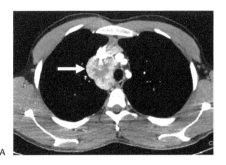 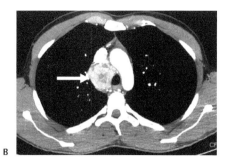 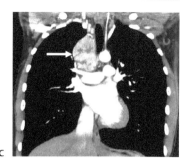

(A–C) Contrast-enhanced CT axial images **(A, B)** and coronal reconstruction image **(C)** show an enhancing and hypervascular mediastinal mass in the right paratracheal region (*arrows*).

■ Differential Diagnosis

- ***Unicentric Castleman disease.***
- *Multicentric Castleman disease.*
- *Hodgkin lymphoma.*
- *Sarcoidosis.*

■ Essential Facts

- Castleman disease represents a group of benign lymphoid disorders characterized by abnormally enlarged lymph nodes.
- The etiology of Castleman disease is not known, but both HIV and human herpesvirus type 8 (HHV-8) infection have been associated with this condition.
- Depending on the anatomic regions affected, the disease can be classified as unicentric or multicentric. In unicentric Castleman disease (UCD), one single abnormally enlarged lymph node or a single region of affected lymph nodes is present (neck, chest, or abdomen). In multicentric Castleman disease (MCD), multiple anatomic regions of groups of lymph nodes are involved.
- There are two subtypes of MCD: one associated with HHV-8; and another form considered idiopathic, in which affected patients are negative for HHV-8. Patients with MCD who are positive for HHV-8 and HIV are typically male (90%) and have a high incidence of Kaposi sarcoma (60%), lymphoma (10%), and increased mortality.
- There are two principal histologic subtypes of Castleman disease, the hyaline vascular and the plasma cell variant. The hyaline vascular variant accounts for the vast majority of UCD. The plasma cell variant can be seen both in the unicentric and multicentric forms. In some cases, a mixture of both histologic patterns is identified.

- Patients with UCD are commonly asymptomatic. Few present with nonspecific symptoms from mechanical compression by the abnormal lymphatic growth, or with systemic symptoms such as fever, fatigue, weight loss, and so forth.
- Surgical removal of the affected lymphadenopathy can be curative in UCD; for MCD, chemotherapy as well as antiinflammatory, immunosuppressive, and cytotoxic therapy have been used.

■ Other Imaging Findings

- Thoracic involvement in UCD is characterized by the presence of a solitary mass or conglomerate of mediastinal lymph nodes with significant enhancement after contrast injection.
- Internal calcification is uncommon but may occur. Larger lesions usually display a more heterogeneous internal density.
- In MCD, abnormally enlarged lymph nodes may affect the neck, mediastinum, pulmonary hila, and axillary lymph nodes.

✓ Pearls and ✗ Pitfalls

- ✓ The most common presentation of Castleman disease is an enhancing hypervascular mediastinal mass (70%).
- ✗ Lymphadenopathy in Castleman disease may show increased metabolic activity, similar to lymphomas and metastatic lymphadenopathy.

Case 80

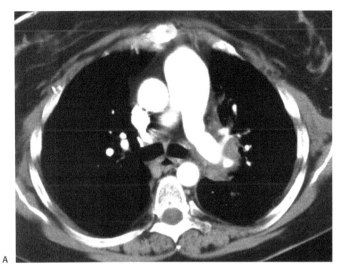

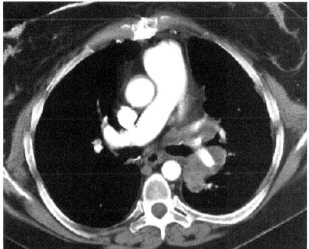

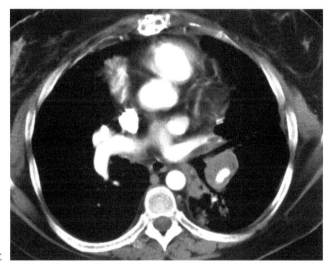

A

B

C

■ Clinical Presentation

A 41-year-old woman with fever, night sweats, and cough, 8 months after bilateral lung transplantation for pulmonary fibrosis.

■ Imaging Findings

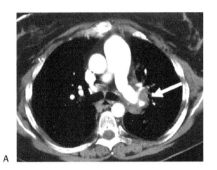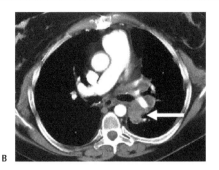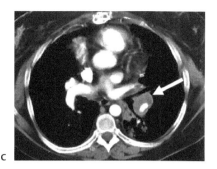

(A–C) Contrast-enhanced CT axial images at three different levels through the pulmonary hila reveal extensive lymphadenopathy in the left hilum (*arrows*) surrounding the left pulmonary artery and bronchi.

■ Differential Diagnosis

- ***Posttransplant lymphoproliferative disorder.***
- *Tuberculosis.*
- *Histoplasmosis.*
- *Sarcoidosis.*

■ Essential Facts

- Posttransplant lymphoproliferative disorder (PTLD) is a heterogeneous common lymphoid disorder, ranging from indolent lymphoid proliferation to aggressive malignancy, that results after solid organ or hematopoietic transplantation in both pediatric and adult patients.
- The majority of cases (65%) are associated with Epstein–Barr virus (EBV) infection.
- The incidence of PTLD is higher in patients < 10 or > 60 years old.
- PTLD may occur in as much as 25% of patients, depending on the type of transplant, degree and duration of immunosuppression, and number of EBV-positive donor lymphocytes in the graft.
- The World Health Organization divides PTLD in four types: early plasmacytic hyperplasia, polymorphic lesions (polyclonal or monoclonal), monomorphic lesions (most common type: usually a diffuse large B-cell lymphoma, Burkitt lymphoma, plasma cell myeloma), and classic Hodgkin-type lymphoma (very rare).
- PTLD is more common after heart, lung, and small bowel transplantation (< 25%) and is relatively rare after kidney and liver transplantation (< 5%).
- The majority of PTLD cases occur in the first year after transplantation, with a second peak after 4 to 5 years.
- Treatment usually includes reduction of the immunosuppressive medication, in addition to rituximab, chemotherapy, and occasionally antiviral medication.

■ Other Imaging Findings

- Imaging manifestations of PTLD include both nodal involvement and extranodal disease.
- In the chest, nodal involvement is the most significant imaging finding with enlarged mediastinal or hilar lymph nodes or as a mediastinal mass, which in the setting of immunosuppression raises concern for opportunistic infection.
- Pulmonary involvement is less common than nodal disease and may present as multiple pulmonary nodules.
- On contrast-enhanced CT imaging, these enlarged lymph nodes tend to be hypoattenuating.
- On fluorodeoxyglucose–positron emission tomography image, increased metabolic activity is commonly found.

✓ Pearls and ✗ Pitfalls

- ✓ The location of PTLD-related tumors varies depending on the type of transplanted organ. In case of heart or lung transplantation, the lung and mediastinum are the most common locations.
- ✗ In the setting of immunosuppression in a posttransplant patient, the presence of multiple pulmonary nodules more commonly represents infection than PTLD.

Case 81

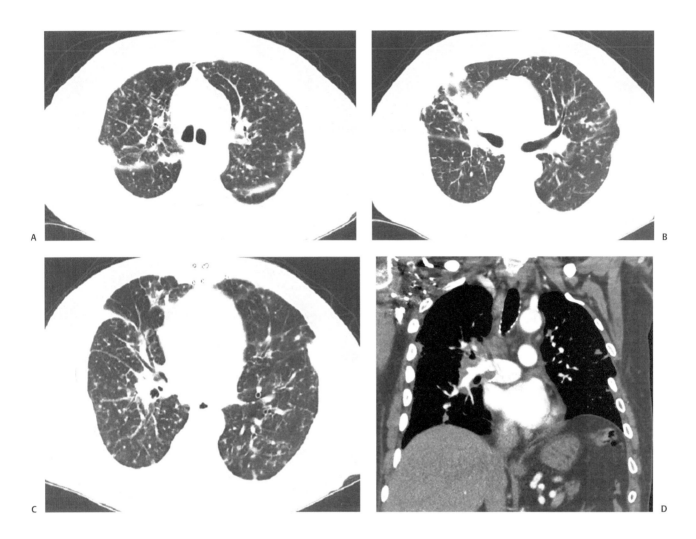

■ Clinical Presentation

A 53-year-old man with a history of bilateral lung transplant 6 months before has cough, fever, and shortness of breath.

■ Imaging Findings

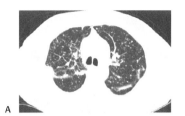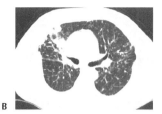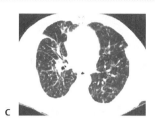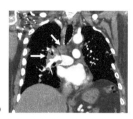

(A–C) Contrast-enhanced chest CT lung window axial images at three different levels show innumerable small pulmonary nodules scattered throughout the bilateral lungs, with patchy areas of air-space disease. (D) Mediastinal window coronal image through the right hilum shows hilar and mediastinal lymphadenopathy (*arrows*).

■ Differential Diagnosis

- ***Coccidioidomycosis.***
- *Histoplasmosis.*
- *Tuberculosis.*

■ Essential Facts

- Coccidioidomycosis (also known as valley fever) results from the inhalation of arthroconidia (spores) of *Coccidioides* spp., which include *Coccidioides immitis* and *C. posadasii.*
- Pulmonary disease, which is the most common form of coccidioidomycosis infection (95%), has a wide spectrum of clinical severity and manifestation ranging from asymptomatic exposure (60%) to symptomatic disease (40%), which includes severe disseminated infection with high mortality.
- *Coccidioides* spp. are soil-dwelling dimorphic fungi that exist only in arid or semiarid areas of the southwestern United States (e.g., California, New Mexico, Arizona, Texas), northern Mexico, and some parts of Central and South America (e.g., Argentina, Bolivia).
- In endemic areas, acute coccidioidomycosis is responsible for up to one third of all cases of community-acquired pneumonia, with most cases occurring in adulthood.
- Agriculture and construction workers and immunosuppressed patients (e.g., HIV-AIDS, solid organ or bone marrow transplantation) have an increased risk for pulmonary coccidioidomycosis infection.
- Primary pulmonary infection usually consists of a lobar or multilobar pneumonia with associated hilar and/or mediastinal lymphadenopathy, after which thin-walled pulmonary nodules or cavities may develop.

- Rupture of peripheral and subpleural cavities may result in hydropneumothorax from a bronchopleural fistula. Associated pleural effusion and empyema are seen in some cases (< 15%).
- Acute respiratory distress syndrome from coccidioidal infection is associated with very high mortality.
- Treatment is antifungal therapy (e.g., fluconazole, itraconazole).

■ Other Imaging Findings

- Primary pulmonary coccidioidomycosis may present with mostly unilateral pulmonary parenchymal opacities and air-space consolidation (75%), similar to a community-acquired pneumonia.
- In about 10% of patients, hilar and mediastinal (paratracheal) lymphadenopathy occur. Cavities and pulmonary nodules are also common (20%). Chronic fibrotic cavitary disease with pleural thickening and extensive pulmonary destruction occurs in a minority of cases (1%).

✓ Pearls and ✗ Pitfalls

- ✓ Several areas of the southwestern United States are considered hyperendemic for *Coccidioides* spp.
- ✗ Miliary disease from hematogenous spread results in development of a miliary pattern of disease, similar to tuberculosis, with multiple small pulmonary nodules and disseminated extrapulmonary disease (1–10%).

Case 82

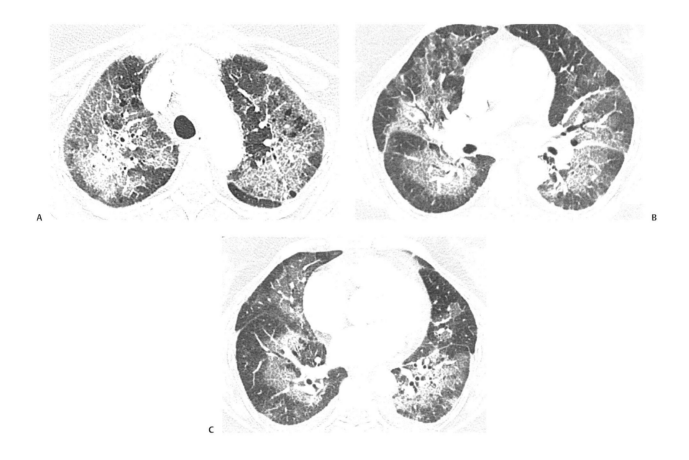

■ Clinical Presentation

A 57-year-old woman with rheumatoid arthritis has worsening dyspnea, cough, and fever.

▪ Imaging Findings

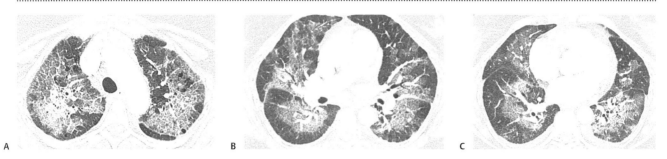

(A–C) Contrast-enhanced CT lung window axial images at the upper, middle, and lower lung zones show patchy ground-glass opacities with interlobular septal thickening, with some denser opacities in a peribronchovascular distribution. There are also small bilateral pleural effusions.

▪ Differential Diagnosis

- *Organizing pneumonia.*
- *Pneumonia.*
- *Nonspecific interstitial pneumonia.*
- *Pulmonary edema.*

▪ Essential Facts

- Organizing pneumonia is characterized pathologically by the presence of plugs of granulation tissue and fibrin exudates with loose collagen-containing fibroblasts in the distal air-space and bronchiolar lumen.
- This pathologic pattern is not specific for any particular disorder and just reflects a type of inflammatory response resulting from different lung injuries, including infectious pneumonia, malignancy, connective tissue disorders, vasculitis, drug toxicity, radiation therapy, and so forth.
- Depending on the cause or underlying condition, organizing pneumonia may be classified into three groups: organizing pneumonia of a known or determined cause (e.g., bacterial pneumonia), organizing pneumonia of undetermined cause but occurring in the context of a specific and relevant condition (e.g., rheumatoid arthritis, Sjögren syndrome, vasculitis, post–lung transplant), and cryptogenic (idiopathic) organizing pneumonia.
- Of organizing pneumonia cases, 60 to 79% are idiopathic. Cough, fever, and dyspnea are the most common clinical manifestations.

- Men and women are affected equally, with most cases presenting in the 5th or 6th decade of life. Organizing pneumonia in children is rare.
- Steroids are commonly used in the treatment of the different types of organizing pneumonia. In the secondary form, treatment of the underlying condition is also performed.

▪ Other Imaging Findings

- The imaging manifestation of organizing pneumonia can be variable, manifesting as multiple alveolar opacities, solitary focal opacity, or diffuse interstitial opacities.
- On high-resolution CT, common imaging findings of organizing pneumonia include patchy peribronchovascular or subpleural ground-glass opacities with interlobular septal thickening forming polygonal arcades (crazy paving). Patchy air-space, masslike consolidation, and lung nodules can also occur.

✓ Pearls and ✗ Pitfalls

- ✓ Organizing pneumonia was formerly known as *bronchiolitis obliterans organizing pneumonia*, but in 2002 the American Thoracic Society/European Respiratory Society International Consensus Panel for the Classification of Idiopathic Interstitial Pneumonia recommended that the term *cryptogenic organizing pneumonia* be used as the preferred clinical term for the idiopathic form of the disease.
- ✗ Organizing pneumonia is a morphologic pattern of injury recognized under the microscope and is not a specific disease or clinical entity.

Case 83

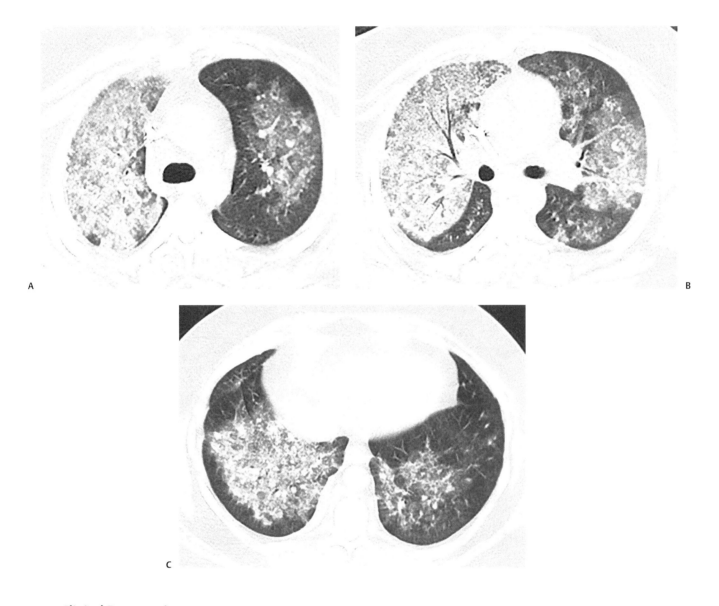

A

B

C

■ Clinical Presentation

A 22-year-old man with hemoptysis in acute renal failure.

■ Imaging Findings

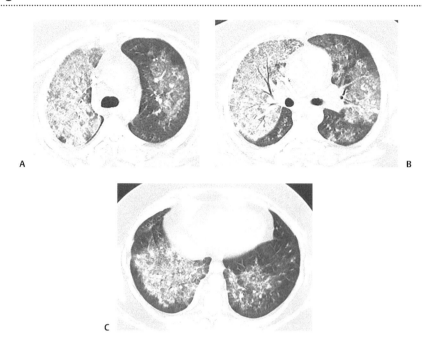

(A–C) Noncontrast CT images of the chest; axial lung window images at different levels. Extensive areas of air-space disease with consolidation and ground-glass opacities are noted in the bilateral lungs, more pronounced in the right lung.

■ Differential Diagnosis

- ***Diffuse alveolar hemorrhage.***
- *Pulmonary edema.*
- *Pneumonia.*
- *Pulmonary alveolar proteinosis.*

■ Essential Facts

- Diffuse alveolar hemorrhage (DAH) results from numerous different conditions with injury to the alveolar microcirculation (capillaries, venules, or arterioles) of the alveolar septal wall resulting in disruption of the alveolar-capillary basement membrane, and bleeding into the alveolar space.
- Hemoptysis is the most common clinical manifestation (70%), often associated with anemia, cough, dyspnea, and hypoxemia. Several diseases in which both the lungs and kidneys are affected (pulmonary renal syndrome) will also manifest with abnormal renal function and hematuria.
- On histopathology examination, three different morphologic patterns are recognized: diffuse alveolar damage (e.g., acute respiratory distress syndrome, cocaine), pulmonary capillaritis (e.g., systemic vasculitis, Goodpasture syndrome, idiopathic pulmonary hemosiderosis), and bland pulmonary hemorrhage (e.g., bleeding disorders).
- Most cases of DAH are secondary to an underlying pathology affecting the lungs. Common conditions include vasculitis (granulomatosis with polyangiitis, formerly Wegener granulomatosis), eosinophilic granulomatosis with polyangiitis (Churg–Strauss syndrome), microscopic polyangiitis, connective tissue disorders (systemic lupus erythematosus, antiphospholipid antibody syndrome), and so forth.
- Management includes supportive therapy as well as treatment of the underlying condition. Glucocorticoids and, in some cases, immunosuppressive therapy are commonly used.

■ Other Imaging Findings

- Initial imaging exams are normal in a substantial number of cases (> 20%).
- Later, ground-glass and air-space opacities develop, characteristically with a central and basal predominance.
- The combination of ground-glass opacities with interlobular septal thickening resulting in a crazy-paving pattern is common, in particular in the subacute stage.
- Patients with chronic recurrent DAH may develop interstitial pulmonary fibrosis.

✓ Pearls and ✗ Pitfalls

- ✓ Of the different histopathologic patterns associated with DAH, pulmonary capillaritis is the most common (88%).
- ✗ DAH is a clinicopathologic syndrome characterized by the accumulation of red blood cells in the alveolar space, originating from the capillaries of the alveolar wall, and is not a specific clinical entity.

Case 84

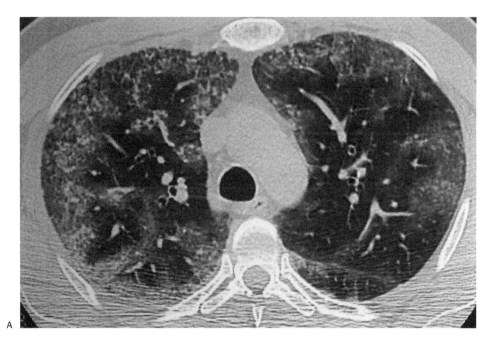

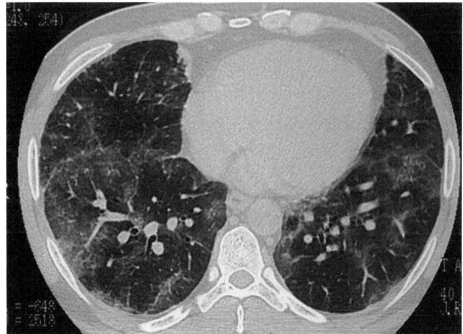

■ Clinical Presentation

A 40-year-old man with chronic cough and eosinophilia in blood.

■ Imaging Findings

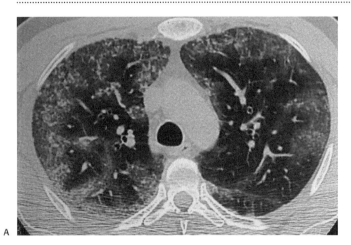
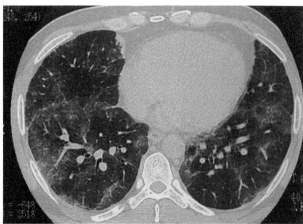

(A, B) Noncontrast chest CT images. Lung window axial images at the upper and lower lung zones show bilateral ground-glass opacities with reticulation/interlobular septal thickening with a predominant peripheral distribution.

■ Differential Diagnosis

- ***Idiopathic chronic eosinophilic pneumonia.***
- *Loeffler syndrome.*
- *Churg–Strauss syndrome (eosinophilic granulomatosis with polyangiitis).*
- *Idiopathic hypereosinophilic syndrome.*

■ Essential Facts

- Idiopathic chronic eosinophilic pneumonia (ICEP) is an uncommon disorder characterized by eosinophilia in the lung parenchyma and blood in patients with respiratory symptoms, and abnormal pulmonary opacities on imaging exams.
- ICEP is an adult disease, extremely rare in children, that more commonly affects females.
- Clinical manifestations are common, including cough, dyspnea, and wheezing, and as much as 50% have asthma.
- Significant eosinophilia on bronchoalveolar lavage (> 40%) is common, associated with mild to moderate peripheral eosinophilia in blood.
- Microscopic examination reveals alveolar and interstitial eosinophils and lymphocytes, with a variable degree of pulmonary fibrosis.
- Corticosteroids are the treatment of choice, usually with good response.

■ Other Imaging Findings

- Characteristic imaging finding in ICEP is peripheral nonsegmental parenchymal ground-glass opacities with reticulation, commonly bilaterally, with a predominant upper lobe distribution.
- This imaging pattern has been commonly described as "photographic negative" of pulmonary edema.
- Additional imaging findings include patchy opacities with a variable degree of air space consolidation.

✓ Pearls and ✗ Pitfalls

✓ Different from other conditions associated with eosinophilia, in ICEP there are no extrathoracic manifestations. There are other conditions that also course with pulmonary opacities and eosinophilia, but those are more commonly associated with extrathoracic disease (e.g., skin, heart, brain, gastrointestinal tract involvement), such as Churg–Strauss syndrome and idiopathic hypereosinophilic syndrome.

✗ The characteristic imaging pattern of peripheral opacities is seen in < 50% of patients with ICEP.

Case 85

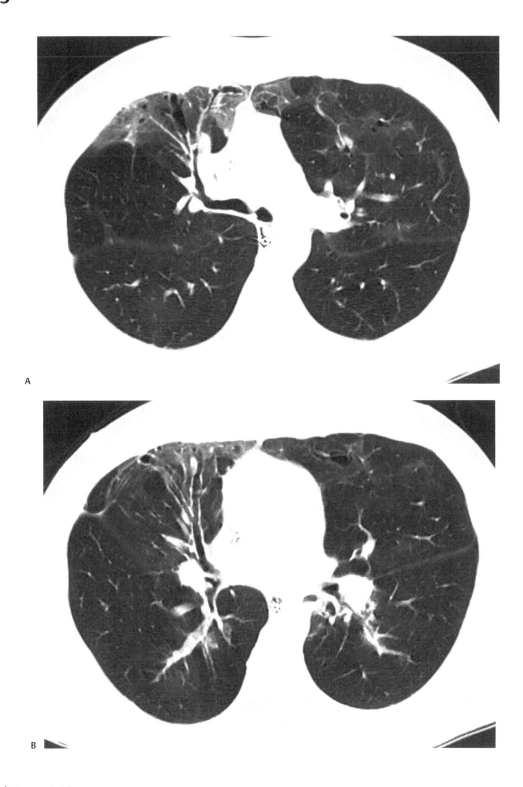

A

B

■ Clinical Presentation

A firefighter who had massive smoke inhalation at a petrochemical refinery fire 4 weeks previously has wheezing and severe respiratory distress.

■ Imaging Findings

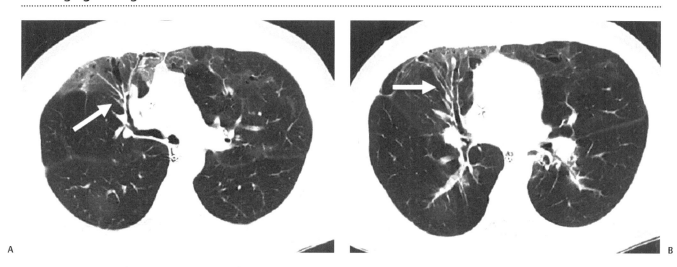

(A, B) Chest CT images, lung window settings; axial images through different levels show mosaic pattern of lung attenuation with areas of air trapping and bronchiectasis (*arrows*).

■ Differential Diagnosis

- ***Inhalational lung injury.***
- *Hypersensitivity pneumonitis.*
- *Respiratory bronchiolitis.*
- *Asthma.*

■ Essential Facts

- Inhalational lung injury results from acute inhalation of smoke, chemical irritants, or products of combustion, which may be associated with thermal injury of the airways.
- Inhalational injury may be classified into three main subtypes depending on whether the primary location of the injury is in the upper respiratory airway, tracheobronchial tree, or lung parenchyma.
- Pulmonary complications following burns and inhalation injury are responsible for significant morbidity and mortality.
- The spectrum of chemical-induced inhalational lung injuries is broad and includes tracheobronchitis, bronchiolitis, permeability pulmonary edema, chemical pneumonitis, organizing pneumonia, acute respiratory distress syndrome/diffuse alveolar damage, and so forth.
- Peak damage to the lung parenchyma is usually delayed days or weeks after the toxic exposure.
- The early acute stage is characterized by loss of surfactant, atelectasis, pulmonary edema, vasoconstriction, and clinically manifest as hypoxemia.

- Most patients do not suffer long-term respiratory impairment; however, irreversible sequelae including tracheobronchial stenosis, bronchiectasis, bronchiolitis obliterans, and interstitial pulmonary fibrosis may occur.
- Treatment is mainly supportive including intubation if needed, aerosolized bronchodilators, mucolytic agents, antibiotics, respiratory therapy, and airway suctioning.

■ Other Imaging Findings

- In the acute phase, chest radiograph may be normal.
- Cases of severe thermal injury and massive smoke inhalation may demonstrate tracheobronchial edema (on CT), atelectasis, and progressive air-space consolidation secondary to acute respiratory distress syndrome.
- High-resolution CT is the imaging modality of choice. Subacute and chronic stage weeks or months after exposure may demonstrate mosaic pattern of lung attenuation, air trapping, and centrilobular nodules secondary to constrictive bronchiolitis, as well as bronchiectasis and bronchiolectasis.

✓ Pearls and ✗ Pitfalls

- ✓ The most common complications following inhalation injury are respiratory tract infection and pneumonia.
- ✗ The diagnosis of lung inhalation injury requires the history of exposure because the clinical and imaging manifestations of inhalation injury are nonspecific and can be seen in several different conditions.

Case 86

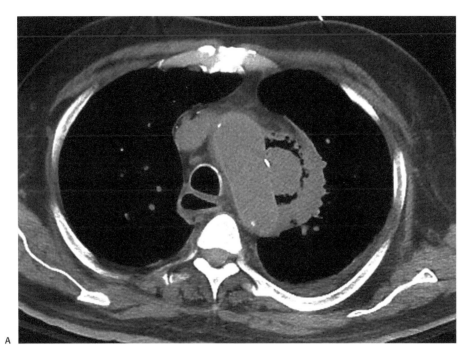

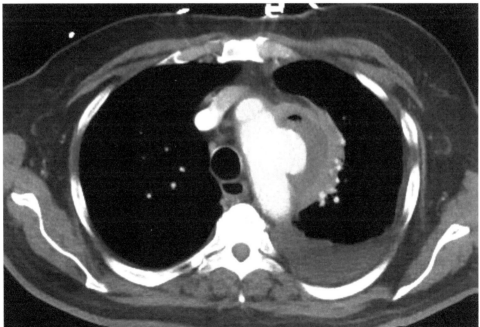

■ **Clinical Presentation**

A 74-year-old man with chest pain and fever.

■ Imaging Findings

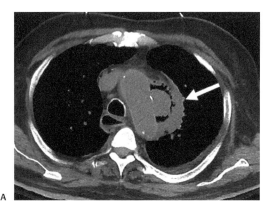 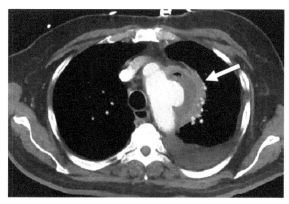

(A) Noncontrast chest CT axial image at the level of the aortic arch demonstrates abnormal bulge on the left-side lateral contour of the aortic arch, within the mediastinum and surrounded by gas (*arrow*). **(B)** Contrast-enhanced chest CT image after 1 week of antibiotics shows the aortic arch saccular aneurysm with a left lateral incomplete fluid rim and a small amount of residual gas (*arrow*). There is a small left-side pleural effusion.

■ Differential Diagnosis

- *Infected ("mycotic") aortic aneurysm.*
- *Atherosclerotic aortic aneurysm.*
- *Posttraumatic aortic pseudoaneurysm.*

■ Essential Facts

- Infected aortic aneurysms can develop from infection of a preexisting aneurysm, usually atherosclerotic, or from a primary aortic wall infection and injury with subsequent aneurysmal dilation.
- The name "mycotic" was coined by Sir William Osler to describe a mushroom-shaped aneurysm in a patient with bacterial endocarditis. His original description did not refer to a fungal etiology. "Mycotic" is confusing because the vast majority of these are bacterial in origin; hence, the term *infected aneurysm* is preferred.
- Infected aneurysms are rare, representing < 3% of all aortic aneurysms; depending on the underlying aortic wall injury, they may represent true aneurysms (involving all three layers of the aortic wall) or false aneurysms (pseudoaneurysms), which represent a contained aortic rupture.
- Risk factors include aortic wall trauma/injury (catheters, medical devices), preexisting infection (endocarditis, pneumonia, spondylodiskitis, urinary tract infection), impaired immune system (diabetes, steroids, chemotherapy, malignancy, AIDS), atherosclerotic disease, and preexisting aneurysm.
- Blood cultures are positive in < 80% of cases, with *Staphylococcus*, *Salmonella*, and *Streptococcus* spp. and gram-negative bacteria (*Pseudomonas*, *Escherichia coli*) being the most common organisms. In endemic areas for tuberculosis infection, *Mycobacterium* tuberculosis is also known to occur, typically from extension of periaortic lymph node infection into the aortic wall.

- Roughly half of infected aortic aneurysms are located in the thoracic aorta, and the other half are located in the abdominal aorta.
- Management of infected aortic aneurysms includes a combination of antibiotics with treatment of the abnormal arterial wall either by surgical debridement of the infected tissue with arterial wall reconstruction or by endovascular therapy.

■ Other Imaging Findings

- Most infected aortic aneurysms are saccular or lobulated in morphology (> 90%); this is different from atherosclerotic aneurysms, which are predominantly fusiform (90%).
- Location also differs because the majority of noninfected atherosclerotic aneurysms are in the infrarenal abdominal aorta, whereas a significant number of infected aortic aneurysms are seen in the thoracic aorta and suprarenal abdominal aorta (70%).
- Imaging findings associated with infected aortic aneurysms include the presence of para-aortic soft tissue mass with a variable degree of rim enhancement, stranding, or fluid (50–70%).
- Vertebral body destruction and paraspinal abscess formation may also occur (5%).
- Infected aortic aneurysms expand more rapidly than atherosclerotic aneurysms.

✓ Pearls and ✗ Pitfalls

- ✓ Aortic wall or periaortic gas is an uncommon finding (7–33%) but is highly suggestive of an infected aneurysm.
- ✗ Differentiation between an infected aortic aneurysm and a noninfected atherosclerotic aneurysm can be difficult. Infected aortic aneurysms often have an atypical morphology and are commonly found in unusual locations for atherosclerotic aneurysm.

Case 87

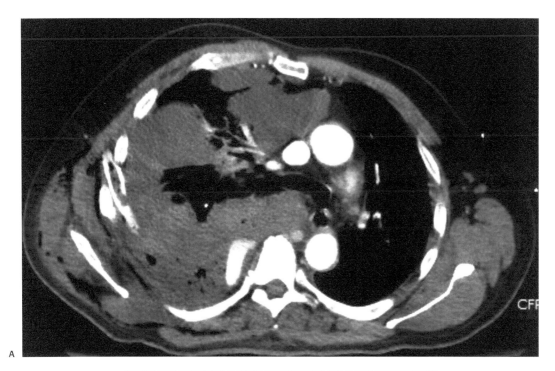

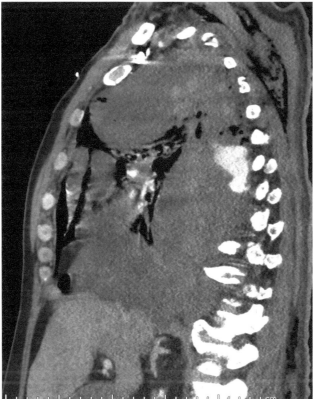

■ Clinical Presentation

A 60-year-old man with shortness of breath, hypotension, and severe chest pain after a motor vehicle accident.

■ Imaging Findings

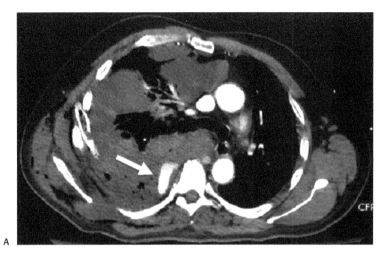 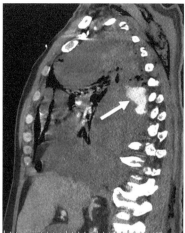

(A, B) Contrast-enhanced chest CT axial **(A)** and coronal **(B)** images. A high-density collection of contrast is appreciated in the posterior right paraspinal region (*arrows*), within a massive right hemothorax.

■ Differential Diagnosis

- ***Hemothorax with active bleeding.***
- *Pleural effusion.*
- *Empyema.*
- *Chylothorax.*

■ Essential Facts

- Thoracic injuries occur in as much as two thirds of polytrauma patients and are responsible for one quarter of all fatalities.
- Hemothorax is a common complication of both blunt thoracic trauma and penetrating injuries and should be suspected in all trauma patients with hemodynamic instability or respiratory insufficiency.
- Approximately 300,000 cases of traumatic hemothorax occur in the United States each year.
- In blunt chest trauma, rib fractures are commonly responsible for bleeding from either an intercostal vessel, internal mammary vessel, or pulmonary parenchymal injury.
- There is correlation between the number of rib fractures and traumatic hemothorax. In the absence of rib fractures, hemothorax is rare, whereas in patients with three or more rib fractures, thoracic bleeding is common.
- Penetrating trauma may cause direct vascular injury without skeletal abnormality.
- Tube thoracostomy is the most common first-line therapeutic approach for the management of an acute hemothorax.
- Surgical intervention after an acute traumatic hemothorax is indicated when initial thoracostomy drainage exceeds 1500 mL, or if there is continuous drainage > 200 mL/h for 4 hours.

■ Other Imaging Findings

- On chest radiograph, blunting of the costophrenic angle may occur with about 200 mL of pleural fluid.
- Layering fluid enough to produce diffuse veil opacity on a supine radiograph usually requires about 1000 mL.
- CT, which has become the standard of care in the evaluation of trauma patients, allows a much better detection and characterization of pleural fluid. In case of doubt, the measurement of fluid density can be useful. On CT imaging, hemothorax density ranges between 35 and 70 Hounsfield units (HU); this is different from serous or nonhemorrhagic effusions, which typically have a fluid density < 15 HU.
- On contrast-enhanced CT image, an arterial blush indicates active bleeding and is considered an indication for urgent intervention.
- Focused assessment with sonography for trauma (FAST) performed at bedside in patients with acute trauma has been reported to have a wide range of sensitivity (12.5–92%) but high specificity (98.4–100%) and good negative predictive value (98%) for the detection of pleural fluid.

✓ Pearls and ✗ Pitfalls

- ✓ In addition to trauma, spontaneous or nontraumatic hemothorax can also occur. Conditions such as aortic dissection; ruptured aortic aneurysm; arteriovenous malformations in the lung; chest wall, pleural, and pulmonary tumors (both primary and metastatic); endometriosis; and bleeding disorders are also known to be associated with spontaneous thoracic bleeding.
- ✗ Not all hemorrhagic fluid collections represent a hemothorax. Pleural fluid will appear hemorrhagic with a hematocrit as low as 5%. A hemothorax should have a hematocrit that is at least 50% of the patient's blood hematocrit.

Case 88

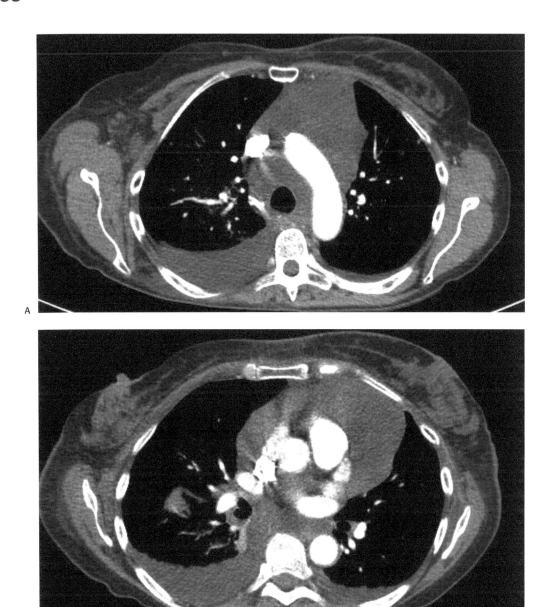

■ Clinical Presentation

A 57-year-old woman with recurrent right-side pleural effusion and chronic low-density mediastinal mass.

■ Imaging Findings

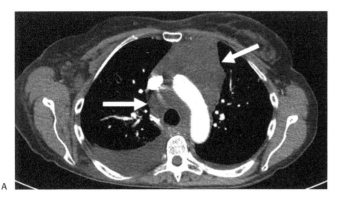 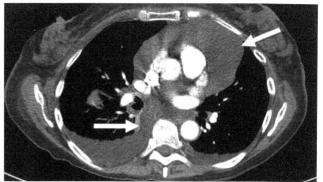

(A, B) Contrast-enhanced CT images of the chest: axial images at the aortic arch (A) and pulmonary trunk (B). A water-density mass is visualized in the anterior, middle, and posterior mediastinum (*arrows*), associated with low-density bilateral pleural effusions.

■ Differential Diagnosis

- *Mediastinal lymphangioma.*
- *Thymic cyst.*
- *Foregut duplication cyst.*
- *Pleuropericardial cyst.*
- *Dermoid tumor.*

■ Essential Facts

- Lymphangiomas are rare benign lesions of lymphatic origin that represent < 5% of all mediastinal tumors.
- According to their histologic appearance, lymphangiomas are classified as simple or capillary lymphangioma, cystic lymphangioma, and cavernous lymphangioma.
- The exact etiology of lymphangiomas is not well known, but they are believed to represent a congenital malformation of the lymphatic system with sequestration of embryonal lymphatic remnants that fail to communicate with the normal lymphatic tissue.
- Most lymphangiomas involve the neck (75%) and axilla or chest wall (20%), with only a few extending to the mediastinum (5–10%).
- The majority of lymphangiomas in children present in the first 2 years of life.
- Most mediastinal lymphangiomas in adults are asymptomatic. Occasional mass effect on adjacent structures may manifest as vocal cord paralysis, stridor, pain, superior vena cava syndrome, or upper extremity edema or paresthesia.
- Uncommon complications include infection, rupture, and hemorrhage.
- Chromosomal and genetic abnormalities such as Turner syndrome, Down syndrome (trisomy 21), and trisomy 13 and 18 have a higher incidence of lymphangiomas.

- In symptomatic patients, surgical resection is commonly performed, with significant recurrence (10–50%), in particular after incomplete resection. Additional treatments include radiation therapy, chemotherapy, and sclerotherapy with percutaneous injection of sclerosing agents, with variable results.

■ Other Imaging Findings

- Most common imaging feature of mediastinal lymphangioma is a thin-walled, nonenhancing, well-circumscribed water-density mass, modeling around adjacent structures with no infiltrative changes and usually with no significant mass effect.
- The mass may appear unilocular or septated and multilocular in appearance, in which case septal enhancement may occur.
- Mediastinal lymphangiomas can involve any mediastinal compartment, but the anterior, superior, and middle mediastinum is the most common presentation. The pericardium and pleura can also be involved.

✓ Pearls and ✗ Pitfalls

- ✓ Cystic lymphangiomas, also referred to as hygromas or cystic hygromas, are the most common type of lymphangioma.
- ✗ Clinical and imaging manifestations of lymphatic disorders can be very complex and misleading when they present as part of lymphangiectasis, diffuse lymphangiomatosis, or lymphatic dysplasia syndrome. In such cases, pleural effusion and chylothorax and pericardial effusion are common manifestations.

Case 89

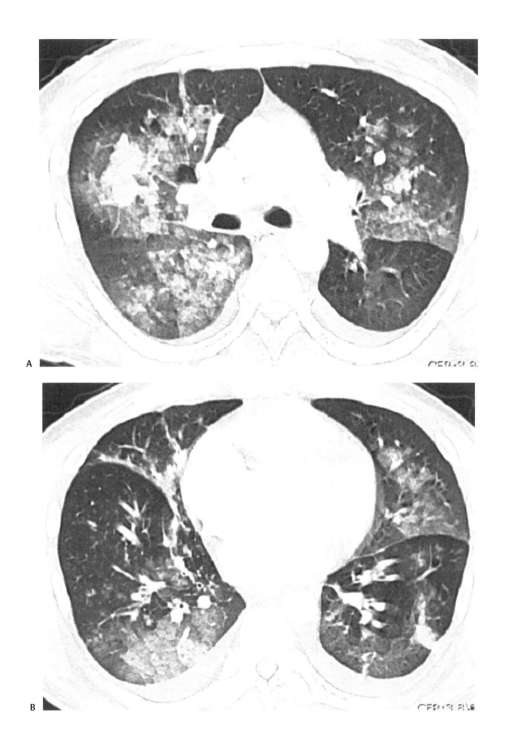

■ Clinical Presentation

Hypoxemia in a 47-year-old woman with immunoglobulin A gammopathy.

■ **Imaging Findings**

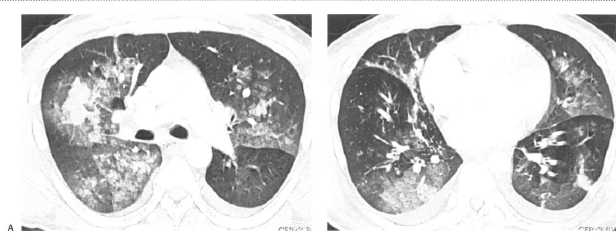

(A, B) Contrast-enhanced CT axial images with lung window settings show multifocal ground-glass opacities with patchy areas of denser consolidation bilaterally with posteriorly layering pleural effusions.

■ **Differential Diagnosis**

- ***Amyloidosis.***
- *Bronchopneumonia.*
- *Malignancy.*
- *Alveolar hemorrhage.*

■ **Essential Facts**

- Amyloidosis represents a heterogeneous group of diseases characterized by abnormal accumulation of extracellular amyloid, an insoluble fibrillary protein aggregate that resists degradation by macrophages.
- There are several clinical and molecular forms of amyloidosis. The two most common types are light-chain (AL) amyloidosis and amyloid A (AA) amyloidosis.
- AL amyloidosis is considered a B-cell dyscrasia in which the abnormal protein is derived from light chain immunoglobulin fragments; it can be associated with multiple myeloma, B-cell lymphoma, or Waldenström macroglobulinemia.
- AL amyloidosis is a systemic disease of older adults, which can present with single organ or multiorgan involvement.
- AA amyloidosis often results from association with a chronic inflammatory or infectious condition (rheumatoid arthritis, Crohn's disease, Sjögren syndrome, tuberculosis, osteomyelitis, leprosy, familial Mediterranean fever) or malignancy (renal cell carcinoma, Hodgkin disease).
- The vast majority of systemic amyloidosis and clinically significant respiratory amyloidosis are due to the AL form (> 90%).
- Thoracic amyloidosis can affect any structure including lung parenchyma, lymph nodes, blood vessels, pleura, heart, and pericardium. Amyloidosis in the lung can appear in three distinct forms: diffuse alveolar-septal amyloidosis, nodular pulmonary amyloidosis, or tracheobronchial amyloidosis.

- Treatment of systemic AL amyloidosis aims to control the underlying plasma cell dyscrasia with chemotherapy and/or hematopoietic stem cell transplantation. Localized amyloidosis usually does not require systemic therapy, and specific situations may benefit from surgical resection.

■ **Other Imaging Findings**

- Tracheobronchial amyloidosis manifests as nodular or diffuse plaque formation with wall thickening and luminal narrowing, which may result in atelectasis and air trapping.
- Nodular pulmonary form presents as single or multiple lobulated or spiculated pulmonary nodules, which commonly calcify (50%). Larger lesions may present with a masslike appearance.
- The diffuse alveolar-septal disease is characterized by a diffuse interstitial process with reticular opacities from interlobular septal thickening, micronodules, ground-glass opacification, and patchy focal areas of denser opacification. Associated hilar and mediastinal lymphadenopathy are common in AL systemic amyloidosis (75%). Affected lymph nodes may demonstrate a significant degree of calcification.
- In some cases, a combination of systemic and localized features may occur.
- Nodular amyloid deposits associated with lung cysts are most commonly seen in patients with Sjögren syndrome.

✓ **Pearls and** ✗ **Pitfalls**

✓ The heart can be affected in several different types of amyloidosis; in particular in the AL systemic disease and in ATTR (transthyretin) or senile form, with significant morbidity and mortality.

✗ Solitary masslike amyloidoma mimicking malignancy is a common presentation of pulmonary amyloidosis (60%).

Case 90

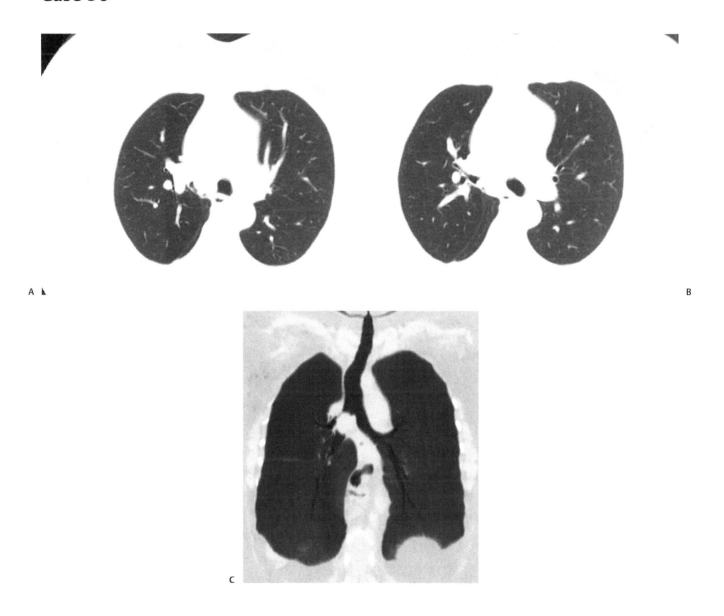

Clinical Presentation

A 47-year-old woman with a history of breast cancer and recent onset of cough and shortness of breath.

■ Imaging Findings

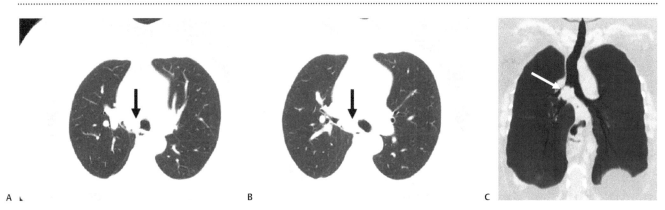

(A–C) Contrast-enhanced chest CT lung window settings axial images **(A, B)** and minimum intensity projection coronal reconstruction image **(C)** show a lobulated soft tissue density endobronchial mass (*arrows*) with complete obstruction of the right mainstem bronchus.

■ Differential Diagnosis

- ***Bronchial metastasis.***
- *Bronchial carcinoid.*
- *Lung cancer.*
- *Foreign body.*

■ Essential Facts

- The lungs are the most common site of distant metastatic disease from extrapulmonary malignancy.
- Tracheobronchial metastasis is equally distributed between the right and left lung, with the majority located in a bronchus (> 90%) and only a few in the trachea (5%).
- The occurrence of bronchial metastases from extrapulmonary malignancy is rare, although the exact incidence is unknown. Metastatic disease represents 2 to 4% of all biopsies in patients with endobronchial tumors.
- A significant number of cases are asymptomatic (25–50%) and incidentally found in staging follow-up CT images in cancer patients. Symptomatic patients commonly manifest with dyspnea, cough and hemoptysis, or postobstructive infection.
- Except for brain tumors (gliomas), virtually all malignant solid tumors, epithelial and mesenchymal, have the capability of producing endobronchial metastases.
- Most common extrapulmonary tumors that present with an endobronchial metastasis include breast cancer (30%), colorectal cancer (25%), renal cell carcinoma (14%), gastric cancer (6%), prostate cancer (4.5%), and melanoma (4.5%).
- Nearly 90% of endobronchial metastases are diagnosed after the originating primary tumor has been identified (metachronous).
- In a minority of cases, the endobronchial metastasis is either synchronous with the primary tumor or diagnosed before (10%).

- Immunohistochemistry may be needed to differentiate between a primary endobronchial tumor and a metastatic deposit.
- Prognosis is generally poor, with average survival between 1 and 2 years in most series.
- Treatment options for endobronchial metastases include surgery, external radiation therapy, chemotherapy, brachytherapy, endobronchial stent, and laser.

■ Other Imaging Findings

- Careful evaluation of the airway patency on axial images and multiplanar reconstructions is critical for the diagnosis of endobronchial lesions.
- On CT, a hilar mass ipsilateral to the endobronchial metastasis is a relatively uncommon imaging finding (16%). Nevertheless, imaging exams are almost always abnormal, demonstrating multiple pulmonary nodules (53%), mediastinal lymphadenopathy (47%), unilateral peripheral lung mass (30%), atelectasis (28%), and/or pleural effusion (23%).

✓ Pearls and ✗ Pitfalls

✓ Most endobronchial metastases are diagnosed late, on average about 4 years after the diagnosis of the primary malignancy.

✗ The differentiation between a primary lung cancer and an endobronchial metastasis can be very difficult. In patients with a past medical history of malignancy, the possibility of metastatic disease should be considered in the presence of any endobronchial tumor. This differentiation is significant because treatment possibilities may be different.

Case 91

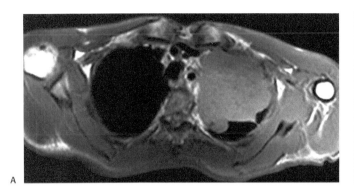

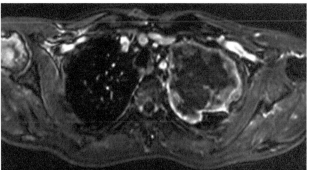

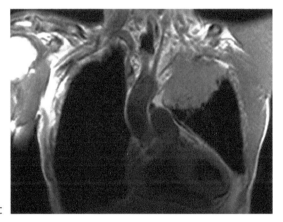

■ Clinical Presentation

A 47-year-old man with left shoulder pain.

■ **Imaging Findings**

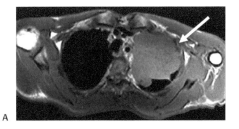 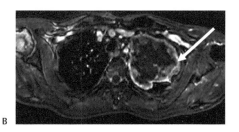 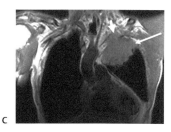

(A–C) Chest MR images: T1-weighted axial image **(A)**, T1-weighted fat-suppressed image after contrast injection **(B)**, and coronal T1-weighted image **(C)**. Axial and coronal images show a large left upper lobe mass (*long arrows*), isointense to muscle on T1-weighted images, and with peripheral contrast enhancement. The coronal image demonstrates left apical chest wall invasion (*short arrow*).

■ **Differential Diagnosis**

- ***Lung cancer with chest wall invasion.***
- *Sarcoma.*
- *Lymphoma.*
- *Mesothelioma.*

■ **Essential Facts**

- Lung cancer remains as the most common cancer worldwide, with more than 1.8 million new cases per year.
- Despite significant improvement in early diagnosis, prevention, and treatment, lung cancer remains as the most common cause of cancer-related deaths in the United States, with about 1.6 million annual deaths.
- Multidetector CT (MDCT) and 18-fluorodeoxyglucose–positron emission tomography (^{18}FDG-PET) are the preferred imaging modalities used for lung cancer staging and treatment planning.
- The routine use of MRI of the chest is not currently recommended for lung cancer staging, but it is considered useful when there is concern for chest wall or brachial plexus invasion in patients with superior sulcus tumors.
- In selective cases, MRI in lung cancer patients may also help in the evaluation of mediastinal invasion, including heart, pericardium, and great vessels, and in the examination of lymph nodes.
- Superior sulcus (Pancoast) tumors, which represent a special group of lung cancer located in the apex of the lung, account about 5% of all lung carcinomas, commonly extend through the soft tissues, and by definition are either T3 or T4 tumors.
- Potentially resectable Pancoast tumors are initially treated with induction chemoradiation therapy, after which the possibility of complete tumor resection is considered.
- Invasion of the brachial plexus above the T1 nerve, destruction of > 50% of a vertebral body, N2 or N3 lymph node involvement, and distant metastatic disease are considered exclusion criteria for surgical resection.

■ **Other Imaging Findings**

- MR and MR angiography of the thoracic inlet have demonstrated better accuracy than CT for the detection of locoregional extension, including parietal pleura, extrapleural fat, vertebral body, spinal canal, brachial plexus, and vascular invasion.
- MR is also better than CT for the differentiation between tumor and adjacent atelectasis, pneumonia, and postradiation changes.

✓ **Pearls and ✗ Pitfalls**

- ✓ Advantages of MRI over CT in the evaluation of cardiothoracic pathology include lack of ionizing radiation, better contrast resolution, and capability for vascular examination without contrast injection.
- ✗ In addition to some absolute contraindications for MR (metallic foreign body near critical structure, ferromagnetic vascular clip), and relative contraindications (several medical devices like pacemaker or automated implantable cardioverter defibrillator, cochlear implants, etc.), MR examination has some disadvantages over CT, including limited detection of calcification, limited use in claustrophobic patients, longer examination time, higher cost, and more limited availability.

Case 92

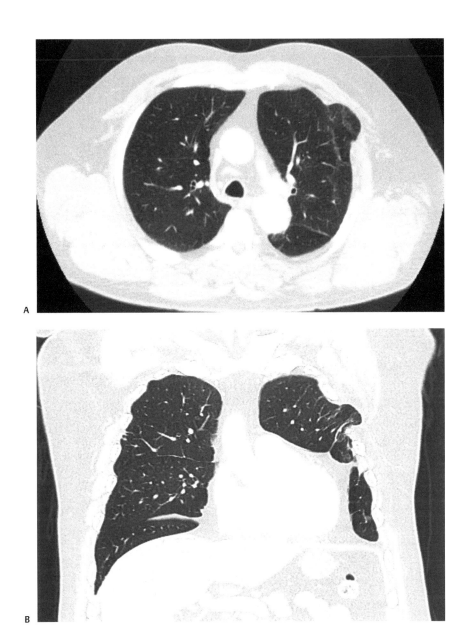

■ Clinical Presentation

A 45-year-old man with left-side chest pain.

■ Imaging Findings

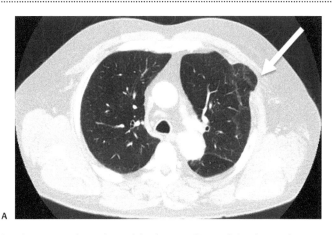 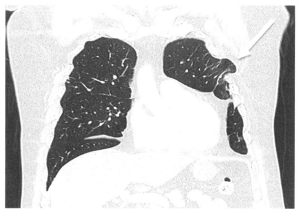

(A, B) Contrast-enhanced CTs of the chest: axial image **(A)** and coronal reconstruction with lung window settings **(B)**. Images show abnormal protrusion of lung parenchyma through a left upper intercostal space (*arrows*). Irregular appearance of a left-side rib next to the herniated lung is a sequela of a remote surgery.

■ Differential Diagnosis

- ***Acquired postsurgical lung hernia.***
- *Acquired posttraumatic lung hernia.*
- *Acquired pathological lung hernia.*
- *Congenital lung hernia.*

■ Essential Facts

- A lung hernia consists of an abnormal protrusion of pulmonary tissue and pleura beyond the confines of the thoracic cavity or chest wall.
- Lung hernias can be classified according to their location (cervical or apical, thoracic, or diaphragmatic) and cause (congenital or acquired).
- The majority of lung hernias are acquired and result from weakness in the chest wall, commonly at the level of an intercostal space; from trauma; from surgery; or (rarely) from a primary lesion in the chest wall (e.g., infection, tumor), cases of which are classified as pathologic lung hernias.
- Acquired hernias may also develop spontaneously with increased intrathoracic pressure in patients with cough or chronic obstructive pulmonary disease. They more commonly present in the apical region and result from the combination of increased intrathoracic pressure and a defect in Sibson's fascia or aponeurosis (membrane suprapleuralis), which is an extension and reinforcement of the endothoracic fascia.
- Clinically, lung hernias may present as a painful lump in the chest wall or may be asymptomatic. Clinical presentation may be acute or delayed months or years after surgery or trauma.
- Incarceration and strangulation may occur, in particular when herniation occurs through a small chest wall defect.

- Management of lung hernias depends on the type of hernia, clinical presentation, and size of the defect. Asymptomatic lung hernias can be observed and followed. Symptomatic hernias in particular, when the chest wall defect is small, are commonly repaired with surgical correction of the chest wall to prevent incarceration and ischemia/necrosis of the herniated lung.

■ Other Imaging Findings

- Chest radiographs may reveal lucency that is characteristic of lung parenchyma projecting into the bony thorax.
- Multidetector CT with multiplanar reconstruction is the preferred imaging modality for the diagnosis and evaluation of lung hernias, demonstrating the abnormal protrusion of lung parenchyma through the chest wall.
- Besides the lung parenchyma herniation, CT often shows abnormal widening of the intercostal space with splaying of the adjacent ribs.

✓ Pearls and ✗ Pitfalls

- ✓ Radiographs or CT images obtained during Valsalva maneuver or during expiration (increased intrathoracic pressure) may show an increase in the size and conspicuity of the herniated lung.
- ✗ In patients with severe pulmonary emphysema, abnormal bulging of the lung through the intercostal space may occur without herniation, usually in a bilateral, symmetrical, and multifocal distribution more pronounced in the midthoracic region.

Case 93

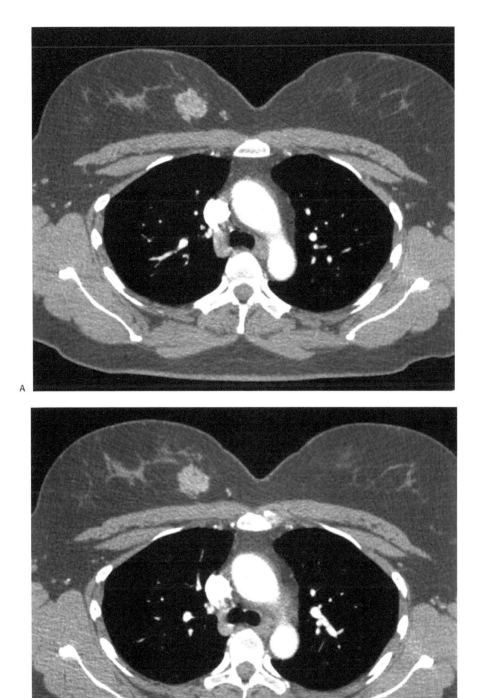

A

B

■ Clinical Presentation

A 44-year-old woman with a history of arterial hypertension who has atypical chest pain. CT ordered to rule out aortic dissection.

■ Imaging Findings

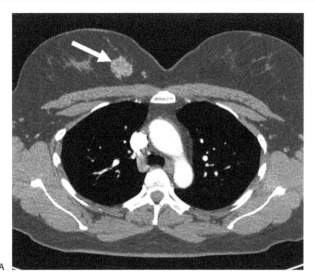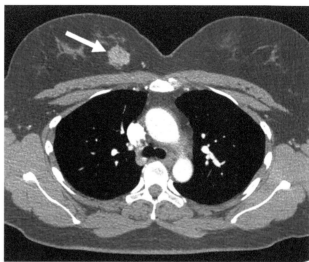

A   B

(**A, B**) Contrast-enhanced CT images of the chest. Axial images at two contiguous levels demonstrate a soft tissue density round mass in the medial aspect of the right breast (*arrows*).

■ Differential Diagnosis

- ***Breast cancer.***
- *Fibroadenoma.*
- *Fibroadenolipoma.*

■ Essential Facts

- Breast cancer is the most common malignancy affecting women in the Western world, with invasive ductal carcinoma being the most common type (> 80%).
- A significant number of breast lesions are detected in asymptomatic patients through screening mammograms.
- Abnormal breast lesions are also identified incidentally on cross-sectional imaging studies (CT, positron emission tomography–CT, MR) for pathologies other than breast.
- During the last decade, there has been a dramatic increase in the utilization of CT in the emergency setting, both in trauma and nontrauma patients.
- In adult female patients, incidental breast lesions are found in 1 to 8% of all chest CT scans obtained for nonmammary indication.
- Roughly one third of all incidental breast masses detected on CT are malignant.
- Tissue diagnosis of this lesion is required to determine the most appropriate treatment option (e.g., surgery, chemotherapy, radiation therapy, hormonal therapy).
- Treatment plans depend on numerous variables such as the biology of the tumor, stage, genomic markers, genetic mutations, and the patient's age.

■ Other Imaging Findings

- Predictive features of breast malignancy on incidental breast lesions include spiculated irregular margin, irregular shape, lobulated contour, and contrast enhancement.
- Pattern of contrast enhancement of breast cancer on CT imaging can be variable and may appear as early arterial enhancement, peripheral rim enhancement, or homogeneous or heterogeneous contrast uptake with or without enhancing internal septations.
- Oval-shape or ellipsoid breast lesions are more likely to be benign.

✓ Pearls and ✗ Pitfalls

- ✓ On CT imaging of incidental breast lesions, the imaging features that have the highest positive predictive value for malignancy are a spiculated margin (76–100%) and irregular shape (58–99%).
- ✗ Breast calcification on CT has a low positive predictive value for malignancy. Nearly all breast calcifications identified on CT images are benign.

Case 94

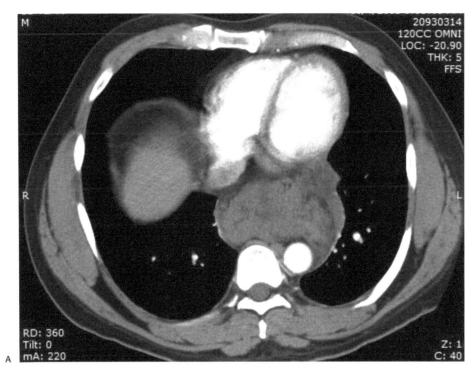

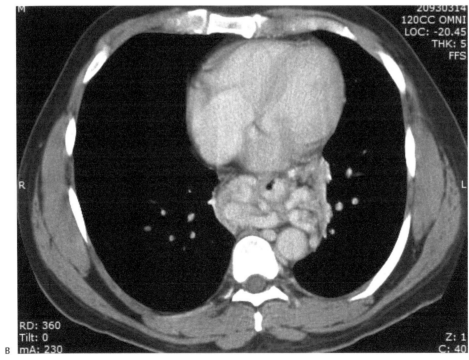

■ Clinical Presentation

A 55-year-old man with hematemesis.

■ Imaging Findings

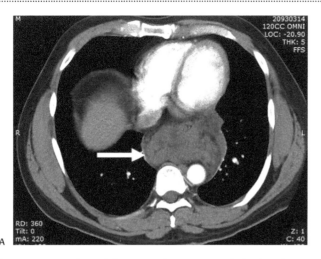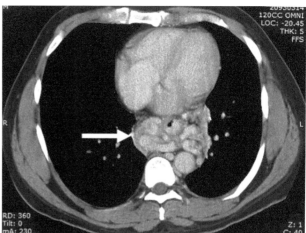

(**A, B**) Contrast-enhanced chest CT axial images at similar levels in the same patient during arterial (**A**) and delayed phase (**B**) show numerous gradually enhancing elongated tortuous vessels surrounding the esophagus (*arrows*).

■ Differential Diagnosis

- ***Esophageal varices.***
- *Hypervascular mediastinal tumor.*
- *Arteriovenous malformation.*

■ Essential Facts

- Esophageal and paraesophageal varices represent abnormally dilated native veins that serve as collateral circulation in case of vascular obstruction or increased resistance in the portal venous system or vena cava obstruction.
- Both are seen in patients with portal hypertension, but bleeding is more likely to occur from esophageal than from paraesophageal varices.
- The prevalence of esophageal varices in patients with cirrhosis is as high as 90%, with bleeding at a rate as high as 30% per year.
- Patients with cirrhosis and portal hypertension are at increased risk for variceal hemorrhage with significant morbidity and mortality.
- Most esophageal varices develop in the lower third of the esophagus and drain into the azygos or hemiazygos venous system.
- Mortality associated with bleeding esophageal varices is as high as 35% at 3 months and 70% at 2 years.
- Small (< 3 mm) esophageal varices detected on CT images are less likely to produce esophageal bleeding. In contrast, large varices (> 5 mm) more likely manifest with bleeding episodes.
- Treatment includes endoscopic band ligation, nonselective β blockers, and transjugular intrahepatic portosystemic shunt.

■ Other Imaging Findings

- The typical CT appearance of esophageal varices is as enhancing nodular thickening of the esophageal wall, whereas paraesophageal varices present as a network of enhancing tubular or serpentine veins surrounding the esophagus, anterior to the aorta and spine, with dilated azygos/hemiazygos vein, vertebral plexus, and coronary (or left gastric) vein.
- Contrast-enhanced CT, including arterial and portal-phase images, has a high sensitivity (> 90%) for the detection of large, clinically significant esophageal varices, and moderate sensitivity (53–60%) for the detection of small varices, with an overall sensitivity around 70%.
- Distension of the distal esophagus with air during contrast-enhanced CT (CT esophagography) improves visualization of esophageal varices.

✓ Pearls and ✗ Pitfalls

- ✓ CT is a good noninvasive imaging tool for the diagnosis of esophageal varices in patients with cirrhosis. Endoscopy is usually recommended for the screening of all patients with cirrhosis, but it is invasive, requires sedation, and is expensive.
- ✗ The differentiation of esophageal and paraesophageal varices on CT can be difficult. Esophageal varices present as dilated subepithelial and submucosal vessels within the esophageal wall, whereas paraesophageal varices are juxtaposed to the outer wall of the esophagus, beyond the adventitia.

Case 95

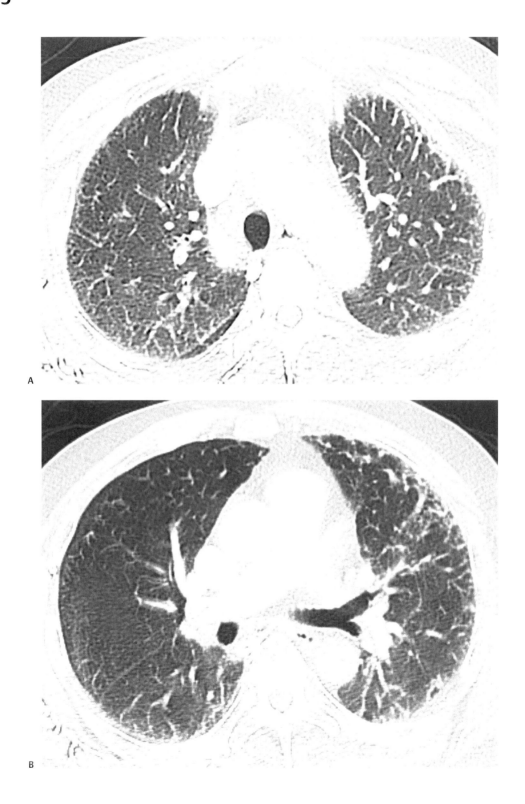

A

B

■ Clinical Presentation

A 53-year-old man with a history of cirrhosis who has shortness of breath and hypoxemia.

■ Imaging Findings

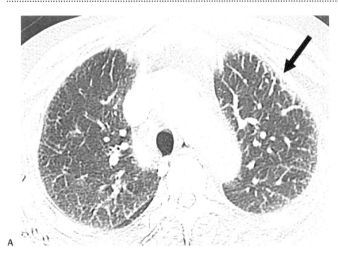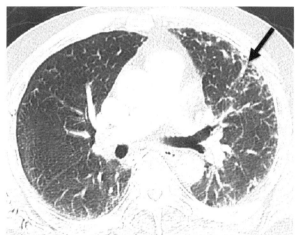

(A, B) Contrast-enhanced chest CT images. Axial images with lung window settings at two different levels show abnormally prominent vessels in the periphery and subpleural region of the lungs, more pronounced in the left side (*arrows*).

■ Differential Diagnosis

- ***Hepatopulmonary syndrome.***
- *Hereditary hemorrhagic telangiectasia (Rendu–Osler–Weber syndrome).*
- *Pulmonary edema.*
- *Lymphangitic carcinomatosis.*

■ Essential Facts

- The hepatopulmonary syndrome consists of a clinical triad of liver disease, pulmonary vascular dilation, and abnormal oxygenation. It is characterized by abnormal arterial oxygenation secondary to abnormal pulmonary vascular dilation, mainly associated with liver cirrhosis or liver dysfunction.
- The most common clinical manifestation of hepatopulmonary syndrome is dyspnea.
- Most cases of hepatopulmonary syndrome are associated with cirrhotic or noncirrhotic portal hypertension, but other acute and chronic liver disease may also manifest with dilation of the pulmonary vasculature and hypoxemia.
- Hepatopulmonary syndrome has been reported in as much as 20% of liver transplant candidates.
- There is no correlation between the severity of hepatopulmonary syndrome and the severity of liver disease, but the presence of hepatopulmonary syndrome worsens the prognosis of patients with cirrhosis.
- On histopathology, the unique feature of hepatopulmonary syndrome is gross dilation of pulmonary capillary vessels with absolute increase in the number of dilated vessels, pleural pulmonary arteriovenous communications, and portopulmonary venous anastomoses.

- A combination of an increased serum concentration of many circulating mediators and increased angiogenesis is likely the responsible mechanism.
- The only effective treatment is liver transplantation, because no other effective medical or pharmacologic treatment is available. Supplemental oxygen therapy is commonly used.

■ Other Imaging Findings

- Intrapulmonary arteriovenous shunting can be demonstrated with echocardiography or with nuclear medicine.
- Contrast-enhanced transthoracic echo with microbubbles demonstrates early opacification of the left ventricle within three to six cardiac contractions after right atrial opacification.
- Injection of technetium-99m–labeled macroaggregated albumin in a peripheral vein for lung perfusion scanning will reveal increased extrapulmonary uptake (brain, kidneys).
- CT may demonstrate increased number and caliber of peripheral pulmonary vessels in the subpleural surface of the lungs that do not taper normally.

✓ Pearls and ✗ Pitfalls

- ✓ Contrast-enhanced echocardiography is the imaging modality of choice for the diagnosis of hepatopulmonary syndrome.
- ✗ Regarding the appearance of microbubbles in the left atrium or left ventricle immediately after reaching the right atrium, the most likely diagnosis is an intracardiac shunt rather than hepatopulmonary syndrome.

Case 96

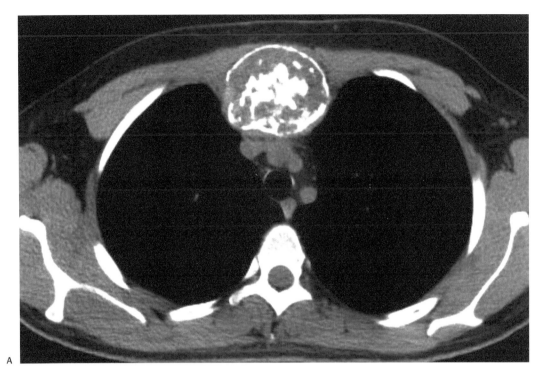

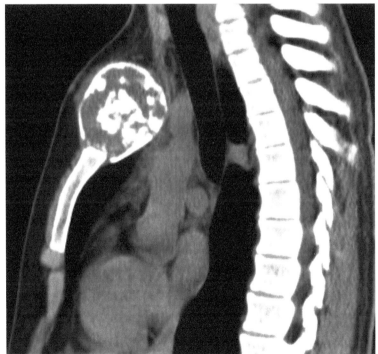

■ Clinical Presentation

A 29-year-old man with painful anterior chest wall bump.

■ Imaging Findings

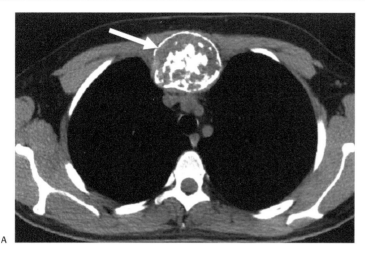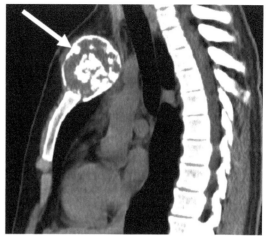

(A, B) Noncontrast chest CT images: axial image **(A)** and midline sagittal reconstruction image with soft tissue window settings **(B)**. Both images reveal an expansile lesion in the sternal manubrium with soft tissue and internal irregular calcified densities (*arrows*).

■ Differential Diagnosis

- ***Chondrosarcoma.***
- *Metastasis.*
- *Lymphoma.*
- *Osteosarcoma.*
- *Ewing sarcoma.*

■ Essential Facts

- Metastatic disease is the most common sternal tumor. The most common primary tumors to present with sternal metastatic lesions are breast and lung cancer, followed by thyroid, kidney, colon, and lymphomas.
- Primary tumors of the sternum are rare and represent around 1% of all primary bone tumors. The majority of these are malignant, and chondrosarcoma is the most common type (30–50%).
- Other primary malignant tumors of the sternum include plasmacytomas, lymphomas, osteosarcomas, Ewing sarcoma, and fibrosarcoma.
- Sternal chondrosarcomas usually present in adults, around the 5th decade of life, as an initially indolent mass in the anterior chest wall. Some patients feel pain as the initial manifestation before a palpable mass becomes evident.
- Although these tumors grow slowly, they may invade locally adjacent structures and metastasize to distant organs. Recurrence rate after surgical resection is not rare, particularly after incomplete excision.

- Overall survival in patients with sternal chondrosarcoma is 66% at 5 years.
- Surgical resection (radical en bloc excision) is the preferred method of treatment because chondrosarcomas do not respond to radiotherapy or chemotherapy. Radical surgical treatment requires chest wall reconstruction to provide stability to the chest and avoid flail chest and prevent deformity.

■ Other Imaging Findings

- Lateral chest radiograph may occasionally demonstrate a sternal mass. On CT, the characteristic imaging presentation is as an expansile sternal lesion with internal stipple calcification or mineralized chondroid matrix, which may appear as ringlike or arclike calcified densities.
- On MR, the tumor has a low signal on T1-weighted images and a high signal on T2-weighted sequences, with patchy enhancement after contrast administration.

✓ Pearls and ✗ Pitfalls

- ✓ All tumors of the sternum should be regarded as malignant until proven otherwise.
- ✗ Anterior chest wall chondrosarcomas do not always arise from the sternum. In some series, the origin from the anterior chondroid segment of a rib is three times more common than origin from the sternum.

Case 97

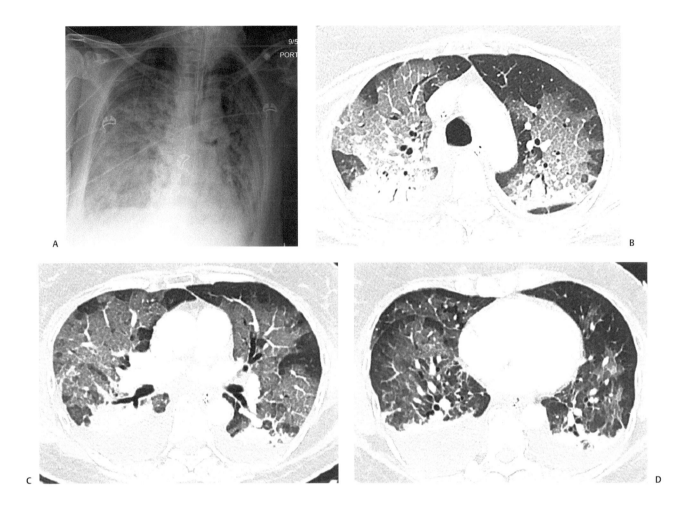

■ Clinical Presentation
··

Worsening hypoxemia and respiratory distress in a 49-year-old woman with a pelvic abscess and sepsis.

■ Imaging Findings

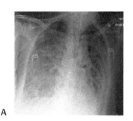 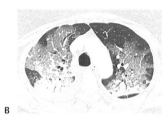 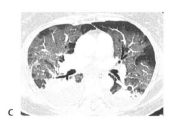 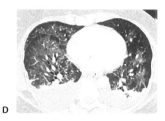

(A) Portable chest radiograph, anteroposterior view, shows extensive alveolar parenchymal opacities with air-space consolidation throughout the bilateral lungs. **(B–D)** Contract-enhanced chest CT images. Axial images with lung window settings at three different levels show predominantly ground-glass opacities throughout the bilateral lungs. There are also bilateral posteriorly layering pleural effusions.

■ Differential Diagnosis

- ***Acute respiratory distress syndrome.***
- *Cardiogenic pulmonary edema.*
- *Acute interstitial pneumonia.*
- *Diffuse alveolar hemorrhage.*

■ Essential Facts

- Acute respiratory distress syndrome (ARDS) is a form of acute diffuse inflammatory alveolar lung injury characterized by increased permeability of the alveolar-capillary membrane, resulting in pulmonary edema with influx fluid and proteins into the alveoli and interstitium, causing impaired gas exchange with hypoxemia (Pao_2:$Fio_2 \leq 200$ mm Hg).
- The diagnosis of ARDS is based on the onset of hypoxemia and abnormal bilateral opacities seen on chest radiographs or chest CT within 1 week of a known risk factor, in a patient with respiratory failure not fully explained by fluid overload or heart failure.
- ARDS is classified into three levels (mild, moderate, or severe) according to the severity of gas-exchange abnormality.
- ARDS is common, with incidence of 80 cases/y/100,000 population, and represents 10% of all admissions to the intensive care unit; it has a mortality rate that remains high, around 50%.
- The precipitating conditions can be pulmonary or extrapulmonary. The more common pulmonary abnormalities responsible for ARDS include pneumonia, aspiration, inhalational injury, trauma (pulmonary contusion), near drowning, and vasculitis. Extrapulmonary conditions include sepsis, noncardiogenic shock, polytrauma, extensive burns, pancreatitis, transfusion, and drugs.
- On histopathology, the hallmark of ARDS is diffuse alveolar damage (DAD) that evolves over a few weeks from an acute exudative phase (1–7 days), to a proliferative intermediate phase (8–14 days), and finally into a chronic fibrotic late phase (> 15 days).
- Management includes mechanical ventilation and support measures.

■ Other Imaging Findings

- The acute exudative phase (initial 48 hours) imaging exams may be normal or may simply demonstrate the underlying pathology (e.g., pneumonia) in cases of pulmonary ARDS.
- After 48 to 72 hours, as the patient clinically deteriorates, bilateral patchy alveolar and interstitial opacities ("crazy paving") and focal consolidation develop, which may progress to diffuse bilateral consolidation.
- Distribution is nonhomogeneous, usually with a gravitational ventrodorsal gradient with denser air-space disease and consolidation in the dependent regions, and more ground-glass densities and better aeration in the nondependent lung.
- Associated pleural effusion is common. Lung cyst may develop, often in patients with mechanical ventilation. Bronchial dilation within areas of ground-glass opacification is also observed in ARDS, which can be reversible.
- Many surviving patients (> 70%) have residual abnormalities on CT, including persistent ground-glass densities, reticulation, air cysts, and in some cases frank interstitial pulmonary fibrosis with traction bronchiectasis.

✓ Pearls and ✗ Pitfalls

✓ A symmetrical pattern and distribution of parenchymal abnormalities on CT between the right and left lung favor an extrapulmonary ARDS. An asymmetrical pattern with, for example, a unilateral focal consolidation or a nondependent consolidation favors pulmonary ARDS.

✗ ARDS and acute interstitial pneumonia (AIP) are not equivalent conditions. Both are similar in their clinical manifestations (hypoxia and respiratory failure) and histopathology (DAD), but they differ in pathophysiology. The majority of cases of ARDS are secondary to a known condition, whereas AIP is idiopathic. Only a minority of ARDS patients have AIP. AIP can be considered an idiopathic form of ARDS.

Case 98

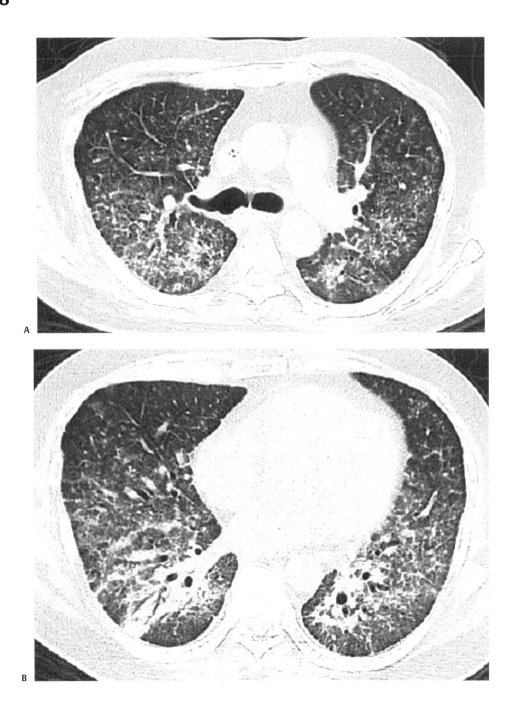

■ Clinical Presentation

A 47-year-old man who is malnourished and immunosuppressed, with eosinophilia, respiratory insufficiency, petechia, purpura, and subcutaneous nodules.

■ **Imaging Findings**

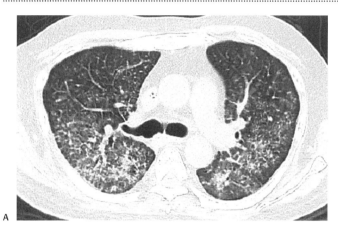 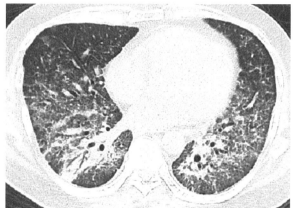

A   B

(A, B) Noncontrast chest CT images. Lung window setting axial images at two different levels demonstrate a complex imaging pattern with reticular and nodular opacities with patchy areas of ground-glass and air-space consolidation bilaterally.

■ **Differential Diagnosis**

- ***Strongyloides hyperinfection.***
- *Bronchopneumonia.*
- *Pulmonary edema.*

■ **Essential Facts**

- Strongyloidiasis, the most important human nematode infection in the United States, is caused by the soil-dwelling helminth *Strongyloides stercoralis*, which is endemic in the Southeastern part of the country (Appalachian Mountains region) and is also highly prevalent in tropical and subtropical regions of the world.
- Strongyloidiasis is caused by the female nematode, which enters the venous system through the skin and migrates to the lungs and later to the gastrointestinal tract of the infected host.
- Hyperinfection syndrome and disseminated disease usually result as a complication of immunosuppression caused by HIV or human T-cell lymphotropic virus type 1 infection, administration of corticosteroids, organ transplantation, chemotherapy, hematologic malignancies, chronic infection, or malnutrition.
- In patients with impaired cell-mediated immunity, *S. stercoralis* nematodes have the ability to produce autoinfection, either by enteral circulation (endoautoinfection) or from the perianal skin (exoautoinfection), with a massive multiplication and migration of infective larvae.
- Hyperinfection syndrome can occur in up to 2.5% of infected patients.

- Pulmonary strongyloidiasis is one of the most important signs of disseminated disease, which can also affect the liver, kidneys, heart, brain, skin, and other organs.
- Eosinophilia in blood (> 5% eosinophils) is commonly seen in infected patients (> 80%).
- The mortality from *S. stercoralis* hyperinfection and disseminated disease can be very high (up to 87%).
- Treatment involves antiparasitic drugs (e.g., ivermectin, albendazole, mebendazole, thiabendazole).

■ **Other Imaging Findings**

- Multifocal nodular or patchy air-space opacities that may progress to dense consolidation.
- Ground-glass opacities in areas with associated alveolar hemorrhage.

✓ **Pearls and ✗ Pitfalls**

✓ Any immunosuppressed patient with eosinophilia who has visited tropical or subtropical regions of the world or areas of the United States endemic for *S. stercoralis* and who presents with signs of systemic disease, including multifocal pulmonary abnormalities, should be evaluated for the possibility of strongyloidiasis.

✗ The diagnosis of strongyloidiasis can be difficult. Sensitivity of available tests such as stool examination (< 50% sensitivity) and enzyme-linked immunosorbent assay (13–68% sensitivity) is relatively low in immunosuppressed patients.

Case 99

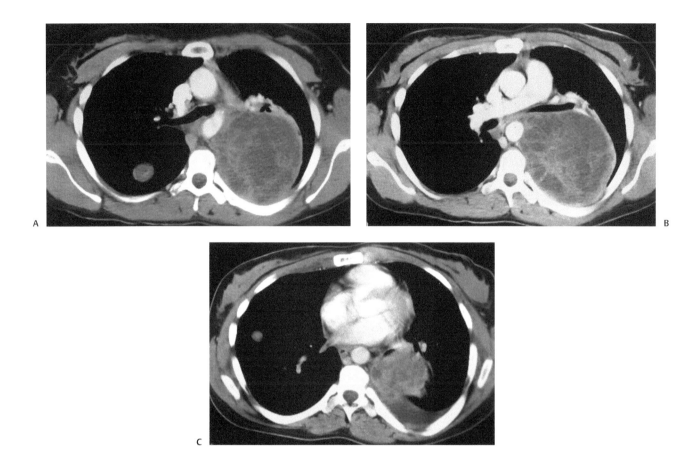

■ Clinical Presentation

A 27-year-old woman with a history of neurofibromatosis who has chest pain.

■ Imaging Findings

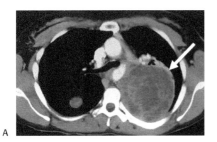 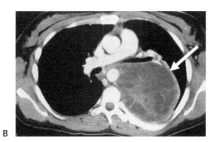 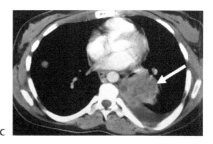

(A–C) Contrast-enhanced chest CT images. Axial images with soft tissue settings at three different levels. There is a large left-side soft tissue density mediastinal or extrapleural mass with irregular areas of contrast enhancement, with a small ipsilateral pleural effusion (*arrows*).

■ Differential Diagnosis

- ***Malignant peripheral nerve sheath tumor.***
- *Schwannoma.*
- *Neurofibroma.*
- *Sympathetic ganglion neoplasm.*

■ Essential Facts

- Malignant peripheral nerve sheath tumors (MPNSTs) are uncommon aggressive sarcomas of neural origin (Schwann cells) that represent 5 to 10% of all soft tissue sarcomas. They arise from a peripheral nerve from a preexisting nerve sheath tumor.
- Around 40% of these tumors are associated with neurofibromatosis type 1 (NF1), which is the most common human cancer genetic predisposition syndrome given its association with a variety of malignancies including MPNST, leukemia, gastrointestinal stromal tumor, and rhabdomyosarcoma. The other 60% are sporadic.
- MPNSTs may develop at any age and have no gender predilection. Sporadic MPNSTs tend to occur in the 5th decade, different from MPNSTs associated with NF1 that tend to occur earlier, at an average age around 30 years.
- Most MPNSTs in the context of NF1 arise from a preexisting plexiform neurofibroma of the nerve roots and nerve plexus of the extremities and pelvis (60%), with a very high incidence from the sciatic nerve.
- Intrathoracic MPNSTs, which are rare (15–20%), may be located in the mediastinum, chest wall, lung, or paraspinal region.

- MPNSTs have poor prognosis due to their large size at the time of diagnosis, local aggressive behavior, and metastatic potential, with an overall 5-year survival rate of < 50%.
- Complete surgical excision, when feasible, is the treatment of choice, followed by adjuvant radiation to reduce local recurrence and neoadjuvant chemotherapy in advanced cases.

■ Other Imaging Findings

- On noncontrast CT imaging, MPNST typically presents as a large soft tissue mass either hypodense or isodense to muscle.
- On noncontrast MR, they are hypointense on T1- and hyperintense on T2-weighted sequences.
- MPNSTs present contrast enhancement on both CT and MR images, with heterogeneous appearance due to necrosis (25%) and calcification (25%).

✓ Pearls and ✗ Pitfalls

- ✓ MPNSTs with rhabdomyoblastic differentiation (skeletal muscle) are known as malignant triton tumors and have worse prognosis than conventional MPNSTs.
- ✗ Differentiation of malignant and benign nerve sheath tumor is difficult. A "target sign" consisting of a central hypodense region on T2-weighted images, which was previously reported as an indicator of MPNST, has not consistently proven reliable in additional studies.

Case 100

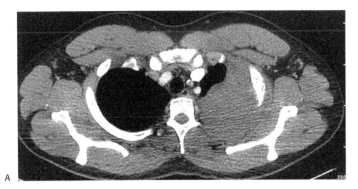
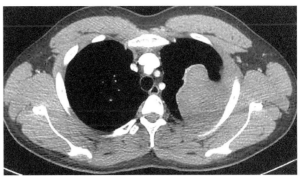
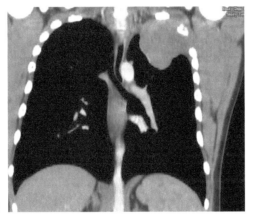

■ Clinical Presentation

A 22-year-old white man with left shoulder pain.

■ Imaging Findings

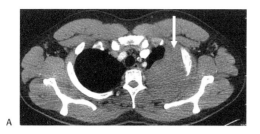 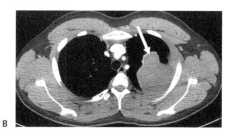 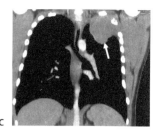

(A–C) Contrast-enhanced chest CT images. **(A, B)** Axial images at two different levels. **(C)** Coronal reconstruction image. These images demonstrate a large, pleural-based soft tissue density pleural or extrapleural mass that partially protrudes through the left-side first intercostal space (*arrows*).

■ Differential Diagnosis

- **Primary primitive neuroectodermal tumor.**
- *Rhabdomyosarcoma.*
- *Fibrosarcoma.*
- *Lymphoma.*

■ Essential Facts

- The Ewing family of tumors (EFT) is a group of cancers of neuroectodermal origin; they start in the bones or nearby soft tissues that share common neuronal immunohistochemical markers and cytogenetic and ultrastructural features. Ewing sarcoma of bone is the most common tumor of this family.
- Extraosseous Ewing sarcoma, also known as extraskeletal Ewing sarcoma, arises from the soft tissues around the bone.
- Peripheral primitive neuroectodermal tumor (PNET or PPNET) may arise from bone or soft tissue and is currently considered, along with classic Ewing sarcoma of bone and extraskeletal Ewing sarcoma, to be part of the Ewing family of tumors. A PNET that arises in the chest wall is also referred to as Askin tumor.
- For EFT, chest wall is the third most common location (20%) after diaphysis of long bones (50%) and the pelvic region (25%).
- Most patients affected with EFT are Caucasians, with very low incidence among black and Asian populations. Males are affected more than females. EFT is more common in the 2nd decade, but 30% arise in adults > 20 years old. The mean age of PNET tumors of the chest wall is 27 years.
- Treatment options depend on tumor extension and include integration of surgical excision, radiation therapy, and chemotherapy.

■ Other Imaging Findings

- Large soft tissue density extrapleural mass, with heterogeneous appearance due to contrast enhancement, hemorrhage, and calcification.
- Necrotic areas may appear as low density/fluid density on CT imaging.
- Associated bone destruction (40%) and chest wall invasion are common.
- Mediastinal invasion may occur with involvement of the heart and great vessels.
- Pleural effusion may occur.
- Heterogeneous appearance on T1-weighted sequences, with intermediate to high signal on T2-weighted images.
- Contrast enhancement of the non-necrotic, nonhemorrhagic tumor after gadolinium injection.

✓ Pearls and ✗ Pitfalls

- ✓ Nearly all cases of EFT have a unique pattern of chromosomal translocation within a single gene (*EWSR1*) locus on chromosome 22q12.
- ✗ On histopathology with light microscopy alone with hematoxylin-eosin–stained sections, the morphologic appearance of EFT and PNET tumors is similar to that of other small, round blue-cell tumors involving bone and soft tissue, including rhabdomyosarcoma, synovial sarcoma, undifferentiated neuroblastoma, mesenchymal chondrosarcoma, small-cell osteosarcoma, and lymphoma. Immunohistochemistry and cytogenetic and molecular genetic studies are required to confirm diagnosis.

Case Questions and Answers

The questions and answers in the following section are numbered as cases 1 through 100. The questions correspond to the respectively numbered case reviews and are intended to be answered after working through the cases.

■ Case 1

1. Which of the following features favors an intralobar sequestration?
   a) Diagnosed as a neonate
   b) Situated in the lower lobes/lung bases
   c) Systemic arterial supply
   d) Pulmonary venous drainage
   e) Communication with the bronchial tree

The correct answer is (**d**). In contradistinction to extralobar sequestrations, intralobar sequestrations have pulmonary venous drainage.

2. Which of the following regarding extralobar sequestrations is true?
   a) Mostly present clinically with recurrent pneumonia
   b) Typically not symptomatic until adulthood
   c) Can be associated with other congenital anomalies such as diaphragmatic hernia
   d) Usually found in the right upper lobe
   e) Only occurs in males

The correct answer is (**c**). Extralobar sequestrations are often associated with other congenital anomalies such as diaphragmatic hernia and congenital heart disease.

■ Case 2

1. What is the most common location of a bronchogenic cyst?
   a) Within the lung parenchyma
   b) In the neck
   c) Abutting the diaphragm
   d) Within the esophageal wall
   e) Near the carina

The correct answer is (**e**). Approximately 85% of bronchogenic cysts occur within 2 cm of the carina.

2. Which of the following regarding bronchogenic cysts is true?
   a) They always have homogeneous water attenuation.
   b) Mild contrast enhancement is expected.
   c) The signal intensity on T1-weighted MR images is variable.
   d) They usually cause symptoms.
   e) Bacterial superinfection is common.

The correct answer is (**c**). The signal intensity on T1-weighted images is variable, depending on the presence of mucus, protein, or hemorrhage within the cyst.

■ Case 3

1. What best describes the vascular anatomy of a pulmonary arteriovenous malformation (AVM)?
   a) Abnormal communication between the bronchial artery and the pulmonary vein
   b) Abnormal communication between the pulmonary artery and the pulmonary vein
   c) Abnormal dilatation of the pulmonary vein
   d) A large dilated pulmonary capillary
   e) Aneurysmal dilatation of the pulmonary artery

The correct answer is (**b**). Pulmonary AVMs are abnormal communications between the pulmonary artery and vein with no intervening capillary network.

2. Which of the following regarding hereditary hemorrhagic telangiectasia is true?
   a) It is inherited as an autosomal-recessive disorder of variable penetrance.
   b) Stroke is the most common presentation.
   c) It may first present with recurrent epistaxis.
   d) Presence of a pulmonary AVM is a mandatory diagnostic criterion.
   e) Bronchoscopy is the preferred diagnostic modality.

The correct answer is (**c**). Recurrent epistaxis is due to abnormal blood vessels in the nasal mucosa and is a common clinical presentation (50–80%).

■ Case 4

1. What is the most common type of congenital pulmonary airway malformation (CPAM)?
   a) Large cyst
   b) Mixed
   c) Small cyst
   d) Microcystic
   e) Macrocystic

The correct answer is (**a**). Large cyst (> 2 cm)–type CPAM is the most common type, comprising 50 to 70% of cases.

2. What is the most common complication of CPAM?
   a) Malignant transformation
   b) Oligohydramnios
   c) Respiratory distress
   d) Recurrent infection
   e) Coexistent congenital anomalies

The correct answer is (**c**). Large CPAMs may compromise respiration and/or cause pulmonary hypoplasia.

■ Case 5

1. Which of the following supports a diagnosis of teratoma?
   a) Elderly patient
   b) Pulmonary nodules
   c) Pericardial effusion
   d) Paraneoplastic syndrome
   e) Internal foci of fat

The correct answer is (**e**). On CT, internal foci of fat are seen in 75%.

2. Which of the following is unexpected in teratomas?
   a) Midline location
   b) Metastatic disease
   c) Calcification
   d) Soft tissue enhancement
   e) Rim enhancement

The correct answer is (**b**). Pulmonary metastases are not expected with most teratomas. The most common type is a mature teratoma, which has benign features.

■ Case 6

1. Which of the following imaging findings related to a solitary pulmonary nodule favor malignancy?
   a) Dense calcification
   b) Smooth margins
   c) Size > 2 cm
   d) Popcorn calcification
   e) Patient < 30 years old

The correct answer is (**c**). In general, the smaller the nodule, the more likely it is to be benign. Even though size > 2 cm is not indicative of malignancy, 80% of benign nodules are < 2 cm in diameter. The other choices all favor benign etiologies.

2. Which of the following regarding solitary pulmonary nodules is true?
   a) Calcified nodules are never malignant.
   b) When > 2 cm, metastases are usually also present.
   c) A spiculated margin favors a malignant etiology.
   d) Stability over 6 months is indicative of a benign etiology.
   e) Several infections can present as solitary pulmonary nodules but are usually cavitary.

The correct answer is (**c**). A nodule with a spiculated margin with distortion of adjacent vessels is likely to be malignant.

■ Case 7

1. Where are the intrathoracic abnormalities found in α_1-antitrypsin (AAT) deficiency typically localized?
   a) Central airways
   b) Upper lobes
   c) Lower lobes
   d) Mediastinum
   e) Pleura

The correct answer is (**c**). Patients with AAT deficiency have panlobular emphysema, which is localized to the lower lobes.

2. What is the etiology of AAT deficiency?
   a) Cigarette smoking
   b) Asbestos exposure
   c) Chronic infection
   d) Drug toxicity
   e) Genetic abnormality

The correct answer is (**e**). AAT deficiency is inherited by autosomal co-dominant transmission. Affected individuals must inherit an abnormal *AAT* gene from each parent.

■ Case 8

1. Where are the intrathoracic abnormalities found in α_1-antitrypsin deficiency typically localized?
   a) Superior mediastinum
   b) Abutting the superior vena cava
   c) Superior segment of the left lower lobe
   d) Lung apex
   e) Right middle lobe

The correct answer is (**d**). A superior sulcus tumor is a non–small-cell lung carcinoma arising from the lung apex and invading the chest wall or soft tissues of the thoracic inlet.

2. Which of the following is *not* a component of Horner syndrome?
    a) Ptosis
    b) Miosis
    c) Anhidrosis
    d) Mydriasis
    e) Sympathetic nerve invasion

The correct answer is (**d**). Mydriasis refers to dilated pupils and is not a component of Horner syndrome.

■ **Case 9**

1. Which of the following imaging findings related to small-cell lung cancer (SCLC) suggest advanced disease?
    a) Collateral neck and chest wall veins
    b) Involvement of the mediastinum
    c) An enlarged supraclavicular lymph node
    d) Hoarseness
    e) Pleural effusion

The correct answer is (**e**). In general, extensive disease is defined by disease beyond the ipsilateral hemithorax, which may include malignant pleural or pericardial effusion or hematogenous metastases.

2. Which of the following regarding SCLC is true?
    a) Has a better prognosis than non–small-cell lung cancer
    b) Is usually treated with surgery
    c) Typically manifests as a peripheral mass
    d) May secrete hormones
    e) Shows slow growth

The correct answer is (**d**). SCLC, like other neuroendocrine tumors, may produce metabolically active substances (e.g., adrenocorticotropic hormone, parathyroid hormone, antidiuretic hormone, calcitonin) that manifest clinically before the lung cancer is diagnosed.

■ **Case 10**

1. Which of the following imaging findings favor malignancy over pneumonia?
    a) Bronchial wall thickening proximal to the lesion
    b) Pleural thickening
    c) Straightening of the interlobar fissure
    d) Deformity of the air-filled bronchus within the area of consolidation
    e) Air bronchograms

The correct answer is (**d**). Deformity of the air-filled bronchus within the area of consolidation (stretching, squeezing, widening of the branching angle) or bulging of the interlobar fissure favor malignancy.

2. Which of the following regarding lepidic predominant adenocarcinoma is true?
    a) Has replaced large-cell carcinoma in the new lung cancer classification scheme
    b) Typically shows avid fluorodeoxyglucose uptake on positron emission tomography scans
    c) Usually presents as multiple dense spiculated nodules
    d) Has a worse prognosis than small-cell carcinoma
    e) May be mistaken for bacterial pneumonia on initial imaging

The correct answer is (**e**). Lepidic predominant adenocarcinoma can present as ground-glass opacity or air-space consolidation, making differentiation from bacterial pneumonia difficult.

■ **Case 11**

1. Which of the following is not a major cause of pulmonary artery aneurysms and pseudoaneurysms?
    a) Tuberculosis (TB)
    b) Syphilis
    c) Atherosclerotic disease
    d) Posttraumatic
    e) Vasculitis

The correct answer is (**c**). As opposed to aneurysms in other vascular territories, atherosclerotic disease typically does not affect the pulmonary arterial circulation and is not a cause of pulmonary artery aneurysms.

2. What is the major complication of a Rasmussen aneurysm?
    a) Chronic infection
    b) Massive hemoptysis
    c) Distal embolization
    d) Pulmonary infarct
    e) Mass effect on the superior vena cava

The correct answer is (**b**). Rasmussen aneurysm usually occurs in a peripheral pulmonary artery due to weakening of the wall from adjacent cavitary TB. Hemoptysis is the usual symptom at initial manifestation.

■ **Case 12**

1. The following imaging findings are all suggestive of active tuberculosis (TB) except for which of the following?
    a) Cavitation
    b) Consolidation
    c) Centrilobular and tree-in-bud opacities
    d) Pleural effusion
    e) Calcified lymph nodes

The correct answer is (**e**). Calcified lymph nodes are more typically related to previous/healed/inactive TB.

2. What is the most common intrathoracic location of postprimary TB?
    a) Lung bases
    b) Upper lobes and superior segments of lower lobe
    c) Mediastinum
    d) Pleural space
    e) Vertebral body

The correct answer is (**b**). In postprimary TB, consolidation and cavitation have a strong predilection for the apical and posterior segments of the upper lobes and superior segments of the lower lobes.

■ **Case 13**

1. Which of the underlying conditions is most commonly seen in allergic bronchopulmonary aspergillosis (ABPA)?
    a) Asthma
    b) Emphysema
    c) Neutropenia
    d) AIDS
    e) Sarcoidosis

The correct answer is (**a**). ABPA is a complication of asthma, in part related to the excessive production of viscous mucus and abnormal mucociliary clearance.

2. Which of the following imaging findings supports a diagnosis of ABPA?
    a) Lymphadenopathy
    b) Lung cysts
    c) Halo sign
    d) Finger-in-glove sign
    e) Pleural effusion

The correct answer is (**d**). The finger-in-glove sign represents the tubular branching pattern of mucoid impaction.

■ **Case 14**

1. Which of the following imaging findings is classically associated with *Klebsiella* pneumonia?
    a) CT halo sign
    b) S sign of golden
    c) V sign of Naclerio
    d) Bulging fissure sign
    e) Comet tail sign

The correct answer is (**d**). The bulging fissure sign represents expansive lobar consolidation and exudate, which displaces the adjacent fissure.

2. Which of the following statements regarding *Klebsiella* pneumonia is false?
    a) Cavitary consolidation is a classic imaging feature.
    b) It most commonly presents in debilitated adults.
    c) It can be nosocomial or community acquired.
    d) It can be associated with a parapneumonic effusion.
    e) It is associated with pneumatoceles, which are a particular type of fluid-filled lung abscess.

The correct answer is (**e**). Pneumatoceles differ from lung abscesses associated with gram-negative or anaerobic bacteria. Pneumatoceles are thin-walled, gas-filled spaces seen in areas of air-space disease and consolidation in patients with pneumonia. They develop from the acute infection and resolve in weeks or months.

■ **Case 15**

1. Which of the following imaging findings is not typically associated with *Varicella* pneumonia?
    a) Miliary pattern of disease
    b) Nodules with a halo sign
    c) Calcified nodules
    d) Ground-glass opacity
    e) Lymphadenopathy

The correct answer is (**e**). Although the imaging findings are nonspecific, a miliary pattern of nodules, some with calcification or with a halo, and ground-glass opacity have all been described in *Varicella* pneumonia. Substantial lymphadenopathy is not expected.

2. Which of the following statements regarding *Varicella* pneumonia is false?
    a) A pleural effusion is not typically present.
    b) In adults, it most commonly affects immunocompromised patients and those with lymphoma.
    c) The radiographic appearance is nonspecific and mimics that of other viral pneumonias.
    d) Pulmonary nodules may calcify and persist.
    e) Lobar consolidation is less common in viral pneumonia than in bacterial infection.

The correct answer is (**a**). Pleural effusion is not exclusively a complication of bacterial pneumonias. A significant amount of parapneumonic pleural fluid can be associated with different viral pneumonias.

■ Case 16

1. Which of the following is the major risk factor for *Pneumocystis* pneumonia?
   a) Immune compromise
   b) Emphysema
   c) Travel to endemic areas
   d) Cystic fibrosis
   e) Asbestos exposure

The correct answer is (**a**). Affected patients usually have profound T-cell immunosuppression.

2. What is the most common imaging feature of *Pneumocystis* pneumonia?
   a) Perihilar and upper lobe ground-glass opacity
   b) Dense consolidation
   c) Lymphadenopathy
   d) Pleural effusions
   e) Solitary pulmonary nodule

The correct answer is (**a**). Although the findings on chest radiograph are often normal or nonspecific, perihilar and upper lung–predominant ground-glass opacity on CT is the most characteristic imaging finding.

■ Case 17

1. Which of the following features best describes the pulmonary manifestations of laryngotracheal papillomatosis?
   a) Pulmonary involvement is far more common than tracheal involvement.
   b) They typically resolve with antibiotic therapy.
   c) They are present in the neonatal period.
   d) They are characterized by well-defined nodules that eventually cavitate.
   e) Nodules grow rapidly.

The correct answer is (**d**). Lung disease is characterized by multiple well-defined perihilar and posteriorly located nodules that eventually cavitate.

2. Which of the following is not a potential complication of pulmonary papillomatosis?
   a) Malignancy
   b) Superinfection
   c) Atelectasis
   d) Respiratory failure
   e) Pulmonary embolism

The correct answer is (**e**). Pulmonary embolism is not a typical complication of pulmonary papillomatosis.

■ Case 18

1. Which of the following supports a diagnosis of angioinvasive aspergillosis?
   a) S sign of Golden
   b) Split pleura sign
   c) Finger-in-glove opacity
   d) CT halo sign
   e) Comet tail sign

The correct answer is (**d**). The halo sign consists of a halo of ground-glass attenuation, which represents alveolar hemorrhage, surrounding a central denser nodule, which corresponds to the focus of infarction. This is highly suggestive of angioinvasive aspergillosis in an immuno-compromised patient.

2. Which of the following favors a diagnosis of angioinvasive aspergillosis?
   a) Lymphadenopathy
   b) Pleural effusion
   c) Thin-walled cyst
   d) Nodules with surrounding hemorrhage
   e) Bronchiectasis

The correct answer is (**d**). A nodule with surrounding hemorrhage describes the CT halo sign and is highly suggestive of angioinvasive aspergillosis.

■ Case 19

1. Which of the following is usually seen in bacterial spondylodiskitis?
   a) High signal intensity of the disk on T1-weighted images
   b) Involvement of the sacrum
   c) Underlying metastatic disease
   d) Inhomogeneous enhancement of the disk and surrounding vertebral bodies
   e) Decreased uptake on fluorodeoxyglucose–positron emission tomography

The correct answer is (**d**). Typical findings of spondylodiskitis on MR images are low signal intensity of the disks and adjacent vertebral bodies on T1-weighted images and hyperintensity on T2-weighted and fat-suppressed sequences. There is typically inhomogeneous enhancement of the disk and surrounding vertebral bodies.

2. In adults, which of the following is a common risk factor for the development of bacterial spondylodiskitis?
   a) Bacterial meningitis
   b) CNS neoplasms
   c) Prior radiation therapy
   d) Trauma
   e) Endocarditis

The correct answer is (**e**). The infectious process is believed to begin at the vertebral body end plate as the consequence of hematogenous dissemination from a distant source (e.g., urinary tract infection, skin, prostatitis, endocarditis).

■ **Case 20**

1. What is the most common organism associated with sternal dehiscence and infection?
   a) *Staphylococcus aureus*
   b) *Streptococcus pneumoniae*
   c) Tuberculosis
   d) *Escherichia coli*
   e) *Pneumocystis*

The correct answer is (**a**); the most common organism isolated is *S. aureus.*

2. Which of the following is true regarding the time course of sternal wound dehiscence and infection?
   a) It is usually a late complication, occurring years after surgery.
   b) Complications usually manifest 1 to 2 weeks after surgery.
   c) Subcutaneous air seen following sternotomy is a specific finding of necrotizing fasciitis.
   d) It can usually be diagnosed at the time of closure.
   e) It only occurs in diabetics.

The correct answer is (**b**). Complications usually manifest 1 to 2 weeks after surgery.

■ **Case 21**

1. Large B-cell lymphoma is typically seen in which demographic?
   a) Young adult females
   b) Elderly men
   c) Infants
   d) Smokers
   e) People with AIDS

The correct answer is (**a**). Large B-cell lymphoma is typically seen in young adult females.

2. Which of the following imaging signs supports the diagnosis of lymphoma?
   a) Superior vena cava invasion
   b) Large soft tissue mass
   c) Calcification
   d) Pulmonary nodules
   e) Osseous lesions

The correct answer is (**b**). The classic finding on CT images is a large anterior mediastinal soft tissue mass.

■ **Case 22**

1. Which of the following findings supports a diagnosis of pleural metastatic disease?
   a) Calcification
   b) Split pleura sign
   c) Masses with angles acute to the chest wall
   d) Pleural effusion
   e) Fat-density lesions

The correct answer is (**d**). A pleural effusion, mostly hemorrhagic, is seen in 60% of patients.

2. What is the most common tumor to metastasize to the pleura?
   a) Small-cell lung cancer
   b) Breast cancer
   c) Non–small-cell lung cancer
   d) Renal cell carcinoma
   e) Glioblastoma multiforme

The correct answer is (**c**). Adenocarcinoma is the most common tumor to metastasize to the pleura, with lung (35%) and breast (25%) cancer accounting for the majority of cases.

■ **Case 23**

1. Which of the following imaging findings would not be expected in leukemia?
   a) Pleural effusion
   b) Lymphadenopathy
   c) Ground-glass opacities
   d) Lung cysts
   e) Subperiosteal nodules

The correct answer is (**d**). Although the imaging findings in leukemia are varied and nonspecific, lung cysts are not expected.

2. Which of the following is true regarding thoracic manifestation of leukemia?
   a) It always presents with discrete pulmonary nodules.
   b) Opportunistic infections are rare.
   c) Most thoracic imaging manifestations of leukemia are only seen on in children.
   d) They often show nonspecific imaging findings such as ground-glass opacities.
   e) Chronic lymphocytic leukemia is the only leukemia variant to show diffuse lymphadenopathy.

The correct answer is (**d**). The most common imaging findings in the lung parenchyma are ground-glass attenuation, centrilobular nodules, and interlobular septal thickening. Lymphocyte infiltration occurs along the interstitium and the alveolar spaces.

■ **Case 24**

1. Which of the following supports a diagnosis of Castleman disease?
   a) Contrast enhancement
   b) Multiple pulmonary nodules
   c) Pericardial effusion
   d) Paraneoplastic syndrome
   e) Internal foci of fat

The correct answer is (**a**). Castleman disease is typically hypervascular and shows avid enhancement.

2. Which of the following is unexpected in Castleman disease?
   a) High T2 signal
   b) Calcification
   c) Mediastinal location
   d) Lymph node hyperplasia
   e) Young adult demographic

The correct answer is (**b**). Calcification is rarely seen (~10% of cases).

■ **Case 25**

1. Which of the following imaging signs are most typical of lymphocytic interstitial pneumonia (LIP)?
   a) Honeycombing
   b) Pleural effusion
   c) Thin-walled cysts
   d) Consolidation
   e) Calcified lymph nodes

The correct answer is (**c**). LIP is most typically associated with randomly distributed thin-walled cysts.

2. LIP is associated with all of the following except . . .
   a) AIDS
   b) Sjögren syndrome
   c) Lupus
   d) Asbestos
   e) Castleman disease

The correct answer is (**d**). Asbestos exposure is not associated with LIP.

■ **Case 26**

1. Which of the following is not a risk factor for reexpansion pulmonary edema (RPE)?
   a) Prolonged pulmonary collapse
   b) Large volume pleural drainage
   c) Young patients
   d) Large pneumothorax
   e) Pulmonary vein stenosis

The correct answer is (**e**). Although pulmonary vein stenosis can lead to unilateral edema, it is not a risk factor for RPE.

2. Which of the following regarding RPE is true?
   a) Pulmonary edema clears within hours.
   b) It is caused by concomitant aspiration.
   c) It mostly occurs in patients with long-standing pulmonary collapse.
   d) It is due to overly aggressive fluid resuscitation.
   e) It is typically not of clinical consequence.

The correct answer is (**c**). More than 80% of cases of RPE occur in patients with prolonged pulmonary collapse (> 72 hours).

■ **Case 27**

1. Which of the following features favors a heroin-induced pulmonary edema?
   a) Fluffy opacities
   b) Large pleural effusions
   c) Cardiomegaly
   d) Large lung volumes
   e) Unilateral opacity

The correct answer is (**a**). Heroin-induced pulmonary edema usually manifests as bilateral perihilar fluffy interstitial and air-space opacities.

2. Which of the following regarding heroin-induced pulmonary edema is true?
   a) It has imaging findings distinct from other causes of noncardiogenic pulmonary edema.
   b) It is only seen with superimposed infection.
   c) It may resolve rapidly.
   d) It is caused by decreased cardiac output.
   e) It is best characterized by septal lines on chest radiograph.

The correct answer is (**c**). The pulmonary edema often resolves rapidly with treatment, mostly within 24 hours.

■ **Case 28**

1. What is the most common manifestation of asbestos exposure?
   a) Pleural plaques
   b) Asbestosis
   c) Mesothelioma
   d) Benign fibrous tumor of the pleura
   e) Pleural effusion

The correct answer is (**a**). Pleural plaques are the most common manifestation of asbestos inhalation and occur 20 to 30 years after first exposure.

2. Pleural plaques have a predilection for which portion of the thorax?
   a) Apices
   b) Costophrenic angles
   c) Visceral pleura
   d) Diaphragmatic dome
   e) Prevascular lymph nodes

The correct answer is (**d**). Pleural plaques arise in the parietal pleura and have a predilection for the diaphragmatic dome and the undersurface of the lower posterolateral ribs.

■ **Case 29**

1. The following imaging findings are all suggestive of mesothelioma except . . .
   a) Volume loss
   b) Pleural effusion
   c) Circumferential pleural thickening
   d) Bilateral disease
   e) Extension into pleural

The correct answer is (**d**). Although pleural plaques are often seen bilaterally, mesothelioma is almost always unilateral.

2. Which of the following statements regarding mesothelioma is true?
   a) Cigarette smoking is a major risk factor.
   b) The latency period from asbestos exposure to diagnosis is short.
   c) The visceral pleura is affected to a greater degree.
   d) Localized fibrous tumor of the pleura is a precursor lesion.
   e) Despite asbestos exposure, calcified pleural plaques are seen in only 20% of cases.

The correct answer is (**e**). Calcified pleural plaques are associated with asbestos exposure but are seen in only 20% of cases of mesothelioma.

■ **Case 30**

1. Which of the following imaging findings supports a diagnosis of silicosis?
   a) Pleural effusion
   b) Eggshell calcification of lymph nodes
   c) Lower lobe consolidation
   d) Thin-walled cysts
   e) Calcified pleural plaques

The correct answer is (**b**). Although not diagnostic of silicosis, eggshell calcification of lymph nodes is commonly seen in this condition.

2. Which of the following best describes the nodules seen in silicosis?
   a) Pleural based
   b) Endobronchial
   c) Centrilobular
   d) Ground-glass
   e) Cavitary

The correct answer is (**c**). The small nodules have a posterior and centrilobular distribution.

■ **Case 31**

1. Which of the following features favors hypersensitivity pneumonitis?
   a) Cavitary nodules
   b) Large pleural effusions
   c) Cardiomegaly
   d) Ground-glass centrilobular nodules
   e) Unilateral opacity

The correct answer is (**d**). Ground-glass opacities and centrilobular ground-glass nodules are the most common imaging findings of hypersensitivity pneumonitis.

2. Which of the following regarding hypersensitivity pneumonitis is true?
   a) Most cases occur after an isolated exposure to an allergen.
   b) It is more common in smokers.
   c) Air trapping often shows on expiratory-phase imaging.
   d) It requires open lung biopsy for diagnosis.
   e) Honeycombing is present in acute cases when severe.

The correct answer is (**c**). Air trapping on expiratory phase HRCT is a hallmark imaging feature.

■ **Case 32**

1. What is the etiology of the opacity in pulmonary alveolar proteinosis?
   a) Hemorrhage
   b) Edema
   c) Tumor
   d) Lipoproteinaceous material
   e) Bacterial pneumonia

The correct answer is (**d**). Pulmonary alveolar proteinosis is characterized by abnormal accumulation of surfactant-like lipoproteinaceous material.

2. Which imaging sign is classically associated with pulmonary alveolar proteinosis?
   a) Crazy-paving
   b) S sign of Golden
   c) Air crescent sign
   d) Westermark sign
   e) Monod sign

The correct answer is (**a**). The combination of smooth septal thickening and ground-glass opacity results in the crazy-paving pattern, which, although highly characteristic, is not pathognomonic of pulmonary alveolar proteinosis.

■ **Case 33**

1. Which of the following imaging findings supports a diagnosis of exogenous lipoid pneumonia?
   a) Pleural effusion
   b) Lymphadenopathy
   c) Low-density consolidation
   d) Bilateral nodules
   e) Ground-glass opacity

The correct answer is (**c**). A consolidation with low density on CT images (−30 to −120 Hounsfield units) is highly suggestive of intrapulmonary fat and lipoid pneumonia.

2. What is the most common cause of lipoid pneumonia?
   a) Lung cancer
   b) Fat embolus
   c) Teratoma
   d) Chronic aspiration of inhalation of oily substances
   e) Asbestos exposure

The correct answer is (**d**). The most common cause of exogenous lipoid pneumonia in the elderly is the aspiration of mineral oil used as a laxative. Inhalation of mineral oil nose drops used for chronic rhinitis also can result in lipoid pneumonia.

■ **Case 34**

1. Which type of bronchiectasis is the commonest and least severe?
   a) Traction
   b) Cylindrical
   c) Cystic
   d) Varicose
   e) Cystic fibrosis

The correct answer is (**b**). Subtypes of bronchiectasis include cylindrical, varicose, and cystic, and these loosely represent a spectrum of severity. Cylindrical is the commonest and least severe.

2. Which imaging sign represents an increased bronchoarterial ratio?
   a) Finger-in-glove
   b) S sign of Golden
   c) Tree-in-bud
   d) Tram-track sign
   e) Signet ring sign

The correct answer is (**e**). The signet ring sign represents the dilated bronchus abutting the accompanying dilated pulmonary artery when seen in cross section. Normally, the diameter of the bronchus should be the same size or smaller than the adjacent pulmonary artery branch.

■ **Case 35**

1. Which of the following is an accepted diagnostic criterion for tracheomalacia (TM)?
   a) Bronchiolar size exceeding that of the adjacent pulmonary artery
   b) Air trapping on expiratory-phase imaging
   c) More than 50% cross-sectional tracheal narrowing on expiration by CT
   d) Anteroposterior diameter of trachea < 2 cm
   e) Visualization of tracheal polyps

The correct answer is (**c**). A diagnostic criterion for TM commonly used on CT imaging and bronchoscopy is > 50% tracheal narrowing (cross-sectional area) during expiration.

2. What is the most common cause of TM in adults?
    a) History of prematurity
    b) History of prolonged intubation
    c) Vascular ring
    d) Relapsing polychondritis
    e) Chronic inflammation

The correct answer is (**e**). Cigarette smoking and general chronic inflammation are major contributors to TM.

■ Case 36

1. Which of the following is the most reliable indirect imaging sign seen in tracheal rupture?
    a) Pneumothorax
    b) Pericardial effusion
    c) Widened mediastinum
    d) Pneumomediastinum
    e) Malpositioned endotracheal tube

The correct answer is (**d**). Pneumomediastinum, often extending into the neck, is the most common imaging sign in tracheal rupture.

2. Which of the following regarding tracheal rupture is true?
    a) The most common site of rupture is through the anterior cartilage.
    b) It is more common in blunt thoracic trauma.
    c) It typically occurs close to the carina.
    d) It is typically not of clinical consequence.
    e) It only occurs with preexisting tracheal anomalies such as tracheal diverticulum.

The correct answer is (**c**). The typical morphology of tracheal rupture is longitudinal/vertical, occurring more commonly in the distal third, close to the carina.

■ Case 37

1. What is the most common origin of a broncholith?
    a) Erosion of a calcified lymph node into the bronchus
    b) Calcified carcinoid tumor
    c) Aspiration from oropharynx
    d) Tracheopathia osteochondroplastica
    e) Relapsing polychondritis

The correct answer is (**a**). A broncholith is typically the result of erosion of a calcified lymph node into the bronchial lumen. It may also occur secondary to in situ calcification of aspirated foreign material. Much rarer causes include extrusion of calcified bronchial cartilage plates and bronchial migration of calcified material such as a pleural plaque or renal stone via a fistula.

2. What is the most common clinical presentation of a broncholith?
    a) Fever
    b) Chronic nonproductive cough
    c) Paraneoplastic syndrome
    d) Chest pain
    e) Pulmonary edema

The correct answer is (**b**). Broncholiths usually present with a chronic nonproductive cough. They can often be removed via bronchoscopy with the aid of laser photocoagulation.

■ Case 38

1. Which of the following imaging signs suggests pulmonary infarct?
    a) Pleural effusion
    b) Peripheral consolidation with central lucency
    c) Large draining vein
    d) Perihilar opacity
    e) Thin-walled cavity

The correct answer is (**b**). Pulmonary infarction is very likely if a peripheral consolidation contains central lucencies.

2. Which of the following statements regarding pulmonary infarction is true?
    a) Pulmonary infarction is commonly seen in patients with pulmonary embolism.
    b) Pulmonary infarction is usually present in the upper lobes.
    c) The opacity related to pulmonary infarct clears rapidly.
    d) Pleuritic chest pain is more commonly seen with infarcts.
    e) It is rare to have coexistent pulmonary hemorrhage.

The correct answer is (**d**). Pleuritic chest pain is more commonly seen with infarcts, presumably related to adjacent pleural inflammatory response.

■ Case 39

1. Which of the following is not associated with right heart strain?
   a) Contrast reflux into the inferior vena cava
   b) Right ventricular dilation
   c) Right ventricle (RV):left ventricle (LV) ratio < 1
   d) Hypotension
   e) D-shaped left ventricular cavity

The correct answer is (**c**). A distended right ventricle, reflected by an increase in RV:LV ratio > 1, is indicative of right heart strain.

2. Which of the following signs helps distinguish tumor embolus from bland embolus?
   a) Vessel enlargement
   b) Central location
   c) Bilaterality
   d) Enhancement
   e) Dyspnea

The correct answer is (**d**). A tumor embolus may show contrast enhancement, whereas conventional bland embolus will not.

■ Case 40

1. For an uncomplicated pneumothorax, what is the preferred location of the tip of a chest tube?
   a) Anterior superior chest
   b) Intrafissural
   c) At the base of the lung
   d) Along the mediastinal margin
   e) Coiled in the dependent portion of the chest

The correct answer is (**a**). In the absence of loculations, air collects in the nondependent portions of the chest. Anterior and superior placement situates the tube in the optimal location for a supine and upright patient.

2. Which of the following is not true with regard to chest tube placement?
   a) Bubbling in the air leak chamber of a water seal drainage system immediately after placement is normal.
   b) Movement of the water column with coughing and respiration can be a sign of a malpositioned tube.
   c) A persistent pneumothorax is indicated by ongoing bubbling of air from a chest drain 48 hours after its insertion.
   d) Tubes placed for free-flowing pleural effusions should extend to the anterior mediastinum.
   e) New subcutaneous emphysema can suggest tube malposition.

The correct answer is (**d**). For the drainage of fluid, a posterior/dependent position is preferred because this is where most fluid will collect with the patient supine and upright.

■ Case 41

1. What is most consistent imaging finding in acute respiratory distress syndrome (ARDS)?
   a) Ground-glass opacity
   b) Pleural effusions
   c) Pneumothorax
   d) Cysts
   e) Consolidation

The correct answer is (**a**). Ground-glass opacity is a nonspecific imaging sign that is commonly seen with ARDS. It likely represents edema and protein within the interstitium and alveoli.

2. Which of the following statements regarding the course and etiology of ARDS is true?
   a) Like cardiogenic pulmonary edema, ARDS can rapidly clear once euvolemia is achieved.
   b) ARDS is most commonly seen with drug reactions.
   c) A pneumothorax almost always occurs once positive-pressure ventilation is initiated.
   d) It is the most severe form of the smoking-related lung disease desquamative interstitial pneumonia (DIP).
   e) The diffuse lung opacity seen in congestive heart failure is not primarily due to elevated pulmonary venous pressure.

The correct answer is (**e**). The pulmonary edema in ARDS is noncardiogenic. The lack of cardiomegaly, septal lines, vascular redistribution, and peribronchial cuffing favor ARDS over cardiogenic edema.

■ Case 42

1. Which of the following is not typically found in Kartagener syndrome?
   a) Situs inversus
   b) Sinusitis
   c) Varicose bronchiectasis
   d) Small centrilobular nodules
   e) Honeycombing

The correct answer is (**e**). Although patients can develop severe chronic lung disease, the hallmark finding is bronchiectasis, not honeycombing.

2. Visualization of a dilated bronchus adjacent to the pulmonary artery in cross section is described by which imaging sign?
   a) Signet ring sign
   b) Finger-in-glove sign
   c) Scimitar sign
   d) Comet tail sign
   e) Sign of Golden

The correct answer is (**a**). Typically, the bronchus is equal to or smaller in diameter than the adjacent pulmonary artery. When dilated and viewed in cross section, the appearance mimics a signet ring.

■ Case 43

1. Which of the following findings support rounded atelectasis?
   a) Adjacent pleural thickening
   b) History of malignancy
   c) Pericardial effusion
   d) Intense fluorodeoxyglucose uptake
   e) "Popcorn" calcification

The correct answer is (**a**). Rounded atelectasis is associated with adjacent pleural thickening.

2. Which of the following is true regarding rounded atelectasis?
   a) Is due to mucus plugging
   b) Usually found at the lung apices
   c) May be associated with asbestos-related pleural disease
   d) Is a premalignant condition
   e) Usually resolves rapidly

The correct answer is (**c**). Rounded atelectasis is most commonly associated with asbestos-related pleural disease, but it may occur with any cause of pleural fibrosis.

■ Case 44

1. In Boerhaave syndrome, from which structure does the mediastinal air originate?
   a) Esophagus
   b) Trachea
   c) Lung
   d) Colon
   e) External to the patient

The correct answer is (**a**). Postemetic perforation of the esophagus results in an air leak into the mediastinum.

2. Which of the following would not be expected in a patient with Boerhaave syndrome?
   a) Subcutaneous emphysema
   b) Chest pain
   c) Vomiting
   d) Odynophagia
   e) Anemia

The correct answer is (**e**). Boerhaave syndrome is not associated with significant hemorrhage.

■ Case 45

1. Which of the following supports the diagnosis of esophageal leiomyoma?
   a) Esophagorespiratory fistula
   b) Calcification
   c) Irregular margins
   d) Lymphadenopathy
   e) Chronic reflux esophagitis

The correct answer is (**b**). The presence of calcification is highly suggestive of a benign entity such as an esophageal leiomyoma.

2. What is the most common location of esophageal leiomyoma?
   a) Distal esophagus
   b) Middle esophagus
   c) Cervical esophagus
   d) Within a diverticulum
   e) In the mediastinum, abutting the esophageal wall

The correct answer is (**a**). The most common location of esophageal leiomyomas is in the distal esophagus ($> 60\%$), followed by the middle third (30%). Involvement of the upper esophagus is uncommon (10%).

■ Case 46

1. What is the most common cause of esophagopulmonary fistula?
   a) Esophageal cancer
   b) Lung cancer
   c) Trauma
   d) Infection
   e) Iatrogenic

The correct answer is (**a**). The majority of esophageal fistulas seen in adult patients result from acquired diseases such as intrathoracic malignancies ($> 60\%$), in particular esophageal cancer (77%) and lung cancer (16%).

2. Which of the following regarding esophagopulmonary fistula is true?
    a) When esophagopulmonary fistula is suspected, administration of oral contrast is contraindicated.
    b) CT is usually sufficient to define fistula anatomy.
    c) Necrotizing pneumonia can mimic and/or complicate esophagopulmonary fistula.
    d) Most commonly, it presents with acute chest pain.
    e) Typically, it is only seen in patients with a history of congenital tracheoesophageal fistula.

The correct answer is (**c**). If necrotizing pneumonia develops, oral contrast may accumulate within the cavity.

■ **Case 47**

1. Which of the following imaging findings supports a diagnosis of end-stage sarcoidosis?
    a) Pleural effusion
    b) Multifocal cavitary masses
    c) Lower lobe predominance
    d) Architectural distortion
    e) Congestive heart failure

The correct answer is (**d**). End-stage disease results in architectural distortion with upper lobe retraction, traction bronchiectasis, honeycombing, and cysts.

2. Which of the following is not an indirect sign of pulmonary hypertension on CT?
    a) Enlargement of the main pulmonary artery > 29 mm
    b) Enlargement of the interlobar pulmonary artery > 16 mm
    c) Right atrial enlargement
    d) Contrast opacification of the azygos vein
    e) Increased right:left ventricle ratio

The correct answer is (**d**). Reflux of contrast into the hepatic veins and inferior vena cava is an indirect sign of elevated right heart pressures but contrast opacification of the azygos vein in and of itself is not indicative of pulmonary hypertension.

■ **Case 48**

1. Which of the following support a diagnosis of persistent left superior vena cava (SVC)?
    a) Dilated coronary sinus
    b) Hypoxia
    c) Double aortic arch
    d) Dextrocardia
    e) Egg-on-a-string appearance on chest radiograph

The correct answer is (**a**). The persistent left SVC drains into the dilated coronary sinus.

2. What is typically the main clinical consequence of a persistent left SVC?
    a) Right heart failure
    b) Severe left-to-right shunt
    c) Mass effect
    d) Can result in complicated venous access with unusual catheter course
    e) Arrhythmia

The correct answer is (**d**). Persistent left SVC can present technical difficulties during venous catheter placement, especially if the right SVC and/or bridging brachiocephalic vein are small or absent.

■ **Case 49**

1. Which of the following supports a diagnosis of Kaposi sarcoma (KS)?
    a) Pericardial effusion
    b) Pneumothorax
    c) Pleural effusions
    d) Calcified nodules
    e) Halo sign

The correct answer is (**c**). Pleural effusions are commonly seen in association with pulmonary KS.

2. Which of the following best describes the typical appearance of nodules seen in KS?
    a) Flame shaped
    b) Popcorn
    c) Cavitary
    d) Well circumscribed
    e) Ground glass

The correct answer is (**a**). Nodules are typically ill defined and may be coalescent. This appearance has been described as "flame shaped."

■ **Case 50**

1. Which of the following supports a diagnosis of acute chest syndrome?
    a) H-type vertebral bodies
    b) Splenic autoinfarction
    c) Cardiomegaly
    d) Pulmonary hypertension
    e) New pulmonary opacity on chest radiograph

The correct answer is (**e**). Acute chest syndrome is defined as the presence of a new pulmonary opacity on chest radiograph in conjunction with at least one other new symptom or sign: chest pain, wheezing, cough, tachypnea, and/or fever higher than 38°C (100.4°F).

2. Which of the following is not a potential source of pulmonary edema in a patient with sickle cell anemia?
   a) Severe anemia
   b) Renal insufficiency
   c) Pancreatitis
   d) Cardiomyopathy
   e) Pulmonary hypertension

The correct answer is (**c**). Pancreatitis is not a common cause of pulmonary edema in patients with sickle cell anemia.

■ **Case 51**

1. Which of the following statements regarding bronchiolitis obliterans (BO) is true?
   a) BO is also known as bronchiolitis obliterans organizing pneumonia.
   b) BO affects the small-caliber cartilaginous airways.
   c) Predominant functional manifestation of BO is restriction with decline in total lung volume.
   d) BO is the histologic hallmark of chronic lung allograft rejection.
   e) None of the above

The correct answer is (**d**). Bronchiolitis obliterans (BO), also known as obliterative bronchiolitis, affects small-caliber noncartilaginous airways, producing airway obstruction. It is considered the histologic hallmark of chronic lung allograft dysfunction or rejection.

■ **Case 52**

1. Which of the following statements regarding restrictive allograft syndrome (RAS) is true?
   a) RAS can result from primary graft dysfunction (PGD), which can result from ischemia-reperfusion injury, airway injury, aspiration, donor-ventilator injury, or cold ischemia.
   b) RAS is an acute form of rejection that is characterized by the presence of perivascular and interstitial mononuclear cell infiltrate.
   c) RAS is the restrictive form of chronic lung allograft dysfunction (CLAD), which from a histopathology standpoint is characterized by pleuroparenchymal fibroelastosis.
   d) RAS is a likely end result of multiple deleterious mechanisms provoked by donor brain death, mechanical ventilation, allograft procurement stage, and ischemia-reperfusion injury.
   e) All of the above

The correct answer is (**c**). RAS is a chronic condition characterized by pleuroparenchymal fibroelastosis, is not associated with PGD, and is not an acute form of rejection. Deleterious mechanisms provoked by factors like donor brain death, mechanical ventilation, issues during donor-lung procurement, and ischemia-reperfusion injury are associated with PGD and not with CLAD/RAS.

■ **Case 53**

1. Which of the following statements best describes the imaging pattern typically seen in combined pulmonary fibrosis and emphysema (CPFE)?
   a) Centrilobular emphysema in the upper lung zone, with interstitial fibrosis in the lower lung zones
   b) Centrilobular emphysema in the lower lung zone, with interstitial fibrosis in the upper lung zones
   c) Panlobular emphysema in the lower lung zone, with interstitial fibrosis in the upper lung zones
   d) Panlobular emphysema in the upper lung zone, with interstitial fibrosis in the middle parahilar lung zones

The correct answer is (**a**). Histologic analysis of open lung biopsy or explanted lungs demonstrates predominantly centrilobular emphysema in the upper lobes and interstitial pulmonary fibrosis in the lower lobes often with usual interstitial pneumonia or nonspecific interstitial pneumonia. Desquamative interstitial pneumonia and respiratory bronchiolitis–associated interstitial lung disease with alveolar fibrosis have also been reported.

■ **Case 54**

1. Which of the following conditions is not part of chILD (childhood interstitial lung disease) syndrome?
   a) Total anomalous venous return
   b) Kartagener syndrome
   c) Tracheoesophageal fistula
   d) All of the above

The correct answer is (**d**). The diagnosis of chILD syndrome is a diagnosis of exclusion which requires the exclusion of the most common conditions associated with diffuse lung disease in children, such as cystic fibrosis, immunodeficiency syndromes, congenital heart disease, bronchopulmonary dysplasia, pulmonary infection, primary ciliary dyskinesia, and recurrent aspiration. Total anomalous venous return is a congenital heart disease that can be associated with interstitial pulmonary edema. Kartagener syndrome is part of the spectrum of ciliary dyskinesia. Tracheoesophageal fistula is associated with chronic aspiration, which produces chronic interstitial lung disease.

■ **Case 55**

1. Which of the following statements regarding Mounier–Kuhn syndrome is true?
   a) Pulmonary function test demonstrates restriction.
   b) Tracheobronchial diverticulosis is more pronounced in the anterior tracheal wall.
   c) Tracheobronchomegaly may be seen as a primary idiopathic disorder or as secondary to other chronic pulmonary diseases.
   d) Cartilaginous inflammation of the tracheal wall is the histopathologic hallmark of this condition.
   e) None of the above

The correct answer is (**c**). In addition to Mounier–Kuhn syndrome, which is considered an idiopathic primary disorder of the tracheobronchial wall, chronic pulmonary conditions, in particular those associated with chronic cough (e.g., pulmonary fibrosis, chronic obstructive pulmonary disease, recurrent infection), can also result in tracheobronchial dilation.

■ **Case 56**

1. Branching peripheral pulmonary calcified densities seen in a patient with usual interstitial pneumonia (UIP) most likely represents which of the following?
   a) Nodular pulmonary ossification (NPO)
   b) Dendriform pulmonary ossification (DPO)
   c) Metastatic pulmonary calcification
   d) Talc granulomas
   e) None of the above

The correct answer is (**b**). Pulmonary fibrosis including UIP pattern can be associated with DPO. NPO is more commonly seen in association with chronic heart disease. Metastatic calcification of the lung and talc granulomas are not associated with pulmonary fibrosis.

■ **Case 57**

1. Which of the following statements better describes Hermansky–Pudlak syndrome?
   a) Autosomal-dominant disorders characterized by early usual interstitial pneumonia (UIP) pattern of interstitial fibrosis in infancy
   b) Hereditary syndrome of oculocutaneous albinism and hemorrhagic diathesis that is commonly associated with pulmonary fibrosis later in life
   c) Autosomal-recessive syndrome characterized by accumulation of thick pulmonary secretions due to a mutation in the *CFTR* gene
   d) Genetic disorder secondary to protease inhibitor deficiency associated with destruction of alveolar walls

The correct answer is (**b**). This autosomal-recessive hereditary disease is characterized by oculocutaneous albinism associated with bleeding disorder and UIP pattern of pulmonary fibrosis late in life. Cystic fibrosis is an autosomal-recessive condition characterized by thick pulmonary secretions due to mutation in the gene for cystic fibrosis transmembrane conductance regulator (CFTR) protein. α_1-Antitrypsin deficiency is a genetic disorder secondary to protease inhibitor (α_1-antitrypsin) deficiency, with destruction of alveolar walls resulting in emphysema.

■ **Case 58**

1. In a patient with a retropharyngeal abscess, which of the following would be the most sensitive imaging sign for the diagnosis of acute descending necrotizing mediastinitis?
   a) Mediastinal widening
   b) Mediastinal gas
   c) Mediastinal fat stranding
   d) Mediastinal fluid collection
   e) None of the above

The correct answer is (**c**). Abnormal stranding and increased density of the mediastinal fat is the most sensitive CT imaging sign of mediastinitis. Other imaging findings such as mediastinal widening, abnormal gas bubbles, and fluid collections may also be present but are considered less sensitive.

■ **Case 59**

1. Which of the following statements better defines a pneumatocele?
   a) An air crescent collection of air that separates the wall of a cavity from an inner mass
   b) A small gas-containing space within the visceral pleura or in the subpleural lung, not larger than 1 cm in diameter
   c) An air-space measuring > 1 cm—usually several centimeters—in diameter, sharply demarcated by a thin wall that is no more than 1 mm in thickness, usually accompanied by emphysematous changes in the adjacent lung parenchyma
   d) A thin-walled, gas-filled space in the lung
   e) A gas-filled space, seen as a lucency or low-attenuation area, within pulmonary consolidation, a mass, or a nodule

The correct answer is (**d**). A collection of air that separates the wall of a cavity from an inner mass represents an air crescent. A small gas-containing space within the visceral pleura or in the subpleural lung, not larger than 1 cm in diameter, is a bleb. An air-space measuring > 1 cm—usually several centimeters—in diameter, sharply demarcated by a thin wall that is no more than 1 mm in thickness, and accompanied by emphysematous changes in the adjacent lung parenchyma, is a bulla. A gas-filled space, seen as a lucency or low-attenuation area, within pulmonary consolidation, a mass, or a nodule is a cavity.

■ Case 60

1. Which of the following is a common combination of congenital anomalies associated with 22q11.2 deletion syndrome?
   a) Hypertelorism, short stature, short webbed neck, pulmonic valve stenosis
   b) Conotruncal anomalies, cleft palate, immunodeficiency, hypocalcemia
   c) Low muscle tone, atrioventricular/endocardial cushion defect, mental disability
   d) Aortic coarctation, bicuspid aortic valve, short stature, partial anomalous pulmonary venous return

The correct answer is (**b**). Hypertelorism, short stature, webbed neck, and pulmonic valve stenosis are findings associated with Noonan syndrome. Low muscle tone, atrioventricular/endocardial cushion defect, and mental disability are common findings of Down syndrome. Aortic coarctation, bicuspid aortic valve, short stature, and partial anomalous venous return can be seen in patients with Turner syndrome.

■ Case 61

1. The typical clinical triad seen in patients with hyperimmunoglobulin E syndrome (HIES) includes which of the following?
   a) Bronchiectasis, sinusitis, situs inversus
   b) Thrombocytopenia, Sjögren syndrome, primary biliary cirrhosis
   c) Thymic aplasia, conotruncal abnormalities, hypocalcemia
   d) Staphylococcal abscesses, recurrent airway infection, increased levels of IgE

The correct answer is (**d**). Bronchiectasis, sinusitis, and situs inversus are associated with ciliary dyskinesia and Kartagener syndrome. Thymic aplasia, conotruncal abnormalities, and hypocalcemia are seen in DiGeorge syndrome. Thrombocytopenia, Sjögren syndrome, and primary biliary cirrhosis can be seen together as a manifestation of autoimmune disorder.

■ Case 62

1. Which of the following hematologic abnormalities is not associated with common variable immune deficiency (CVID)?
   a) Autoimmune neutropenia
   b) Autoimmune thrombocytopenic purpura
   c) Autoimmune hemolytic anemia
   d) Pernicious anemia
   e) Henoch–Schönlein purpura

The correct answer is (**e**). Henoch–Schönlein purpura, which more commonly affects children, results from a systemic small-vessel vasculitis and is not associated with CVID.

■ Case 63

1. Which of the following is the most likely diagnosis in a patient with altered mental status and fever who develops a complex pleural effusion with numerous small air-fluid levels?
   a) Bronchopleural fistula
   b) Bronchopleurocutaneous fistula
   c) Barotrauma
   d) Multiloculated empyema from anaerobic bacteria
   e) None of the above

The correct answer is (**d**). Anaerobes associated with pleuropulmonary disease are usually derived from the oropharyngeal flora, are commonly seen in patients with aspiration, and when associated with empyema may manifest as multiloculated pleural effusion with gas bubbles and loculated air-fluid levels.

■ Case 64

1. Which of the following is the most likely diagnosis for a newly diagnosed calcified lung mass in a 17-year-old girl with a history of gastric wall tumor and hypertension?
   a) Pulmonary chondroma
   b) Metastatic osteosarcoma
   c) Teratoma
   d) Mucinous adenocarcinoma
   e) Pulmonary hamartoma

The correct answer is (**a**). This patient likely has a pulmonary chondroma. The history of a gastric tumor and hypertension along with a calcified lung mass in a young female patient suggests the possibility of Carney triad (pulmonary chondroma, gastrointestinal stromal tumor, and extra-adrenal paraganglioma).

■ **Case 65**

1. Which of the following is the most common combination of malignancies associated with Gardner syndrome?
   a) Hepatoblastoma, adrenal carcinoma, medulloblastoma
   b) Colorectal cancer, small bowel cancer, pancreatic cancer, papillary thyroid carcinoma
   c) Cholangiocarcinoma, gastric cancer, adrenal carcinoma
   d) Fibroma, sebaceous cyst, lipoma
   e) All of the above

The correct answer is (**b**). The most common malignancy associated with Gardner syndrome is colorectal cancer, followed by cancer of the small bowel, cancer of the pancreas, and papillary thyroid carcinoma. Several other malignancies have been associated with Gardner syndrome but are less common (hepatoblastoma, adrenal carcinoma, gliomas, cholangiocarcinomas, medulloblastoma). Fibromas, sebaceous cysts, and lipomas are common nonmalignant abnormalities in Gardner syndrome.

■ **Case 66**

1. Which of the following imaging features favor a thrombus over a pulmonary artery sarcoma?
   a) Large endoluminal filling defect involving the bilateral pulmonary arteries
   b) Internal calcification and contrast enhancement
   c) Increased diameter of the affected vessel
   d) Low metabolic activity on fluorodeoxyglucose–positron emission tomography (FDG-PET)
   e) None of the above

The correct answer is (**d**). The presence of a large endoluminal filling defect in the pulmonary vasculature with internal calcification, contrast enhancement, and increased diameter of the affected vessel suggest a pulmonary artery sarcoma. Low metabolic activity on FDG-PET favors a thrombus.

■ **Case 67**

1. Which of the following combinations of hemodynamic findings is expected in a patient with pulmonary capillary hemangiomatosis (PCH)?
   a) Mean pulmonary artery pressure (mPAP) = 35 mm Hg; pulmonary capillary wedge pressure (PCWP) = 20 mm Hg
   b) mPAP = 20 mm Hg; PCWP = 20 mm Hg
   c) mPAP = 20 mm Hg; PCWP = 10 mm Hg
   d) mPAP = 35 mm Hg; PCWP = 10 mm Hg
   e) None of the above

The correct answer is (**d**). From a hemodynamic standpoint, both PCH and pulmonary veno-occlusive disease are characterized by pulmonary arterial hypertension (mPAP $\geq$ 25 mm Hg), with normal or low PCWP ($\leq$ 15 mm Hg).

■ **Case 68**

1. Which of the following is the most common anatomic location of congenital lobar overinflation?
   a) Right upper lobe
   b) Right middle lobe
   c) Right lower lobe
   d) Left upper lobe
   e) Left lower lobe

The correct answer is (**d**). About 50% of cases of congenital lobar overinflation are seen in the left upper lobe. The second most common location is in the right middle lobe. Lower lobe involvement is less common.

■ **Case 69**

1. Regarding malignant tracheal tumors, which of the following statements is true?
   a) Adenoid cystic carcinoma predominantly affects elderly male current or former smokers.
   b) Endotracheal carcinoid is the most common tracheal tumor in children.
   c) Mucoepidermoid carcinoma usually manifests as a long segment of tracheal narrowing.
   d) Squamous cell carcinoma may be associated with synchronous or metachronous carcinomas of the oropharynx, larynx, or lung.
   e) None of the above

The correct answer is (**d**). As much as 40% of squamous cell carcinomas of the trachea are associated with carcinomas of the upper airway or lung parenchyma.

■ **Case 70**

1. In a trauma patient with bilateral rib fractures and extensive parenchymal opacities, a chest radiograph 2 weeks after injury reveals worsening air-space consolidation in the left lower lobe. Which of the following is the least likely diagnosis?
   a) Laceration
   b) Atelectasis
   c) Pneumonia
   d) Contusion
   e) Aspiration

The correct answer is (**d**). Pulmonary contusion commonly resolves after 7 to 10 days. A persistent or worsening opacity after 10 days in a trauma patient raises concern for infection, atelectasis, or aspiration. A pulmonary laceration may also persist for an extended time.

■ Case 71

1. Which of the following combinations is commonly seen in Morgagni hernias?
   a) Posterior right side associated with pulmonary hypoplasia
   b) Posterior left side associated with rib fractures
   c) Anterior right side with fat density
   d) Anterior left side containing stomach
   e) All of the above

The correct answer is (**c**). The majority of Morgagni hernias occur in the right side and contain omentum, which has a predominantly fat density with small-caliber vessels that can be tracked from the anterior mediastinum to the abdomen through the anterior diaphragmatic defect.

■ Case 72

1. Which of the following findings would be expected in a patient with diffuse idiopathic pulmonary neuroendocrine cell hyperplasia (DIPNECH)?
   a) Hilar and mediastinal lymphadenopathy
   b) Forced expiratory volume in 1 second of 40% predicted
   c) Calcified pulmonary nodules
   d) Pleural effusion
   e) All of the above

The correct answer is (**b**). DIPNECH is associated with airway obstruction, with mosaic pattern of lung attenuation on CT images, and with obstructive changes on pulmonary function tests. Neither hilar/mediastinal lymphadenopathy nor pleural effusion is a common finding in DIPNECH. Tumorlets and carcinoids associated with DIPNECH do not calcify.

■ Case 73

1. In a young patient with congenital bronchiectasis, which of the following findings would be inconsistent with Williams–Campbell syndrome?
   a) Normal trachea and mainstem bronchi
   b) Fourth, fifth, and sixth bronchial generation cystic and cylindrical bronchiectasis
   c) Situs inversus, varicoid bronchiectasis, and sinusitis
   d) Cystic bronchiectasis with expiratory collapse
   e) All of the above

The correct answer is (**c**). Situs inversus totalis, varicoid bronchiectasis, and sinusitis are characteristic of primary ciliary dyskinesia with Kartagener syndrome.

■ Case 74

1. Which of the following findings is more likely to be seen in people who abuse intravenous (IV) drugs and have endocarditis and pulmonary septic embolism?
   a) Pulmonic valve stenosis
   b) Tricuspid valve regurgitation
   c) Tricuspid valve stenosis
   d) Pulmonic valve insufficiency
   e) None of the above

The correct answer is (**b**). Most commonly affected cardiac valve in IV drug abuse–related endocarditis is the tricuspid valve, with resultant regurgitation. The pulmonic valve is less commonly affected in endocarditis, and when compromised, insufficiency is more common than stenosis.

■ Case 75

1. Regarding solitary fibrous tumor of the pleura (SFTP), which of the following statements is true?
   a) It is currently considered to represent a benign form of mesothelioma.
   b) It is commonly associated with asbestos exposure.
   c) It arises from the mesothelial layer of the parietal pleura.
   d) Hypoglycemia and periosteal hypertrophy are known paraneoplastic manifestations.
   e) None of the above

The correct answer is (**d**). Paraneoplastic syndromes associated with SFTP include refractory hypoglycemia (Doege–Potter syndrome), clubbing, and hypertrophic pulmonary osteoarthropathy (Pierre Marie–Bamberger syndrome). These paraneoplastic manifestations occur in 4 to 20% of cases and are more commonly associated with large tumors.

■ Case 76

1. Which of the following imaging findings favors a primary thoracic sarcoma?
   a) Multiple pulmonary masses with mediastinal lymphadenopathy
   b) Large (10 cm) nonenhancing cavitary mass
   c) Calcified, solid, and cystic mediastinal mass
   d) Large 10-cm single mass with pleural effusion and no lymphadenopathy
   e) None of the above

The correct answer is (**d**). Primary thoracic sarcomas commonly present as a large (> 5 cm) soft tissue density solid mass with pleural effusion and no associated lymphadenopathy.

■ Case 77

1. Which of the following is commonly associated with primary effusion lymphoma (PEL)?
   a) Multicenter Castleman disease
   b) Kaposi sarcoma
   c) Epstein–Barr virus (EBV) infection
   d) All of the above
   e) None of the above

The correct answer is (**d**). PEL is commonly associated with human herpesvirus type 8 (HHV-8) infection in HIV-positive individuals with AIDS. Preexisting Kaposi sarcoma and multicenter Castleman disease are common and are additional manifestations of HHV-8 infection. Coinfection with EBV is also very common (> 90%).

■ Case 78

1. Regarding the imaging evaluation of fibrosing mediastinitis, which of the following statements is true?
   a) Multidetector CT (MDCT) is the best imaging modality for the evaluation of visceral involvement.
   b) On MR image, the focal form demonstrates high signal intensity on T2-weighted sequences.
   c) On 18-fluorodeoxyglucose–positron emission tomography (FDG-PET), fibrosing mediastinitis, as with most inflammatory pathologies, consistently exhibits increased metabolic activity.
   d) Conventional radiographs, when abnormal, demonstrate increased density in the posterior mediastinum.
   e) None of the above

The correct answer is (**a**). Currently, MDCT is considered the imaging modality of choice for the evaluation of fibrosing mediastinitis. MDCT is better than MR for the demonstration of internal calcification and complications from visceral encasement. FDG-PET exhibits a variable degree of metabolic activity. The most common manifestations on conventional radiography are mediastinal widening and abnormalities in the middle mediastinum.

■ Case 79

1. Which of the following is associated with multicentric Castleman disease?
   a) HIV infection
   b) Human herpesvirus type 8 (HHV-8) infection
   c) Kaposi sarcoma
   d) Lymphoma
   e) All of the above

The correct answer is (**e**). Multicentric Castleman disease may occur in association with HHV-8 infection, HIV infection, Kaposi sarcoma, and lymphoma.

■ Case 80

1. Which of the following is a common finding expected in a heart-lung transplant patient with posttransplant lymphoproliferative disorder (PTLD)?
   a) Hilar and mediastinal hypoattenuating lymphadenopathy
   b) Recurrent pleural effusion
   c) Lymphangitic spread in the bilateral lungs
   d) Paraspinal and extrapleural mass lesions
   e) None of the above

The correct answer is (**a**). In the case of heart or lung transplantation, the lung-hila and mediastinum is the most common location of PTLD; nodal involvement is the most significant imaging finding with hypoattenuating enlarged mediastinal-hilar lymph nodes or mediastinal mass.

■ Case 81

1. Which of the following statements regarding coccidioidomycosis infection is true?
   a) The lungs are the target organ of primary infection.
   b) Suppression of cellular immunity is a significant risk factor.
   c) Disseminated disease may manifest as a miliary pattern with numerous small pulmonary nodules.
   d) Air-space disease and consolidation with lymphadenopathy are common imaging findings.
   e) All of the above

The correct answer is (**e**). The lungs are the primary target organ in *Coccidioides* spp. infection. Airborne spores reach the lung parenchyma, inducing air-space consolidation, and manifest as a community-acquired pneumonia. Concomitant lymphadenopathy is common. In a minority of cases, as in patients with suppressed cellular immunity, disseminated multinodular miliary disease may occur.

■ Case 82

1. Which of the following statements regarding organizing pneumonia is false?
   a) Cryptogenic organizing pneumonia (COP) is considered an idiopathic interstitial pneumonia.
   b) The most common cause of COP is previous pulmonary infection.
   c) When organizing pneumonia is seen in association with connective tissue disease, it is considered secondary organizing pneumonia.
   d) Men and women are equally affected, typically in the 5th or 6th decade of life.
   e) All of the above

The correct answer is (**b**). By definition, the etiology of COP is unknown. Organizing pneumonia after a pulmonary infection is considered a secondary form of this condition.

■ Case 83

1. Which of the following is considered the most common cause of diffuse alveolar hemorrhage (DAH) in adults?
   a) Idiopathic pulmonary hemosiderosis and mitral stenosis
   b) Henoch–Schönlein purpura and pulmonary capillary hemangiomatosis
   c) Behçet syndrome and pulmonary veno-occlusive disease
   d) Granulomatosis with polyangiitis (GPA) and Goodpasture syndrome
   e) None of the above

The correct answer is (**d**). GPA and Goodpasture syndrome are two of the most common conditions associated with DAH. Idiopathic pulmonary hemosiderosis is also a cause of DAH but is not the most common and often presents in childhood. All other conditions listed are also associated with DAH but are not the most common.

■ Case 84

1. Which of the following statements regarding idiopathic chronic eosinophilic pneumonia (ICEP) is correct?
   a) Less than 50% of affected patients present with the "characteristic" pattern of peripheral pulmonary opacities.
   b) Most patients present with significant extrapulmonary involvement.
   c) Coexistent parasitic infection is the norm.
   d) Microscopic examination of the lung reveals eosinophilic granulomatosis with polyangiitis.
   e) None of the above

The correct answer is (**a**). The so-called characteristic pattern of peripheral ground-glass opacities is seen in only a minority of cases. Different from other conditions associated with eosinophilia, extrapulmonary involvement in ICEP is uncommon. Parasitic infection is commonly seen associated with pulmonary eosinophilia but not with the idiopathic form of the disease. Eosinophilic granulomatosis with polyangiitis is the histopathologic finding of Churg–Strauss syndrome, not of ICEP.

■ Case 85

1. Which of the following is not commonly seen in acute inhalation lung injury?
   a) Tracheal stenosis
   b) Organizing pneumonia
   c) Constrictive bronchiolitis
   d) Alveolar hemorrhage
   e) Diffuse panbronchiolitis

The correct answer is (**e**). Tracheobronchial inhalational injury may induce acute edema with residual stenosis. Organizing pneumonia, constrictive bronchiolitis, and alveolar hemorrhage are all known complication of acute inhalation injury. Diffuse panbronchiolitis is a rare idiopathic disorder characterized by cellular bronchiolitis and chronic sinusitis, is more commonly seen in Asian individuals, and is not associated with acute inhalation injury.

■ Case 86

1. Which of the following findings is not suggestive of an infected aortic aneurysm?
   a) Fusiform shape and calcified wall in the infrarenal abdominal aorta
   b) Saccular and lobulated wall
   c) Intramural or periaortic gas
   d) Periaortic stranding
   e) All of the above

The correct answer is (**a**). Fusiform shape and calcified wall in the infrarenal abdominal aorta are characteristic imaging findings of an atherosclerotic aneurysm.

Case 87

1. A 65-year-old male patient presents with chest pain after a motor vehicle accident. CT images of his chest and abdomen reveal large right-side pleural effusion, a cirrhotic liver, and evidence of portal hypertension. Which of the following findings suggests that the pleural effusion is more likely to be a traumatic hemothorax rather than effusion related to his underlying cirrhosis?
   a) Focused assessment with sonography for trauma (FAST) ultrasound positive for anechoic fluid
   b) CT density = 12 Hounsfield units (HU)
   c) Multiple right-side rib fractures
   d) 7% hematocrit on the pleural fluid

The correct answer is (c). Multiple rib fractures ipsilateral to a pleural fluid collection in a trauma patient suggests hemothorax. FAST ultrasound is positive in the presence of nontraumatic pleural effusions. Low-density fluid (< 15 HU) and low hematocrit level on the pleural fluid suggest that it is not an acute traumatic hemothorax.

Case 88

1. Which of the following imaging features is expected in a mediastinal unilocular lymphangioma?
   a) Anechoic on ultrasound
   b) Average density of 5 and 7 Hounsfield units before and after contrast injection on CT
   c) Isointense to muscle on T1- weighted images and hyperintense on T2-weighted images on MR
   d) No metabolic activity on fluorodeoxyglucose–positron emission tomography (FDG-PET) scans
   e) All of the above

The correct answer is (e). Cystic hygromas are characterized by a cystic-looking mass with water or near-water density on CT, which is typically isointense to muscle on T1-weighted and hyperintense on T2-weighted sequences. Cystic lymphangiomas display no metabolic activity on FDG-PET scans.

Case 89

1. Which of the following statements regarding amyloidosis is true?
   a) Amyloidosis is less commonly a primary disease than secondary to other pathologic processes.
   b) In the lung parenchyma, the nodular form is characterized by multiple nodules that rarely calcify.
   c) Tracheobronchial involvement is always focal and localized.
   d) Cardiac involvement in amyloidosis is only seen in the senile form of the disease.
   e) None of the above

The correct answer is (a). Amyloidosis secondary to other pathologies is more common in clinical practice than the primary form of the disease. The nodular form of pulmonary amyloidosis may calcify in a substantial number of cases. Generalized tracheobronchial involvement with long-segment wall thickening and narrowing is common. The heart can be involved in several forms of amyloidosis in addition to the senile form.

Case 90

1. Which of the following statements regarding tracheobronchial metastasis is true?
   a) Tracheal involvement is common.
   b) Most are diagnosed about the same time of the primary tumor.
   c) They are not commonly seen in association with other signs of disseminated disease.
   d) Common primary malignancies include breast, colon, and kidney.
   e) None of the above

The correct answer is (d). Breast, colorectal, and kidney cancer are common sources of endobronchial metastases. Most are bronchial in location, rarely tracheal, and are typically seen in patients with advanced disease.

Case 91

1. Which of the following is not an appropriate indication for MRI in a patient with lung cancer?
   a) Possible mediastinal invasion in a patient with pericardial effusion
   b) Follow-up of an indeterminate 8-mm pulmonary nodule
   c) Upper lobe mass in a patient with ipsilateral blepharoptosis and miosis
   d) Postradiation follow-up in a patient with postobstructive opacity
   e) All of the above

The correct answer is (b). MRI is not the imaging modality of choice in the follow-up of an indeterminate nodule in a patient with known lung cancer. Evaluation of the mediastinum, heart, and pericardium; evaluation of the thoracic inlet and apical chest wall in a patient with an upper lobe/apical mass and Horner syndrome; and differentiation between tumor, atelectasis, and postobstructive pneumonia are all appropriate indications for MRI in a patient with lung cancer.

■ **Case 92**

1. Which of the following thoracotomies is more likely to be associated with development of a lung hernia as a postoperative complication?
   a) Midline
   b) Clamshell
   c) Anterolateral
   d) Posterolateral
   e) Both c and d are correct.

The correct answer is (**e**). Acquired postsurgical lung hernias may occur after either anterolateral or posterolateral thoracotomies, in particular after rib resection. Lung hernias do not present after midline or clamshell sternotomy.

■ **Case 93**

1. Which of the following imaging features in an incidental breast mass detected in a female trauma patient is more concerning for malignancy?
   a) Calcifications
   b) Oval shape
   c) Spiculated shape
   d) No contrast enhancement
   e) None of the above

The correct answer is (**c**). Spiculated and lobulated contour as well as contrast enhancement are imaging features that suggest malignancy. Oval or ellipsoid shape, smooth contour, calcification, and no contrast enhancement are CT imaging features that favor a benign lesion.

■ **Case 94**

1. Which of the following imaging findings is more likely a good predictor of upper gastrointestinal bleeding in a patient with portal hypertension?
   a) Esophageal varices > 5 mm in diameter
   b) Paraesophageal varices >10 mm in diameter
   c) Collateral flow through the azygos and hemiazygos veins
   d) Dilated coronary (left gastric) vein >10 mm
   e) None of the above

The correct answer is (**a**). Large esophageal varices (> 5 mm) are considered high risk for esophageal bleeding. Dilated paraesophageal varices, which commonly drain to the azygos and hemiazygos veins, and to the coronary (left gastric) vein, have lower tendency to bleed than esophageal varices.

■ **Case 95**

1. Which of the following statements regarding hepatopulmonary syndrome is false?
   a) It can be seen in noncirrhotic patients.
   b) Intrapulmonary arteriovenous shunting is the underlying abnormality responsible for the clinical manifestations.
   c) Pulmonary perfusion scan with technetium-99m–labeled macroaggregated albumin is the imaging modality of choice.
   d) CT reveals dilated and prominent peripheral pulmonary vessels.
   e) All of the above

The correct answer is (**c**). Pulmonary perfusion scan with technetium-99m–labeled macroaggregated albumin may reveal extrapulmonary uptake, but the imaging modality of choice is contrast-enhanced echocardiography. All other statements are true.

■ **Case 96**

1. Which of the following is the least likely diagnosis in a 55-year-old patient with a sternal tumor?
   a) Chondroma
   b) Chondrosarcoma
   c) Metastasis
   d) Plasmacytoma

The correct answer is (**a**). Primary benign tumors of the sternum are very rare. Metastasis is the most common sternal tumor. Among primary sternal malignancies, chondrosarcoma is the most common. Other primary sternal malignancies include osteosarcoma, plasmacytoma, lymphoma, and Ewing sarcoma.

■ **Case 97**

1. Which of the following CT findings is not expected in a 35-year-old man with acute respiratory distress syndrome (ARDS) secondary to intra-abdominal sepsis?
   a) Crazy-paving opacities in a bilateral distribution
   b) Bibasilar-dependent air-space consolidation
   c) Air cyst and dilated bronchi
   d) Cardiomegaly
   e) All of the above

The correct answer is (**d**). The presence of cardiomegaly in a patient with imaging findings in the lung parenchyma similar to those seen in ARDS favors cardiogenic pulmonary edema over ARDS. Crazy-paving abnormalities, bibasilar-dependent consolidation, air cysts, and dilated bronchi are commonly seen in ARDS.

■ Case 98

1. Which of the following is a good combination for
    Strongyloides stercoralis hyperinfection syndrome?
    a) Eosinophilia in blood and multifocal nodular and
        patchy pulmonary opacities in a patient after renal
        transplantation
    b) Neutrophilia in blood and lobar consolidation in a
        patient with diabetes
    c) Lymphocytosis in blood and apical lung cavitary
        lesion in a patient who is HIV positive
    d) Neutropenia in blood and cavitary nodule with
        ground-glass halo in a patient following lung
        transplantation
    e) None of the above

The correct answer is (**a**). Eosinophilia in blood and
multifocal nodular and patchy pulmonary opacities in a
patient after renal transplant should raise the possibility
of *S. stercoralis* infection. Neutrophilia in blood and lobar
consolidation in a patient with diabetes suggests bacterial
pneumonia. Lymphocytosis in blood and apical lung cavitary lesion in a patient with HIV suggests the possibility of
tuberculosis. Neutropenia in blood and a cavitary nodule
with ground-glass halo in a patient after lung transplant
can be seen in angioinvasive aspergillosis.

■ Case 99

1. Which of the following names is commonly used to
    refer to a malignant peripheral nerve sheath tumor
    (MPNST) with rhabdomyoblastic differentiation?
    a) Neurofibrosarcoma
    b) Malignant triton tumor
    c) Malignant schwannoma
    d) Primitive neuroectodermal tumor
    e) None of the above

The correct answer is (**b**). MPNST with rhabdomyoblastic
differentiation (skeletal muscle) is known as malignant triton tumor, and has a worse prognosis than a conventional
MPNST.

■ Case 100

1. Which of the following statements regarding
    peripheral primitive neuroectodermal tumors (PNET)
    is true?
    a) PNET typically arise in the central nervous system
        in children.
    b) The most common location is in the chest wall.
    c) Ewing sarcoma of bone, extraskeletal Ewing
        sarcoma, PNET, and Askin tumor are part of the
        Ewing sarcoma family of tumors.
    d) Histopathologic differentiation between the
        different types of round-blue small-cell tumors
        can be accomplished with light microscopy and
        hematoxylin-eosin staining.
    e) None of the above

The correct answer is (**c**). The Ewing sarcoma family of
tumors comprises a spectrum of neoplastic diseases with
similar histologic and immunohistochemical characteristics and a nonrandom chromosomal translocation, and it
includes the classic Ewing sarcoma of bone, extraskeletal
Ewing sarcoma, PNET, and malignant small-cell tumor of
the chest wall (Askin tumor).

Further Readings

■ Case 1

Hertzenberg C, Daon E, Kramer J. Intralobar pulmonary sequestration in adults: three case reports. J Thorac Dis 2012;4(5):516–519

Walker CM, Wu CC, Gilman MD, Godwin JD II, Shepard JA, Abbott GF. The imaging spectrum of bronchopulmonary sequestration. Curr Probl Diagn Radiol 2014;43(3):100–114

Zylak CJ, Eyler WR, Spizarny DL, Stone CH. Developmental lung anomalies in the adult: radiologic-pathologic correlation. Radiographics 2002;22(Spec No):S25–S43

■ Case 2

Berrocal T, Madrid C, Novo S, Gutiérrez J, Arjonilla A, Gómez-León N. Congenital anomalies of the tracheobronchial tree, lung, and mediastinum: embryology, radiology, and pathology. Radiographics 2004;24(1):e17

Jeung M-Y, Gasser B, Gangi A, et al. Imaging of cystic masses of the mediastinum. Radiographics 2002;22(Spec No): S79–S93

■ Case 3

Engelke C, Schaefer-Prokop C, Schirg E, Freihorst J, Grubnic S, Prokop M. High-resolution CT and CT angiography of peripheral pulmonary vascular disorders. Radiographics 2002;22(4):739–764

Frazier AA, Galvin JR, Franks TJ, Rosado-De-Christenson ML. From the archives of the AFIP: pulmonary vasculature: hypertension and infarction. Radiographics 2000;20(2): 491–524, quiz 530–531, 532

Minai OA, Rigelsky C, Eng C, Arroliga AC, Stoller JK. Long-term outcome in a patient with pulmonary hypertension and hereditary hemorrhagic telangiectasia. Chest 2007;131(4):984–987

■ Case 4

Biyyam DR, Chapman T, Ferguson MR, Deutsch G, Dighe MK. Congenital lung abnormalities: embryologic features, prenatal diagnosis, and postnatal radiologic-pathologic correlation. Radiographics 2010;30(6):1721–1738

Paterson A. Imaging evaluation of congenital lung abnormalities in infants and children. Radiol Clin North Am 2005;43(2):303–323

■ Case 5

Rosado-de-Christenson ML, Templeton PA, Moran CA. From the archives of the AFIP. Mediastinal germ cell tumors: radiologic and pathologic correlation. Radiographics 1992;12(5):1013–1030

Strollo DC, Rosado-de-Christenson ML. Primary mediastinal malignant germ cell neoplasms: imaging features. Chest Surg Clin N Am 2002;12(4):645–658

Whitten CR, Khan S, Munneke GJ, Grubnic S. A diagnostic approach to mediastinal abnormalities. Radiographics 2007;27(3):657–671

■ Case 6

Erasmus JJ, Connolly JE, McAdams HP, Roggli VL. Solitary pulmonary nodules: part I. Morphologic evaluation for differentiation of benign and malignant lesions. Radiographics 2000;20(1):43–58

MacMahon H, Naidich DP, Goo JM, et al. Guideline for management of incidental pulmonary nodules detected on CT images: from the Fleischner Society 2017. Radiology 2017;284(1):228–243

■ Case 7

King MA, Stone JA, Diaz PT, Mueller CF, Becker WJ, Gadek JE. Alpha 1-antitrypsin deficiency: evaluation of bronchiectasis with CT. Radiology 1996;199(1):137–141

Needham M, Stockley RA. Alpha1-antitrypsin deficiency. 3: clinical manifestations and natural history. Thorax 2004;59(11):986–991

■ Case 8

Bruzzi JF, Komaki R, Walsh GL, et al. Imaging of non-small cell lung cancer of the superior sulcus: part 1: anatomy, clinical manifestations, and management. Radiographics 2008;28(2):551–560, quiz 620

Bruzzi JF, Komaki R, Walsh GL, et al. Imaging of non-small cell lung cancer of the superior sulcus: part 2: initial staging and assessment of resectability and therapeutic response. Radiographics 2008;28(2):561–572

■ **Case 9**

Chong S, Lee KS, Chung MJ, Han J, Kwon OJ, Kim TS. Neuroendocrine tumors of the lung: clinical, pathologic, and imaging findings. Radiographics 2006;26(1):41–57, discussion 57–58

Irshad A, Ravenel JG. Imaging of small-cell lung cancer. Curr Probl Diagn Radiol 2004;33(5):200–211

■ **Case 10**

Kim TH, Kim SJ, Ryu YH, et al. Differential CT features of infectious pneumonia versus bronchioloalveolar carcinoma (BAC) mimicking pneumonia. Eur Radiol 2006;16(8):1763–1768

Travis WD, Brambilla E, Noguchi M, et al. International Association for the Study of Lung Cancer/American Thoracic Society/European Respiratory Society International multidisciplinary classification of lung adenocarcinoma. J Thorac Oncol 2011;6(2):244–285

■ **Case 11**

Castañer E, Gallardo X, Rimola J, et al. Congenital and acquired pulmonary artery anomalies in the adult: radiologic overview. Radiographics 2006;26(2):349–371

Nguyen ET, Silva CIS, Seely JM, Chong S, Lee KS, Müller NL. Pulmonary artery aneurysms and pseudoaneurysms in adults: findings at CT and radiography. AJR Am J Roentgenol 2007;188(2):W126-W134

■ **Case 12**

Burrill J, Williams CJ, Bain G, Conder G, Hine AL, Misra RR. Tuberculosis: a radiologic review. Radiographics 2007;27(5):1255–1273

Nachiappan AC, Rahbar K, Shi X, et al. Pulmonary tuberculosis: role of radiology in diagnosis and management. Radiographics 2017;37(1):52–72

■ **Case 13**

Franquet T, Müller NL, Giménez A, Guembe P, de La Torre J, Bagué S. Spectrum of pulmonary aspergillosis: histologic, clinical, and radiologic findings. Radiographics 2001;21(4):825–837

Martinez S, Heyneman LE, McAdams HP, Rossi SE, Restrepo CS, Eraso A. Mucoid impactions: finger-in-glove sign and other CT and radiographic features. Radiographics 2008;28(5):1369–1382

■ **Case 14**

Lipchik RJ, Kuzo RS. Nosocomial pneumonia. Radiol Clin North Am 1996;34(1):47–58

Walker CM, Abbott GF, Greene RE, Shepard JA, Vummidi D, Digumarthy SR. Imaging pulmonary infection: classic signs and patterns. AJR Am J Roentgenol 2014;202(3): 479–492

■ **Case 15**

Franquet T. Imaging of pulmonary viral pneumonia. Radiology 2011;260(1):18–39

Kim EA, Lee KS, Primack SL, et al. Viral pneumonias in adults: radiologic and pathologic findings. Radiographics 2002;22(Spec No):S137–S149

■ **Case 16**

Franquet T, Giménez A, Hidalgo A. Imaging of opportunistic fungal infections in immunocompromised patient. Eur J Radiol 2004;51(2):130–138

Kanne JP, Yandow DR, Meyer CA. *Pneumocystis jiroveci* pneumonia: high-resolution CT findings in patients with and without HIV infection. AJR Am J Roentgenol 2012;198(6):W555-W561

■ **Case 17**

Kramer SS, Wehunt WD, Stocker JT, Kashima H. Pulmonary manifestations of juvenile laryngotracheal papillomatosis. AJR Am J Roentgenol 1985;144(4):687–694

Kuhlman JE, Reyes BL, Hruban RH, et al. Abnormal air-filled spaces in the lung. Radiographics 1993;13(1):47–75

Prince JS, Duhamel DR, Levin DL, Harrell JH, Friedman PJ. Nonneoplastic lesions of the tracheobronchial wall: radiologic findings with bronchoscopic correlation. Radiographics 2002;22(Spec No):S215–S230

■ **Case 18**

Franquet T, Müller NL, Giménez A, Guembe P, de La Torre J, Bagué S. Spectrum of pulmonary aspergillosis: histologic, clinical, and radiologic findings. Radiographics 2001;21(4):825–837

Pinto PS. The CT halo sign. Radiology 2004;230(1):109–110

■ **Case 19**

Hong SH, Choi J-Y, Lee JW, Kim NR, Choi JA, Kang HS. MR imaging assessment of the spine: infection or an imitation? Radiographics 2009;29(2):599–612

Ledermann HP, Schweitzer ME, Morrison WB, Carrino JA. MR imaging findings in spinal infections: rules or myths? Radiology 2003;228(2):506–514

■ **Case 20**

Boiselle PM, Mansilla AV, Fisher MS, McLoud TC. Wandering wires: frequency of sternal wire abnormalities in patients with sternal dehiscence. AJR Am J Roentgenol 1999;173(3):777–780

Jolles H, Henry DA, Roberson JP, Cole TJ, Spratt JA. Mediastinitis following median sternotomy: CT findings. Radiology 1996;201(2):463–466

■ **Case 21**

Fishman EK, Kuhlman JE, Jones RJ. CT of lymphoma: spectrum of disease. Radiographics 1991;11(4):647–669

Strollo DC, Rosado de Christenson ML, Jett JR. Primary mediastinal tumors. Part 1: tumors of the anterior mediastinum. Chest 1997;112(2):511–522

Whitten CR, Khan S, Munneke GJ, Grubnic S. A diagnostic approach to mediastinal abnormalities. Radiographics 2007;27(3):657–671

■ **Case 22**

Dynes MC, White EM, Fry WA, Ghahremani GG. Imaging manifestations of pleural tumors. Radiographics 1992;12(6):1191–1201

Wang ZJ, Reddy GP, Gotway MB, et al. Malignant pleural mesothelioma: evaluation with CT, MR imaging, and PET. Radiographics 2004;24(1):105–119

■ **Case 23**

Heyneman LE, Johkoh T, Ward S, Honda O, Yoshida S, Müller NL. Pulmonary leukemic infiltrates: high-resolution CT findings in 10 patients. AJR Am J Roentgenol 2000;174(2):517–521

Okada F, Ando Y, Kondo Y, Matsumoto S, Maeda T, Mori H. Thoracic CT findings of adult T-cell leukemia or lymphoma. AJR Am J Roentgenol 2004;182(3):761–767

■ **Case 24**

Johkoh T, Müller NL, Ichikado K, et al. Intrathoracic multicentric Castleman disease: CT findings in 12 patients. Radiology 1998;209(2):477–481

McAdams HP, Rosado-de-Christenson M, Fishback NF, Templeton PA. Castleman disease of the thorax: radiologic features with clinical and histopathologic correlation. Radiology 1998;209(1):221–228

■ **Case 25**

Lynch DA, Travis WD, Müller NL, et al. Idiopathic interstitial pneumonias: CT features. Radiology 2005;236(1):10–21

Mueller-Mang C, Grosse C, Schmid K, Stiebellehner L, Bankier AA. What every radiologist should know about idiopathic interstitial pneumonias. Radiographics 2007;27(3):595–615

■ **Case 26**

Genofre EH, Vargas FS, Teixeira LR, et al. Reexpansion pulmonary edema. J Pneumol 2003;29(2):101–106

Sohara Y. Reexpansion pulmonary edema. Ann Thorac Cardiovasc Surg 2008;14(4):205–209

■ **Case 27**

Hagan IG, Burney K. Radiology of recreational drug abuse. Radiographics 2007;27(4):919–940

Sporer KA, Dorn E. Heroin-related noncardiogenic pulmonary edema: a case series. Chest 2001;120(5):1628–1632

■ Case 28

Roach HD, Davies GJ, Attanoos R, Crane M, Adams H, Phillips S. Asbestos: when the dust settles an imaging review of asbestos-related disease. Radiographics 2002;22(Spec No):S167–S184

Walker CM, Takasugi JE, Chung JH, et al. Tumorlike conditions of the pleura. Radiographics 2012;32(4):971–985

■ Case 29

Miller BH, Rosado-de-Christenson ML, Mason AC, Fleming MV, White CC, Krasna MJ. From the archives of the AFIP. Malignant pleural mesothelioma: radiologic-pathologic correlation. Radiographics 1996;16(3):613–644

Roach HD, Davies GJ, Attanoos R, Crane M, Adams H, Phillips S. Asbestos: when the dust settles an imaging review of asbestos-related disease. Radiographics 2002;22(Spec No):S167–S184

Wang ZJ, Reddy GP, Gotway MB, et al. Malignant pleural mesothelioma: evaluation with CT, MR imaging, and PET. Radiographics 2004;24(1):105–119

■ Case 30

Chong S, Lee KS, Chung MJ, Han J, Kwon OJ, Kim TS. Pneumoconiosis: comparison of imaging and pathologic findings. Radiographics 2006;26(1):59–77

Kim K-I, Kim CW, Lee MK, et al. Imaging of occupational lung disease. Radiographics 2001;21(6):1371–1391

■ Case 31

Hanak V, Golbin JM, Hartman TE, Ryu JH. High-resolution CT findings of parenchymal fibrosis correlate with prognosis in hypersensitivity pneumonitis. Chest 2008;134(1):133–138

Hirschmann JV, Pipavath SN, Godwin JD. Hypersensitivity pneumonitis: a historical, clinical, and radiologic review. Radiographics 2009;29(7):1921–1938

Matar LD, McAdams HP, Sporn TA. Hypersensitivity pneumonitis. AJR Am J Roentgenol 2000;174(4):1061–1066

■ Case 32

Johkoh T, Itoh H, Müller NL, et al. Crazy-paving appearance at thin-section CT: spectrum of disease and pathologic findings. Radiology 1999;211(1):155–160

Rossi SE, Erasmus JJ, Volpacchio M, Franquet T, Castiglioni T, McAdams HP. "Crazy-paving" pattern at thin-section CT of the lungs: radiologic-pathologic overview. Radiographics 2003;23(6):1509–1519

■ Case 33

Baron SE, Haramati LB, Rivera VT. Radiological and clinical findings in acute and chronic exogenous lipoid pneumonia. J Thorac Imaging 2003;18(4):217–224

Laurent F, Philippe JC, Vergier B, et al. Exogenous lipoid pneumonia: HRCT, MR, and pathologic findings. Eur Radiol 1999;9(6):1190–1196

■ Case 34

Hartman TE, Primack SL, Lee KS, Swensen SJ, Müller NL. CT of bronchial and bronchiolar diseases. Radiographics 1994;14(5):991–1003

Ooi GC, Khong PL, Chan-Yeung M, et al. High-resolution CT quantification of bronchiectasis: clinical and functional correlation. Radiology 2002;225(3):663–672

Ouellette H. The signet ring sign. Radiology 1999;212(1):67–68

■ Case 35

Boiselle PM, Feller-Kopman D, Ashiku S, Weeks D, Ernst A. Tracheobronchomalacia: evolving role of dynamic multislice helical CT. Radiol Clin North Am 2003;41(3):627–636

Carden KA, Boiselle PM, Waltz DA, Ernst A. Tracheomalacia and tracheobronchomalacia in children and adults: an in-depth review. Chest 2005;127(3):984–1005

■ Case 36

Dissanaike S, Shalhub S, Jurkovich GJ. The evaluation of pneumomediastinum in blunt trauma patients. J Trauma 2008;65(6):1340–1345

Kaewlai R, Avery LL, Asrani AV, Novelline RA. Multidetector CT of blunt thoracic trauma. Radiographics 2008;28(6):1555–1570

■ Case 37

Conces DJ Jr, Tarver RD, Vix VA. Broncholithiasis: CT features in 15 patients. AJR Am J Roentgenol 1991;157(2):249–253

Seo JB, Song KS, Lee JS, et al. Broncholithiasis: review of the causes with radiologic-pathologic correlation. Radiographics 2002;22(Spec No):S199–S213

■ Case 38

Araoz PA, Gotway MB, Harrington JR, Harmsen WS, Mandrekar JN. Pulmonary embolism: prognostic CT findings. Radiology 2007;242(3):889–897

Frazier AA, Galvin JR, Franks TJ, Rosado-De-Christenson ML. From the archives of the AFIP: pulmonary vasculature: hypertension and infarction. Radiographics 2000;20(2):491–524, quiz 530–531, 532

Revel MP, Triki R, Chatellier G, et al. Is it possible to recognize pulmonary infarction on multisection CT images? Radiology 2007;244(3):875–882

■ Case 39

Araoz PA, Gotway MB, Harrington JR, Harmsen WS, Mandrekar JN. Pulmonary embolism: prognostic CT findings. Radiology 2007;242(3):889–897

Frazier AA, Galvin JR, Franks TJ, Rosado-De-Christenson ML. From the archives of the AFIP: pulmonary vasculature: hypertension and infarction. Radiographics 2000;20(2): 491–524, quiz 530–531, 532

Ghaye B, Ghuysen A, Bruyere PJ, D'Orio V, Dondelinger RF. Can CT pulmonary angiography allow assessment of severity and prognosis in patients presenting with pulmonary embolism? What the radiologist needs to know. Radiographics 2006;26(1):23–39, discussion 39–40

■ Case 40

Hunter TB, Taljanovic MS, Tsau PH, Berger WG, Standen JR. Medical devices of the chest. Radiographics 2004;24(6): 1725–1746

Swain FR, Martinez F, Gripp M, Razdan R, Gagliardi J. Traumatic complications from placement of thoracic catheters and tubes. Emerg Radiol 2005;12(1–2):11–18

■ Case 41

Collins J, Stern EJ. Ground-glass opacity at CT: the ABCs. AJR Am J Roentgenol 1997;169(2):355–367

Lynch DA, Travis WD, Müller NL, et al. Idiopathic interstitial pneumonias: CT features. Radiology 2005;236(1):10–21

Unger JM, Peters ME, Hinke ML. Chest case of the day. AJR Am J Roentgenol 1986;146(5):1080–1086

Ware LB, Matthay MA. The acute respiratory distress syndrome. N Engl J Med 2000;342(18):1334–1349

■ Case 42

Hartman TE, Primack SL, Lee KS, Swensen SJ, Müller NL. CT of bronchial and bronchiolar diseases. Radiographics 1994;14(5):991–1003

Milliron B, Henry TS, Veeraraghavan S, Little BP. Bronchiectasis: mechanisms and imaging clues of associated common and uncommon diseases. Radiographics 2015;35(4):1011–1030

Nadel HR, Stringer DA, Levison H, Turner JA, Sturgess JM. The immotile cilia syndrome: radiological manifestations. Radiology 1985;154(3):651–655

Ouellette H. The signet ring sign. Radiology 1999;212(1): 67–68

■ Case 43

Lynch DA, Gamsu G, Ray CS, Aberle DR. Asbestos-related focal lung masses: manifestations on conventional and high-resolution CT scans. Radiology 1988;169(3): 603–607

Partap VA. The comet tail sign. Radiology 1999;213(2): 553–554

■ Case 44

Ghanem N, Altehoefer C, Springer O, et al. Radiological findings in Boerhaave's syndrome. Emerg Radiol 2003;10(1):8–13

Young CA, Menias CO, Bhalla S, Prasad SR. CT features of esophageal emergencies. Radiographics 2008;28(6):1541–1553

■ Case 45

Jang KM, Lee KS, Lee SJ, et al. The spectrum of benign esophageal lesions: imaging findings. Korean J Radiol 2002;3(3):199–210

Yang PS, Lee KS, Lee SJ, et al. Esophageal leiomyoma: radiologic findings in 12 patients. Korean J Radiol 2001;2(3):132–137

■ **Case 46**

Chauhan SS, Long JD. Management of tracheoesophageal fistulas in adults. Curr Treat Options Gastroenterol 2004;7(1):31–40

Giménez A, Franquet T, Erasmus JJ, Martínez S, Estrada P. Thoracic complications of esophageal disorders. Radiographics 2002;22(Spec No):S247–S258

■ **Case 47**

Frazier AA, Galvin JR, Franks TJ, Rosado-De-Christenson ML. From the archives of the AFIP: pulmonary vasculature: hypertension and infarction. Radiographics 2000;20(2):491–524, quiz 530–531, 532

Koyama T, Ueda H, Togashi K, Umeoka S, Kataoka M, Nagai S. Radiologic manifestations of sarcoidosis in various organs. Radiographics 2004;24(1):87–104

Miller BH, Rosado-de-Christenson ML, McAdams HP, Fishback NF. Thoracic sarcoidosis: radiologic-pathologic correlation. Radiographics 1995;15(2):421–437

Traill ZC, Maskell GF, Gleeson FV, High-Resolution CT. High-resolution CT findings of pulmonary sarcoidosis. AJR Am J Roentgenol 1997;168(6):1557–1560

■ **Case 48**

Goyal SK, Punnam SR, Verma G, Ruberg FL. Persistent left superior vena cava: a case report and review of literature. Cardiovasc Ultrasound 2008;6:50

Sonavane SK, Milner DM, Singh SP, Abdel Aal AK, Shahir KS, Chaturvedi A. Comprehensive imaging review of the superior vena cava. Radiographics 2015;35(7):1873–1892

■ **Case 49**

Restrepo CS, Martínez S, Lemos JA, et al. Imaging manifestations of Kaposi sarcoma. Radiographics 2006;26(4):1169–1185

Wolff SD, Kuhlman JE, Fishman EK. Thoracic Kaposi sarcoma in AIDS: CT findings. J Comput Assist Tomogr 1993;17(1):60–62

■ **Case 50**

Leong CS, Stark P. Thoracic manifestations of sickle cell disease. J Thorac Imaging 1998;13(2):128–134

Lonergan GJ, Cline DB, Abbondanzo SL. Sickle cell anemia. Radiographics 2001;21(4):971–994

■ **Case 51**

Gunn MLD, Godwin JD, Kanne JP, Flowers ME, Chien JW. High-resolution CT findings of bronchiolitis obliterans syndrome after hematopoietic stem cell transplantation. J Thorac Imaging 2008;23(4):244–250

Konen E, Gutierrez C, Chaparro C, et al. Bronchiolitis obliterans syndrome in lung transplant recipients: can thin-section CT findings predict disease before its clinical appearance? Radiology 2004;231(2):467–473

Meyer KC, Raghu G, Verleden GM, et al. An international ISH / ATS / ERS clinical practice guideline: diagnosis and management of bronchiolitis obliterans syndrome. Eur Respir J 2014;14:441479–441503

Todd JL, Palmer SM. Bronchiolitis obliterans syndrome: the final frontier for lung transplantation. Chest 2011;140(2):502–508

■ **Case 52**

Ofek E, Sato M, Saito T, et al. Restrictive allograft syndrome post lung transplantation is characterized by pleuroparenchymal fibroelastosis. Mod Pathol 2013;26(3):350–356

Sato M, Waddell TK, Wagnetz U, et al. Restrictive allograft syndrome (RAS): a novel form of chronic lung allograft dysfunction. J Heart Lung Transplant 2011;30(7):735–742

Verleden GM, Raghu G, Meyer KC, Glanville AR, Corris P. A new classification system for chronic lung allograft dysfunction. J Heart Lung Transplant 2014;33(2):127–133

Vos R, Verleden SE, Verleden GM. Chronic lung allograft dysfunction: evolving practice. Curr Opin Organ Transplant 2015;20(5):483–491

■ **Case 53**

Cottin V, Nunes H, Brillet P-Y, et al; Groupe d'Etude et de Recherche sur les Maladies Orphelines Pulmonaires (GERM O P). Combined pulmonary fibrosis and emphysema: a distinct underrecognised entity. Eur Respir J 2005;26(4):586–593

Cottin V. The impact of emphysema in pulmonary fibrosis. Eur Respir Rev 2013;22(128):153–157

Jankowich MD, Rounds SIS. Combined pulmonary fibrosis and emphysema syndrome: a review. Chest 2012;141(1):222–231

Papiris SA, Triantafillidou C, Manali ED, et al. Combined pulmonary fibrosis and emphysema. Expert Rev Respir Med 2013;7(1):19–31, quiz 32

■ **Case 54**

Guillerman RP, Brody AS. Contemporary perspectives on pediatric diffuse lung disease. Radiol Clin North Am 2011;49(5):847–868

Hime NJ, Zurynski Y, Fitzgerald D, et al. Childhood interstitial lung disease: a systematic review. Pediatr Pulmonol 2015;50(12):1383–1392

Kurland G, Deterding RR, Hagood JS, et al; American Thoracic Society Committee on Childhood Interstitial Lung Disease (chILD) and the chILD Research Network. An official American Thoracic Society clinical practice guideline: classification, evaluation, and management of childhood interstitial lung disease in infancy. Am J Respir Crit Care Med 2013;188(3):376–394

Lee EY. Interstitial lung disease in infants: new classification system, imaging technique, clinical presentation and imaging findings. Pediatr Radiol 2013;43(1):3–13, quiz 128–129

Vece TJ, Young LR. Update on diffuse lung disease in children. Chest 2016;149(3):836–845

■ **Case 55**

Krustins E. Mounier-Kuhn syndrome: a systematic analysis of 128 cases published within last 25 years. Clin Respir J 2016;10(1):3–10

Krustins E, Kravale Z, Buls A. Mounier-Kuhn syndrome or congenital tracheobronchomegaly: a literature review. Respir Med 2013;107(12):1822–1828

Payandeh J, McGillivray B, McCauley G, Wilcox P, Swiston JR, Lehman A. A clinical classification scheme for tracheobronchomegaly (Mounier-Kuhn syndrome). Lung 2015;193(5):815–822

Shin MS, Jackson RM, Ho K-J. Tracheobronchomegaly (Mounier-Kuhn syndrome): CT diagnosis. AJR Am J Roentgenol 1988;150(4):777–779

■ **Case 56**

Fernández Crisosto CA, Quercia Arias O, Bustamante N, Moreno H, Uribe Echevarría A. [Diffuse pulmonary ossification associated with idiopathic pulmonary fibrosis]. Arch Bronconeumol 2004;40(12):595–598

Friedrich T, Steinecke R, Horn LC, Eichfeld U. [Idiopathic pulmonary ossification]. RoFo Fortschr Geb Rontgenstr Nuklearmed 1998;169(3):267–273

Lara JF, Catroppo JF, Kim DU, da Costa D. Dendriform pulmonary ossification, a form of diffuse pulmonary ossification: report of a 26-year autopsy experience. Arch Pathol Lab Med 2005;129(3):348–353

Peros-Golubicić T, Tekavec-Trkanjec J. Diffuse pulmonary ossification: an unusual interstitial lung disease. Curr Opin Pulm Med 2008;14(5):488–492

Reddy TL, von der Thüsen J, Walsh SL. Idiopathic dendriform pulmonary ossification. J Thorac Imaging 2012;27(5):W108-W110

■ **Case 57**

Avila NA, Brantly M, Premkumar A, Huizing M, Dwyer A, Gahl WA. Hermansky-Pudlak syndrome: radiography and CT of the chest compared with pulmonary function tests and genetic studies. AJR Am J Roentgenol 2002;179(4):887–892

Berkmen YM, Dsouza BM. Case 124: Hermansky-Pudlak syndrome. Radiology 2007;245(2):595–599

Hurford MT, Sebastiano C. Hermansky-pudlak syndrome: report of a case and review of the literature. Int J Clin Exp Pathol 2008;1(6):550–554

Kelil T, Shen J, O'Neill AC, Howard SA. Hermansky-pudlak syndrome complicated by pulmonary fibrosis: radiologic-pathologic correlation and review of pulmonary complications. J Clin Imaging Sci 2014;4:59

■ **Case 58**

Corsten MJ, Shamji FM, Odell PF, et al. Optimal treatment of descending necrotising mediastinitis. Thorax 1997;52(8):702–708

Endo S, Murayama F, Hasegawa T, et al. Guideline of surgical management based on diffusion of descending necrotizing mediastinitis. Jpn J Thorac Cardiovasc Surg 1999;47(1):14–19

Katabathina VS, Restrepo CS, Martinez-Jimenez S, Riascos RF. Nonvascular, nontraumatic mediastinal emergencies in adults: a comprehensive review of imaging findings. Radiographics 2011;31(4):1141–1160

Kiernan PD, Hernandez A, Byrne WD, et al. Descending cervical mediastinitis. Ann Thorac Surg 1998;65(5): 1483–1488

Makeieff M, Gresillon N, Berthet JP, et al. Management of descending necrotizing mediastinitis. Laryngoscope 2004;114(4):772–775

Pinto A, Scaglione M, Scuderi MG, Tortora G, Daniele S, Romano L. Infections of the neck leading to descending necrotizing mediastinitis: role of multi-detector row computed tomography. Eur J Radiol 2008;65(3):389–394

■ Case 59

Cho HJ, Jeon YB, Ma DS, Lee JN, Chung M. Traumatic pulmonary pseudocysts after blunt chest trauma: prevalence, mechanisms of injury, and computed tomography findings. J Trauma Acute Care Surg 2015;79(3):425–430

Hansell DM, Bankier AA, MacMahon H, McLoud TC, Müller NL, Remy J. Fleischner Society: glossary of terms for thoracic imaging. Radiology 2008;246(3):697–722

Houtman S, Janssen R. Traumatic pneumatocele. Neth J Cri Care 2012;16(6):224–225

Quigley MJ, Fraser RS. Pulmonary pneumatocele: pathology and pathogenesis. AJR Am J Roentgenol 1988;150(6): 1275–1277

Shen H-N, Lu FL, Wu H-D, Yu CJ, Yang PC. Management of tension pneumatocele with high-frequency oscillatory ventilation. Chest 2002;121(1):284–286

Ulutas H, Celik MR, Ozgel M, Soysal O, Kuzucu A. Pulmonary pseudocyst secondary to blunt or penetrating chest trauma: clinical course and diagnostic issues. Eur J Trauma Emerg Surg 2015;41(2):181–188

■ Case 60

Chaoui R, Kalache KD, Heling KS, Tennstedt C, Bommer C, Körner H. Absent or hypoplastic thymus on ultrasound: a marker for deletion 22q11.2 in fetal cardiac defects. Ultrasound Obstet Gynecol 2002;20(6):546–552

Digilio M, Marino B, Capolino R, Dallapiccola B. Clinical manifestations of Deletion 22q11.2 syndrome (DiGeorge/Velo-Cardio-Facial syndrome). Images Paediatr Cardiol 2005;7(2):23–34

Felman AH, Cohen MD. Thymus. In: Radiology of the Pediatric Chest: Clinical and Pathological Correlations. New York: McGraw-Hill Book Company; 1987.

Goldmuntz E, Clark BJ, Mitchell LE, et al. Frequency of 22q11 deletions in patients with conotruncal defects. J Am Coll Cardiol 1998;32(2):492–498

Momma K. Cardiovascular anomalies associated with chromosome 22q11.2 deletion syndrome. Am J Cardiol 2010;105(11):1617–1624

Ziolkowska L, Kawalec W, Turska-Kmiec A, et al. Chromosome 22q11.2 microdeletion in children with conotruncal heart defects: frequency, associated cardiovascular anomalies, and outcome following cardiac surgery. Eur J Pediatr 2008;167(10):1135–1140

■ Case 61

Alkadhi H, Wildermuth S, Russi EW, Marincek B, Boehm T. Imaging in hyper-IgE syndrome. Respiration 2006;73(3): 365–366

Jhaveri KS, Sahani DV, Shetty PG, Shroff MM. Hyperimmunoglobulinaemia E syndrome: pulmonary imaging features. Australas Radiol 2000;44(3):328–330

Szczawinska-Poplonyk A, Kycler Z, Pietrucha B, Heropolitanska-Pliszka E, Breborowicz A, Gerreth K. The hyperimmunoglobulin E syndrome—clinical manifestation diversity in primary immune deficiency. Orphanet J Rare Dis 2011;6:76

■ Case 62

Bondioni MP, Soresina A, Lougaris V, Gatta D, Plebani A, Maroldi R. Common variable immunodeficiency: computed tomography evaluation of bronchopulmonary changes including nodular lesions in 40 patients. Correlation with clinical and immunological data. J Comput Assist Tomogr 2010;34(3):395–401

Cunningham-Rundles C. The many faces of common variable immunodeficiency. Hematology (Am Soc Hematol Educ Program) 2012;2012(1):301–305

Maarschalk-Ellerbroek LJ, de Jong PA, van Montfrans JM, et al. CT screening for pulmonary pathology in common variable immunodeficiency disorders and the correlation with clinical and immunological parameters. J Clin Immunol 2014;34(6):642–654

Maglione PJ, Overbey JR, Radigan L, et al. Pulmonary radiologic findings in CVID: clinical and immunological correlations. Ann Allergy Asthma Immunol 2014;113(4):452–459

■ Case 63

Brook I, Frazier EH. Aerobic and anaerobic microbiology of empyema. A retrospective review in two military hospitals. Chest 1993;103(5):1502–1507

Lois M, Noppen M. Bronchopleural fistulas: an overview of the problem with special focus on endoscopic management. Chest 2005;128(6):3955–3965

Stern EJ, Sun H, Haramati LB. Peripheral bronchopleural fistulas: CT imaging features. AJR Am J Roentgenol 1996;167(1):117–120

Tsubakimoto M, Murayama S, Iraha R, Kamiya H, Tsuchiya N, Yamashiro T. Can peripheral bronchopleural fistula demonstrated on computed tomography be treated conservatively? A retrospective analysis. J Comput Assist Tomogr 2016;40(1):86–90

Yuksekkaya R, Ozturk B, Celikyay F, Sade R, Kupeli M, Yeginsu A. Multidetector computed tomography findings of central bronchopleural fistulas as sequelae of tuberculosis, chemo radiation and trauma: a report of three cases. Respir Med Case Rep 2013;9:21–26

■ Case 64

Lott S, Schmieder M, Mayer B, et al. Gastrointestinal stromal tumors of the esophagus: evaluation of a pooled case series regarding clinicopathological features and clinical outcome. Am J Cancer Res 2014;5(1):333–343

Shinagare AB, Zukotynski KA, Krajewski KM, et al. Esophageal gastrointestinal stromal tumor: report of 7 patients. Cancer Imaging 2012;12:100–108

Winant AJ, Gollub MJ, Shia J, Antonescu C, Bains MS, Levine MS. Imaging and clinicopathologic features of esophageal gastrointestinal stromal tumors. AJR Am J Roentgenol 2014;203(2):306–314

■ Case 65

Abbas AE, Deschamps C, Cassivi SD, et al. Chest-wall desmoid tumors: results of surgical intervention. Ann Thorac Surg 2004;78(4):1219–1223, discussion 1219–1223

Allen PJ, Shriver CD. Desmoid tumors of the chest wall. Semin Thorac Cardiovasc Surg 1999;11(3):264–269

Souza FF, Fennessy FM, Yang Q, van den Abbeele AD. Case report. PET/CT appearance of desmoid tumour of the chest wall. Br J Radiol 2010;83(986):e39–e42

■ Case 66

Chong S, Kim TS, Kim B-T, Cho EY, Kim J. Pulmonary artery sarcoma mimicking pulmonary thromboembolism: integrated FDG PET/CT. AJR Am J Roentgenol 2007;188(6):1691–1693

Cox JE, Chiles C, Aquino SL, Savage P, Oaks T. Pulmonary artery sarcomas: a review of clinical and radiologic features. J Comput Assist Tomogr 1997;21(5):750–755

Huo L, Moran CA, Fuller GN, Gladish G, Suster S. Pulmonary artery sarcoma: a clinicopathologic and immunohistochemical study of 12 cases. Am J Clin Pathol 2006;125(3):419–424

Restrepo CS, Betancourt SL, Martinez-Jimenez S, Gutierrez FR. Tumors of the pulmonary artery and veins. Semin Ultrasound CT MR 2012;33(6):580–590

Wong HH, Gounaris I, McCormack A, et al. Presentation and management of pulmonary artery sarcoma. Clin Sarcoma Res 2015;5(1):3

■ Case 67

Chaisson NF, Dodson MW, Elliott CG. Pulmonary capillary hemangiomatosis and pulmonary veno-occlusive disease. Clin Chest Med 2016;37(3):523–534

Frazier AA, Franks TJ, Mohammed T-LH, Ozbudak IH, Galvin JR. From the Archives of the AFIP: pulmonary veno-occlusive disease and pulmonary capillary hemangiomatosis. Radiographics 2007;27(3):867–882

O'Keefe MCO, Post MD. Pulmonary capillary hemangiomatosis: a rare cause of pulmonary hypertension. Arch Pathol Lab Med 2015;139(2):274–277

■ Case 68

Arnaud D, Varon J, Surani S. An unusual presentation of Congenital lobar emphysema. Case Rep Pulmonol 2017;2017:6719617

Caliskan T, Okutan O, Ciftci F, et al. Congenital lobar emphysema diagnosed in adult age: A case report. Eurasian J Pulmonol 2014;16:50–53

Sadaqat M, Malik JA, Karim R. Congenital lobar emphysema in an adult. Lung India 2011;28(1):67–69

Sasieta HC, Nichols FC, Kuzo RS, Boland JM, Utz JP. Congenital lobar emphysema in an adult. Am J Respir Crit Care Med 2016;194(3):377–378

■ **Case 69**

Macchiarini P. Primary tracheal tumours. Lancet Oncol 2006;7(1):83–91

Ngo A-VH, Walker CM, Chung JH, et al. Tumors and tumor-like conditions of the large airways. AJR Am J Roentgenol 2013;201(2):301–313

Shroff GS, Ocazionez D, Vargas D, et al. Pathology of the trachea and central bronchi. Semin Ultrasound CT MR 2016;37(3):177–189

Webb BD, Walsh GL, Roberts DB, Sturgis EM. Primary tracheal malignant neoplasms: the University of Texas MD Anderson Cancer Center experience. J Am Coll Surg 2006;202(2):237–246

■ **Case 70**

Cohn SM. Pulmonary contusion: review of the clinical entity. J Trauma 1997;42(5):973–979

Cohn SM, Dubose JJ. Pulmonary contusion: an update on recent advances in clinical management. World J Surg 2010;34(8):1959–1970

Ganie FA, Lone H, Lone GN, et al. Lung contusion: a clinico-pathological entity with unpredictable clinical course. Bull Emerg Trauma 2013;1(1):7–16

■ **Case 71**

Aghajanzadeh M, Khadem S, Khajeh Jahromi S, Gorabi HE, Ebrahimi H, Maafi AA. Clinical presentation and operative repair of Morgagni hernia. Interact Cardiovasc Thorac Surg 2012;15(4):608–611

Anthes TB, Thoongsuwan N, Karmy-Jones R. Morgagni hernia: CT findings. Curr Probl Diagn Radiol 2003;32(3):135–136

Arora S, Haji A, Ng P. Adult Morgagni hernia: the need for clinical awareness, early diagnosis and prompt surgical intervention. Ann R Coll Surg Engl 2008;90(8):694–695

Eren S, Ciriş F. Diaphragmatic hernia: diagnostic approaches with review of the literature. Eur J Radiol 2005;54(3):448–459

Sandstrom CK, Stern EJ. Diaphragmatic hernias: a spectrum of radiographic appearances. Curr Probl Diagn Radiol 2011;40(3):95–115

■ **Case 72**

Chassagnon G, Favelle O, Marchand-Adam S, De Muret A, Revel MP. DIPNECH: when to suggest this diagnosis on CT. Clin Radiol 2015;70(3):317–325

Foran PJ, Hayes SA, Blair DJ, Zakowski MF, Ginsberg MS. Imaging appearances of diffuse idiopathic pulmonary neuroendocrine cell hyperplasia. Clin Imaging 2015;39(2):243–246

Rossi G, Cavazza A, Spagnolo P, et al. Diffuse idiopathic pulmonary neuroendocrine cell hyperplasia syndrome. Eur Respir J 2016;47(6):1829–1841

Wirtschafter E, Walts AE, Liu ST, Marchevsky AM. Diffuse idiopathic pulmonary neuroendocrine cell hyperplasia of the lung (DIPNECH): current best evidence. Lung 2015;193(5):659–667

■ **Case 73**

George J, Jain R, Tariq SM. CT bronchoscopy in the diagnosis of Williams-Campbell syndrome. Respirology 2006;11(1):117–119

Jones QC, Wathen CG. Williams-Campbell syndrome presenting in an adult. BMC Case Rep 2012;2012: bcr2012006775

McAdams HP, Erasmus J. Chest case of the day. Williams-Campbell syndrome. AJR Am J Roentgenol 1995;165(1):190–191

Noriega Aldave AP, William Saliski D. The clinical manifestations, diagnosis and management of Williams-Campbell syndrome. N Am J Med Sci 2014;6(9):429–432

■ **Case 74**

Dodd JD, Souza CA, Müller NL. High-resolution MDCT of pulmonary septic embolism: evaluation of the feeding vessel sign. AJR Am J Roentgenol 2006;187(3):623–629

Goswami U, Brenes JA, Punjabi GV, LeClaire MM, Williams DN. Associations and outcomes of septic pulmonary embolism. Open Respir Med J 2014;8:28–33

Iwasaki Y, Nagata K, Nakanishi M, et al. Spiral CT findings in septic pulmonary emboli. Eur J Radiol 2001;37(3):190–194

Ye R, Zhao L, Wang C, Wu X, Yan H. Clinical characteristics of septic pulmonary embolism in adults: a systematic review. Respir Med 2014;108(1):1–8

■ Case 75

Chick JFB, Chauhan NR, Madan R. Solitary fibrous tumors of the thorax: nomenclature, epidemiology, radiologic and pathologic findings, differential diagnoses, and management. AJR Am J Roentgenol 2013;200(3): W238-W248

Sureka B, Thukral BB, Mittal MK, Mittal A, Sinha M. Radiological review of pleural tumors. Indian J Radiol Imaging 2013;23(4):313–320

Zhu Y, Du K, Ye X, Song D, Long D. Solitary fibrous tumors of pleura and lung: report of twelve cases. J Thorac Dis 2013;5(3):310–313

■ Case 76

Dillman JR, Pernicano PG, McHugh JB, et al. Cross-sectional imaging of primary thoracic sarcomas with histopathologic correlation: a review for the radiologist. Curr Probl Diagn Radiol 2010;39(1):17–29

Foran P, Colleran G, Madewell J, O'Sullivan PJ. Imaging of thoracic sarcomas of the chest wall, pleura, and lung. Semin Ultrasound CT MR 2011;32(5):365–376

Koenigkam-Santos M, Sommer G, Puderbach M, et al. Primary intrathoracic malignant mesenchymal tumours: computed tomography features of a rare group of chest neoplasms. Insights Imaging 2014;5(2):237–244

■ Case 77

Chen Y-B, Rahemtullah A, Hochberg E. Primary effusion lymphoma. Oncologist 2007;12(5):569–576

Patel S, Xiao P. Primary effusion lymphoma. Arch Pathol Lab Med 2013;137(8):1152–1154

■ Case 78

Devaraj A, Griffin N, Nicholson AG, Padley SPG. Computed tomography findings in fibrosing mediastinitis. Clin Radiol 2007;62(8):781–786

Koksal D, Bayiz H, Mutluay N, et al. Fibrosing mediastinitis mimicking bronchogenic carcinoma. J Thorac Dis 2013;5(1):E5–E7

McNeeley MF, Chung JH, Bhalla S, Godwin JD. Imaging of granulomatous fibrosing mediastinitis. AJR Am J Roentgenol 2012;199(2):319–327

Rossi SE, McAdams HP, Rosado-de-Christenson ML, Franks TJ, Galvin JR. Fibrosing mediastinitis. Radiographics 2001;21(3):737–757

■ Case 79

Bonekamp D, Horton KM, Hruban RH, Fishman EK. Castleman disease: the great mimic. Radiographics 2011;31(6):1793–1807

Fajgenbaum DC, van Rhee F, Nabel CS. HHV-8-negative, idiopathic multicentric Castleman disease: novel insights into biology, pathogenesis, and therapy. Blood 2014;123(19):2924–2933

Madan R, Chen JH, Trotman-Dickenson B, Jacobson F, Hunsaker A. The spectrum of Castleman's disease: mimics, radiologic pathologic correlation and role of imaging in patient management. Eur J Radiol 2012;81(1):123–131

Talat N, Schulte K-M. Castleman's disease: systematic analysis of 416 patients from the literature. Oncologist 2011;16(9):1316–1324

■ Case 80

Al-Mansour Z, Nelson BP, Evens AM. Post-transplant lymphoproliferative disease (PTLD): risk factors, diagnosis, and current treatment strategies. Curr Hematol Malig Rep 2013;8(3):173–183

Camacho JC, Moreno CC, Harri PA, Aguirre DA, Torres WE, Mittal PK. Posttransplantation lymphoproliferative disease: proposed imaging classification. Radiographics 2014;34(7):2025–2038

LaCasce AS. Post-transplant lymphoproliferative disorders. Oncologist 2006;11(6):674–680

■ Case 81

Jude CM, Nayak NB, Patel MK, Deshmukh M, Batra P. Pulmonary coccidioidomycosis: pictorial review of chest radiographic and CT findings. Radiographics 2014;34(4):912–925

Spinello IM, Munoz A, Johnson RH. Pulmonary coccidioidomycosis. Semin Respir Crit Care Med 2008;29(2):166–173

Thompson GR III. Pulmonary coccidioidomycosis. Semin Respir Crit Care Med 2011;32(6):754–763

■ Case 82

Cordier J-F. Cryptogenic organising pneumonia. Eur Respir J 2006;28(2):422–446

Cordier J-F. Organising pneumonia. Thorax 2000;55(4): 318–328

Feinstein MB, DeSouza SA, Moreira AL, et al. A comparison of the pathological, clinical and radiographical, features of cryptogenic organising pneumonia, acute fibrinous and organising pneumonia and granulomatous organising pneumonia. J Clin Pathol 2015;68(6):441–447

Schlesinger C, Koss MN. The organizing pneumonias: an update and review. Curr Opin Pulm Med 2005;11(5): 422–430

Shaw M, Collins BF, Ho LA, Raghu G. Rheumatoid arthritis-associated lung disease. Eur Respir Rev 2015;24(135):1–16

■ Case 83

Collard HR, Schwarz MI. Diffuse alveolar hemorrhage. Clin Chest Med 2004;25(3):583–592, vii

Lara AR, Schwarz MI. Diffuse alveolar hemorrhage. Chest 2010;137(5):1164–1171

Lichtenberger JP III, Digumarthy SR, Abbott GF, Shepard JA, Sharma A. Diffuse pulmonary hemorrhage: clues to the diagnosis. Curr Probl Diagn Radiol 2014;43(3):128–139

■ Case 84

Jeong YJ, Kim K-I, Seo IJ, et al. Eosinophilic lung diseases: a clinical, radiologic, and pathologic overview. Radiographics 2007;27(3):617–637, discussion 637–639

Katre RS, Sunnapwar A, Restrepo CS, et al. Cardiopulmonary and gastrointestinal manifestations of eosinophilic-associated diseases and idiopathic hypereosinophilic syndromes: multimodality imaging approach. Radiographics 2016;36(2):433–451

Marchand E, Cordier J-F. Idiopathic chronic eosinophilic pneumonia. Orphanet J Rare Dis 2006;1:11

■ Case 85

Akira M, Suganuma N. Acute and subacute chemical-induced lung injuries: HRCT findings. Eur J Radiol 2014;83(8):1461–1469

Rabinowitz PM, Siegel MD. Acute inhalation injury. Clin Chest Med 2002;23(4):707–715

Rehberg S, Maybauer MO, Enkhbaatar P, Maybauer DM, Yamamoto Y, Traber DL. Pathophysiology, management and treatment of smoke inhalation injury. Expert Rev Respir Med 2009;3(3):283–297

Walker PF, Buehner MF, Wood LA, et al. Diagnosis and management of inhalation injury: an updated review. Crit Care 2015;19:351

■ Case 86

Lee W-K, Mossop PJ, Little AF, et al. Infected (mycotic) aneurysms: spectrum of imaging appearances and management. Radiographics 2008;28(7):1853–1868

Lin MP, Chang SC, Wu RH, Chou CK, Tzeng WS. A comparison of computed tomography, magnetic resonance imaging, and digital subtraction angiography findings in the diagnosis of infected aortic aneurysm. J Comput Assist Tomogr 2008;32(4):616–620

Macedo TA, Stanson AW, Oderich GS, Johnson CM, Panneton JM, Tie ML. Infected aortic aneurysms: imaging findings. Radiology 2004;231(1):250–257

Yang CY, Liu KL, Lee CW, Tsang YM, Chen SJ. Mycotic aortic aneurysm presenting initially as an aortic intramural air pocket. AJR Am J Roentgenol 2005;185(2):463–465

■ Case 87

Boersma WG, Stigt JA, Smit HJM. Treatment of haemothorax. Respir Med 2010;104:1583–1587

Broderick SR. Hemothorax. Etiology, diagnosis and management. Thorac Surg Clin 2013;23:89–96

Liu F, Huang YC, Ng Y-B, Liang JH. Differentiate pleural effusion from hemothorax after blunt chest trauma: comparison of computed tomography attenuation values. J Acute Med 2016;6:1–6

Meyer DM. Hemothorax related to trauma. Thorac Surg Clin 2007;17:47–55

■ Case 88

Charruau L, Parrens M, Jougon J, et al. Mediastinal lymphangioma in adults: CT and MR imaging features. Eur Radiol 2000;10(8):1310–1314

Faul JL, Berry GJ, Colby TV, et al. Thoracic lymphangiomas, lymphangiectasis, lymphangiomatosis, and lymphatic dysplasia syndrome. Am J Respir Crit Care Med 2000;161(3 Pt 1):1037–1046

Fokkema JPI, Paul MA, Vrouenraets BC. Mediastinal lymphangioma in an adult. Ann R Coll Surg Engl 2014;96(5): e24–e25

Khobta N, Tomasini P, Trousse D, Maldonado F, Chanez P, Astoul P. Solitary cystic mediastinal lymphangioma. Eur Respir Rev 2013;22(127):91–93

Park JG, Aubry M-C, Godfrey JA, Midthun DE. Mediastinal lymphangioma: Mayo Clinic experience of 25 cases. Mayo Clin Proc 2006;81(9):1197–1203

Vargas D, Suby-Long T, Restrepo CS. Cystic lesions of the mediastinum. Semin Ultrasound CT MR 2016;37(3):212–222

■ **Case 89**

Aylwin ACB, Gishen P, Copley SJ. Imaging appearance of thoracic amyloidosis. J Thorac Imaging 2005;20(1):41–46

Czeyda-Pommersheim F, Hwang M, Chen SS, Strollo D, Fuhrman C, Bhalla S. Amyloidosis: modern cross-sectional imaging. Radiographics 2015;35(5):1381–1392

Khoor A, Colby TV. Amyloidosis of the lung. Arch Pathol Lab Med 2017;141(2):247–254

Lee AY, Godwin JD, Pipavath SNJ. Case 182: pulmonary amyloidosis. Radiology 2012;263(3):929–932

Takahashi N, Glockner J, Howe BM, Hartman RP, Kawashima A. Taxonomy and imaging manifestations of systemic amyloidosis. Radiol Clin North Am 2016;54(3):597–612

■ **Case 90**

Dursun AB, Demirag F, Bayiz H, Sertkaya D. Endobronchial metastases: a clinicopathological analysis. Respirology 2005;10(4):510–514

Katsimbri PP, Bamias AT, Froudarakis ME, Peponis IA, Constantopoulos SH, Pavlidis NA. Endobronchial metastases secondary to solid tumors: report of eight cases and review of the literature. Lung Cancer 2000;28(2):163–170

Marchioni A, Lasagni A, Busca A, et al. Endobronchial metastasis: an epidemiologic and clinicopathologic study of 174 consecutive cases. Lung Cancer 2014;84(3):222–228

Sørensen JB. Endobronchial metastases from extrapulmonary solid tumors. Acta Oncol 2004;43(1):73–79

■ **Case 91**

Foroulis CN, Zarogoulidis P, Darwiche K, et al. Superior sulcus (Pancoast) tumors: current evidence on diagnosis and radical treatment. J Thorac Dis 2013;5(Suppl 4):S342–S358

Hochhegger B, Marchiori E, Sedlaczek O, et al. MRI in lung cancer: a pictorial essay. Br J Radiol 2011;84(1003): 661–668

Manenti G, Raguso M, D'Onofrio S, et al. Pancoast tumor: the role of magnetic resonance imaging. Case Rep Radiol 2013;2013:479120

Sommer G, Stieltjes B. Magnetic resonance imaging for staging of non-small-cell lung cancer-technical advances and unmet needs. J Thorac Dis 2015;7(7):1098–1102

■ **Case 92**

Choe CH, Kahler JJ. Herniation of the lung: a case report. J Emerg Med 2014;46(1):28–30

Detorakis EE, Androulidakis E. Intercostal lung herniation—the role of imaging. J Radiol Case Rep 2014;8(4):16–24

Gross RI, Eversgerd JL. The image of trauma. Transthoracic lung herniation due to blunt trauma. J Trauma 2006;60(5):1149

Moncada R, Vade A, Gimenez C, et al. Congenital and acquired lung hernias. J Thorac Imaging 1996;11(1):75–82

Weissberg D, Refaely Y. Hernia of the lung. Ann Thorac Surg 2002;74(6):1963–1966

Zia Z, Bashir O, Ramjas GE, Kumaran M, Pollock JG, Pointon K. Intercostal lung hernia: radiographic and MDCT findings. Clin Radiol 2013;68(7):e412–e417

■ **Case 93**

Harish MG, Konda SD, MacMahon H, Newstead GM. Breast lesions incidentally detected with CT: what the general radiologist needs to know. Radiographics 2007;27(Suppl 1): S37–S51

Hussain A, Gordon-Dixon A, Almusawy H, Sinha P, Desai A. The incidence and outcome of incidental breast lesions detected by computed tomography. Ann R Coll Surg Engl 2010;92(2):124–126

Monzawa S, Washio T, Yasuoka R, Mitsuo M, Kadotani Y, Hanioka K. Incidental detection of clinically unexpected breast lesions by computed tomography. Acta Radiol 2013;54(4):374–379

Moyle P, Sonoda L, Britton P, Sinnatamby R. Incidental breast lesions detected on CT: what is their significance? Br J Radiol 2010;83(987):233–240

■ **Case 94**

Bandali MF, Mirakhur A, Lee EW, et al. Portal hypertension: imaging of portosystemic collateral pathways and associated image-guided therapy. World J Gastroenterol 2017;23(10):1735–1746

Kim SH, Kim YJ, Lee JM, et al. Esophageal varices in patients with cirrhosis: multidetector CT esophagography—comparison with endoscopy. Radiology 2007;242(3):759–768

Kim YJ, Raman SS, Yu NC, To'o KJ, Jutabha R, Lu DS. Esophageal varices in cirrhotic patients: evaluation with liver CT. AJR Am J Roentgenol 2007;188(1):139–144

Somsouk M, To'o K, Ali M, et al. Esophageal varices on computed tomography and subsequent variceal hemorrhage. Abdom Imaging 2014;39(2):251–256

■ **Case 95**

Lee KN, Lee HJ, Shin WW, Webb WR. Hypoxemia and liver cirrhosis (hepatopulmonary syndrome) in eight patients: comparison of the central and peripheral pulmonary vasculature. Radiology 1999;211(2):549–553

Leung AN. Case 63: hepatopulmonary syndrome. Radiology 2003;229(1):64–67

McAdams HP, Erasmus J, Crockett R, Mitchell J, Godwin JD, McDermott VG. The hepatopulmonary syndrome: radiologic findings in 10 patients. AJR Am J Roentgenol 1996;166(6):1379–1385

Meyer CA, White CS, Sherman KE. Diseases of the hepatopulmonary axis. Radiographics 2000;20(3):687–698

Rodríguez-Roisin R, Krowka MJ. Hepatopulmonary syndrome—a liver-induced lung vascular disorder. N Engl J Med 2008;358(22):2378–2387

■ **Case 96**

Martini N, Huvos AG, Burt ME, et al. Predictors of survival in malignant tumors of the sternum. J Thorac Cardiovasc Surg 1996;111(1):96–105, discussion 105–106

Restrepo CS, Martinez S, Lemos DF, et al. Imaging appearances of the sternum and sternoclavicular joints. Radiographics 2009;29(3):839–859

Waisberg DR, Abrão FC, Fernandez A, Terra RM, Pêgo-Fernandes PM, Jatene FB. Surgically-challenging chondrosarcomas of the chest wall: five-year follow-up at a single institution. Clinics (Sao Paulo) 2011;66(3):501–503

■ **Case 97**

Ranieri VM, Rubenfeld GD, Thompson BT, et al; ARDS Definition Task Force. Acute respiratory distress syndrome: the Berlin Definition. JAMA 2012;307(23):2526–2533

Sheard S, Rao P, Devaraj A. Imaging of acute respiratory distress syndrome. Respir Care 2012;57(4):607–612

Zompatori M, Ciccarese F, Fasano L. Overview of current lung imaging in acute respiratory distress syndrome. Eur Respir Rev 2014;23(134):519–530

■ **Case 98**

Basile A, Simzar S, Bentow J, et al. Disseminated Strongyloides stercoralis: hyperinfection during medical immunosuppression. J Am Acad Dermatol 2010;63(5):896–902

Kassalik M, Mönkemüller K. Strongyloides stercoralis hyperinfection syndrome and disseminated disease. Gastroenterol Hepatol (N Y) 2011;7(11):766–768

Qu TT, Yang Q, Yu M-H, Wang J. A fatal strongyloides stercoralis hyperinfection syndrome in a patient with chronic kidney disease. A case report and literature review. Medicine (Baltimore) 2016;95(19):e3638

Vadlamudi RS, Chi DS, Krishnaswamy G. Intestinal strongyloidiasis and hyperinfection syndrome. Clin Mol Allergy 2006;4:8

■ **Case 99**

Farid M, Demicco EG, Garcia R, et al. Malignant peripheral nerve sheath tumors. Oncologist 2014;19(2):193–201

Kamran SC, Shinagare AB, Howard SAH, Hornick JL, Ramaiya NH. A–Z of malignant peripheral nerve sheath tumors. Cancer Imaging 2012;12:475–483

Kamran SC, Shinagare AB, Howard SAH, et al. Intrathoracic malignant peripheral nerve sheath tumors: imaging features and implications for management. Radiol Oncol 2013;47(3):230–238

■ Case 100

Benbrahim Z, Arifi S, Daoudi K, et al. Askin's tumor: a case report and literature review. World J Surg Oncol 2013;11:10

Demir A, Gunluoglu MZ, Dagoglu N, et al. Surgical treatment and prognosis of primitive neuroectodermal tumors of the thorax. J Thorac Oncol 2009;4(2):185–192

Foran P, Colleran G, Madewell J, O'Sullivan PJ. Imaging of thoracic sarcomas of the chest wall, pleura, and lung. Semin Ultrasound CT MR 2011;32(5):365–376

Gladish GW, Sabloff BM, Munden RF, Truong MT, Erasmus JJ, Chasen MH. Primary thoracic sarcomas. Radiographics 2002;22(3):621–637

Index

Locators refer to case number. Locators in boldface indicate primary diagnosis.